Essentials of
Metabolic Diseases
and Endocrinology

Essentials of Metabolic Diseases and Endocrinology

Habeeb Bacchus, Ph.D., M.D., F.A.C.P.
Associate Professor of Medicine
Loma Linda University School of Medicine;
Associate Chief of Medicine
Riverside General Hospital

University Park Press
Baltimore · London · Tokyo

UNIVERSITY PARK PRESS
International Publishers in Science and Medicine
Chamber of Commerce Building
Baltimore, Maryland 21202

Typeset by The Composing Room of Michigan, Inc.
Manufactured in the United States of America by Universal Lithographers,
Inc., and The Maple Press Co.

Library of Congress Cataloging in Publication Data
Bacchus, Habeeb, 1928–
Essentials of metabolic diseases and endocrinology.
Includes index.
1. Metabolism, Disorders of. 2. Endocrinology.
I. Title. [DNLM: 1. Metabolic diseases. 2. Endo-
crine diseases. WD200 B116e]
RC627.54.B3   616.3'9   75-37804
ISBN 0-8391-0866-4

Contents

Preface   ix
Dedication   x

1. **Intermediary Metabolism: Interrelations among Carbohydrate, Fat, and Protein Metabolism**   1

    Embden-Meyerhof Pathway   2
    Pentose Phosphate Pathway   3
    Glycogen Biosynthesis   5
    Glycogen Breakdown   6
    Polyol Pathway   7
    Glycolysis and Gluconeogenesis   8
    Krebs Citric Acid Cycle   11
    Fat Metabolism   14
    Amino Acid Metabolism   22

2. **Clinical Disorders of Carbohydrate Metabolism**   27

    Gluconeogenesis   29
    Role of Kidney in Glucose Homeostasis   30
    Role of Central Nervous System in Glucose Homeostasis   30
    Role of Red Cell Mass in Glucose Homeostasis   30
    Endocrine Factors in Control of Carbohydrate Homeostasis   30
    Insulin and Intermediary Metabolism   31
    Glucagon and Intermediary Metabolism   33
    Hormonal Control of Carbohydrate Metabolism   33
    Tests of Carbohydrate Metabolism   34
    Diabetes Mellitus   37
    Hypoglycemic Syndromes   63
    Insulin Resistance Phenomena in Diabetic Patients   67
    Carbohydrate Metabolism in Erythrocytes   69
    Glycogen Storage Diseases   74

3. **Lipid Metabolism**   81

    Dietary Lipids   82
    Bile Acid Metabolism   87
    Lipid Transport in Serum   100
    Cholesterol Metabolism   118
    Fatty Acid Synthesis and Degradation   121
    Triglyceride Metabolism   122
    Phospholipid Metabolism   124
    Sulfatide Metabolism   138
    Ganglioside Metabolism   141
    Other Lipid Storage Disorders   148

4. Clinical Disorders of Protein and Amino Acid Metabolism   151

    Protein Metabolism   151
    Protein Synthesis   156
    Disorders of Amino Acid Metabolism   161

5. Clinical Disorders of Purine and Pyrimidine Metabolism   189

    Purine Metabolism   189
    Uric Acid: Metabolic and Clinical Aspects   193
    Gout and Hyperuricemic States   195
    Acute Gouty Arthritis   197
    Hereditary Diseases with Hyperuricemia   199
    Secondary Hyperuricemia   200
    Treatment of Hyperuricemia   201
    Treatment of Acute Gouty Arthritis   203
    Prophylactic Management of Acute Gouty Arthritis   203
    Hereditary Xanthinuria   204
    Clinical Disorders of Pyrimidine Metabolism   204

6. Clinical Disorders of the Connective Tissue Complex   207

    Collagen   207
    Elastin   214
    Glycoproteins   215
    Acid Mucopolysaccharides   217
    Genetic Mucopolysaccharidoses   223
    Inherited Disorders of Connective Tissues   227
    Other Disorders of Connective Tissue Metabolism   232

7. Clinical Disorders of Porphyrin Metabolism   235

    Physical and Chemical Properties   235
    Heme Structure and Function   236
    Biosynthesis of Heme and Porphyrins   236
    Control of Heme Biosynthesis   238
    Descriptions of Clinical Disorders of Porphyrin
        Metabolism   240

8. Clinical Disorders of Bilirubin Metabolism   255

    Heme Degradation and Bilirubin Metabolism   255
    Enzymatic Degradation of Heme to Bilirubin   256
    Bilirubin Transport in Plasma   257
    Clinical Disorders of Bilirubin Metabolism   259
    Drug Effects in Bilirubin Metabolism   267

9. The Vitamins   269

    Vitamin A   269
    Vitamin D   271
    Vitamin E   272
    Vitamin K   273
    Thiamin   274
    Niacin   276

Riboflavin   278
Pantothenic Acid   279
Pyridoxine   280
Biotin   282
Folic Acid   283
Vitamin C   284
Vitamin B_{12} 286

10. **Trace Minerals   289**

Copper   289
Zinc   290
Manganese   291

11. **Mechanisms of Hormone Actions   293**

Processes Propagated by Release of Membrane
    Adenylate Cyclase   293
Processes Propagated by Participation of
    Cytosol and Nuclear Receptors   296

12. **Hypothalamic-Hypophysiotropic-Neurohypophysial
System   299**

Hypothalamic-Neurohypophysial System   299
Vasopressin: Physiological Considerations   303

13. **Anterior Pituitary   311**

Control of Anterior Pituitary Gland   311
Hormones Produced by Anterior Pituitary   312

14. **Thyroid Gland   329**

Synthesis of Thyroid Hormones   330
Biosynthetic Processes in Thyroid Hormone Production   330
Metabolic Effects of Thyroid Hormones   334
Physiological Effects of Thyroid Hormones   335
Long-Acting Thyroid Stimulator   341
Hyperthyroidism   341
Hypothyroidism   354
Thyroid Cancer   359

15. **The Adrenal Cortex   361**

Regulation of Glucocorticoid Secretion   361
Regulation of Mineralocorticoid Secretion   362
Renin-Angiotensin Mechanism   362
Biosynthesis of Adrenal Cortical Hormones   363
Transport of Adrenocortical Hormones   365
Further Considerations on Synthesis of Androgens by
    Adrenal Cortex   366
Steroid Hormone Production in Fetal Adrenals   366
Biological Actions of Adrenocortical Hormones   366
Catabolism of Adrenocortical Secretions   369

Clinical Disorders of Adrenocortical Function   372
Clinical Syndromes Caused by Biosynthetic Defects in
   Adrenal Cortex   383
Idiopathic Hirsutism   390
Feminizing Adrenocortical Tumors   390
Laboratory Diagnosis of Adrenocortical Hyperplasia with
   Biosynthetic Defects   390
Summary of Diagnostic Procedures   391

16. **Adrenal Medulla and Chromaffin System   395**

Biosynthesis of Catecholamines   395
Metabolism of Catecholamines   397
Biological Effects of Catecholamines   397
Clinical Disorders of Chromaffin System   398

17. **Testes   403**

Endocrine Activity of Testis   404
Actions of Testosterone and Androgenic Derivatives   406

18. **The Ovaries   417**

Menstrual Cycle   418
Steriod Synthesis in Ovaries   419
Steroidogenesis during Pregnancy   421
Steroidogenesis in Fetoplacental Unit   422
Other Endocrine Changes in Pregnancy   426
Endocrine Changes in Maternal System in Pregnancy   426
Endocrine Changes in Parturition   427
Endocrine Control of Mammary Growth and Lactation   427
Clinical Investigation of Ovarian Disorders   428
Endocrine Disorders of Ovaries   429

19. **The Parathyroids   439**

Biological Actions of PTH   440
Interrelationships among Metabolic Actions of PTH,
   Calcitonin, and Vitamin D   442
Influence of Interplay among PTH, CT, and 1,25-DHCC
   on Calcium Homeostasis   446
Clinical Disorders of Parathyroid Function   447
Hyperparathyroidism   448
Hypoparathyroidism   458

20. **Special Topics   463**

Metabolic Bone Disease   463
Obesity   466
Endocrine Hypertension   469
Disorders of Sexual Differentiation   469
Sexual Precocity in Males   488
Sexual Precocity in Females   494

Index   499

Preface

The intent of these chapters is to summarize the important aspects of metabolic diseases and endocrinology in a concise manner utilizing schemes and diagrams to explain pathogenesis, disease mechanisms, and natural histories of the various disorders. Abnormalities in metabolic pathways are emphasized in an attempt to direct attention to rational methods of treatment. The information presented in this book is based on a course in metabolic diseases presented at this and other teaching institutions over the past several years. The material was collected from the more encyclopedic standard books in the field as well as from authoritative articles and reviews in specialty journals. Accordingly, the references include only excellent review articles. Highly controversial data are authenticated by specific references. It is hoped that this book will serve as a course book from which the important and relevant aspects of metabolic diseases and endocrinology may be effectively presented. The book should also serve as an up-to-date substantive review of this field for medical students, house staff, and subspecialists for clinical practice as well as for board examinations.

I should like to thank Doctors Fred Palmer and Laird Seaich, formerly Fellows in Endocrinology, for reading the manuscript, and in general for serving as a sounding board, especially for controversial material. I am deeply indebted to Mrs. Lucille Innes of the Audiovisual Service at Loma Linda University for the artwork. The secretarial assistance of Alice Hickman, Carmel Danieri, and Robbie Cleek is gratefully acknowledged. I should also like to thank Paul Brookes, production manager, and Betsy Webb, production editor, for their meticulous attention during the editing and production of this book.

Habeeb Bacchus, Ph.D., M.D., F.A.C.P.

To my students, who hoped I would,
To my friends, who thought I should,
And to my wife, who knew I could,
Write this book.

1 Intermediary Metabolism: Interrelations among Carbohydrate, Fat, and Protein Metabolism

The pathways of carbohydrate synthesis and degradation, as well as the tricarboxylic acid cycle, occupy a central locus in intermediary metabolism and energy production. These pathways also provide intermediates which serve as starting points for several essential biosynthetic and degradation pathways. Carbohydrate is the major substrate for this series of pathways, and is the major energy-producing foodstuff for man and most animals. In discussing these pathways major emphasis will be placed on the mechanisms controlling the various enzymatic reactions. The importance of such control mechanisms in the efficient operation of intermediary metabolism will become evident (1–3).

Glucose is the chief substrate for the enzymes operating in the Embden-Meyerhof (anaerobic glycolysis), the hexose monophosphate shunt (pentose phosphate pathway), and the citric acid cycle. Entrance of glucose into the cell depends on the type of cell—in some cases the carbohydrate is freely diffusible across the cell membrane, whereas in others insulin is necessary for transmembrane transfer of the carbohydrate. This effect of insulin relates to the physicochemical features of C-1–2 of the carbohydrate molecule. Glucose is phosphorylated to glucose-6-P (G-6-P) (the first step in the Embden-Meyerhof reaction). The cell membrane is now impermeable to this phosphorylated carbohydrate. The fates of the intracellular G-6-P are:

1. the Embden-Meyerhof pathway (anaerobic glycolysis)
2. the hexose monophosphate shunt (pentose phosphate pathway)
3. storage as glycogen for rapid utilization later
4. release as glucose and inorganic phosphate (via phosphatase) as a means of maintaining blood glucose levels
5. formation of uronic acids by utilizing the initial steps of alternative 3 above

EMBDEN-MEYERHOF PATHWAY

The Embden-Meyerhof (EM) pathway (anaerobic glycolysis) (Figure 1.1) is a relatively efficient series of reactions in which an initial investment of two high energy phosphate bonds results in a net gain of two adenosine triphosphates (ATPs) per mole of hexose metabolized. This pathway generates high energy phosphates under anaerobic conditions. In this manner, an energy source for muscle, particularly myocardium, functioning often under highly anaerobic conditions, is provided. Lactate is the final product of this anaerobic pathway. Most of the enzymes involved in the Embden-Meyerhof pathway are located in the cytosol of mammalian cells.

Pyruvate, an intermediate in the Embden-Meyerhof pathway, has several alternative fates, including anaerobic conversion to lactate and anaplerotic sequences which provide intermediates either for gluconeogenesis or for generation of the citric acid cycle. The anaerobic conversion to lactate is catalyzed by the enzyme lactic dehydrogenase (L-lactate:NAD oxidoreductase). The enzyme has a molecular weight of 140,000, made up of 4 inactive units of 35,000 each. Under anaerobic conditions (e.g., rapid muscle contraction), reduction of pyruvate to lactate provides for reoxidation of NADH without need for aerobic oxidation. The lactate is aerobically metabolized by reversal of the reaction, the only fate open to it. Lactate oxidation requires rapid removal of pyruvate by oxidizing reactions, providing relatively low concentrations of pyruvate. This latter condition prevails under highly aerobic conditions with rapid oxidative decarboxylation of pyruvate.

The anaplerotic reactions in which pyruvate is involved are as follows. Oxidative decarboxylation to acetyl-CoA is catalyzed by an enzyme complex in mammalian mitochondria, the pyruvate dehydrogenase complex. This complex is made up of three distinct enzymes, viz., pyruvate decarboxylase, lipoic dehydrogenase, and lipoic transacetylase. Carboxylation of pyruvate by the "malic enzyme" in the presence of NADPH and Mn^{++} results in the production of L-malate. Malate is then dehydrogenated in the citric acid cycle to form oxalacetate. Carboxylation of pyruvate is

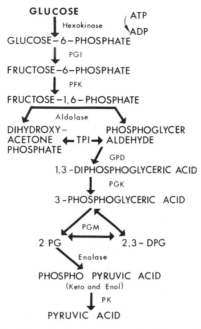

Figure 1.1. The Embden-Meyerhof reaction, a series of anaerobic reactions by which glucose is metabolized to pyruvate. A net gain of 2 moles of high-energy phosphate bonds is achieved for each mole of glucose metabolized, equivalent to 58,000 cal.

catalyzed by pyruvate carboxylase, a mitochondrial enzyme requiring ATP with biotin as cofactor. The end product of this reaction is oxalacetate. Acetyl-CoA also serves as an activator of this enzyme.

PENTOSE PHOSPHATE PATHWAY

The pentose phosphate pathway (hexose monophosphate (HMP) shunt) (Figure 1.2) plays a significant role in carbohydrate metabolism. All details of the quantities of carbohydrate utilized by this pathway are not yet clear. Muscle does not oxidize a high proportion of glucose by this pathway. A higher percentage of glucose is degraded by this pathway by tissues such as the liver, mammary tissue, testes, adipose tissue, and adrenal glands. These organs are subject to hormonal as well as other control mechanisms and the proportions of EM and HMP pathways may be altered under certain conditions. This pathway aids in providing several carbohydrate intermediates needed in cellular metabolism, such as ribose, deoxyribose, glucosamine, uronic acids, neuraminic acids, as well as significant amounts of energy.

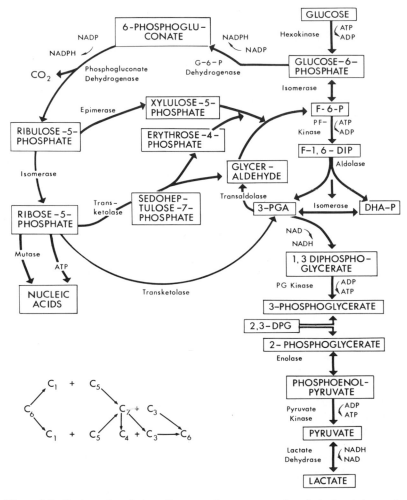

Figure 1.2. Pentose phosphate pathway, or hexose monophosphate shunt, is a major alternative degradation pathway for glucose 6-phosphate in several highly developed tissues. The interconversions of fragments ranging from 7 carbon atoms to 3 carbon atoms are shown.

Glucose-6-phosphatase, a microsomal enzyme catalyzing the irreversible reaction:

$$G\text{-}6\text{-}P + H_2O \rightarrow Glucose + P_i$$

is present in the liver, kidney, and intestinal mucosa. In the pancreatic islet cells, it has been localized in the cisternae of the endoplastic reticulum. Nuclear membrane glucose-6-phosphatase is also capable of cleaving inorganic pyrophosphate hydrolytically and of transferring PO_4 from inorganic pyrophosphate to glucose to form G-6-P. Animal experiments reveal a 3-fold increase in this enzyme after a 48-hr fast; the level returns to normal by 124 hr. In experimental diabetes, this enzyme increases and returns to normal with insulin therapy. This enzyme is also increased after cortisol administration, as well as in hereditary fructose intolerance where a marked deficiency of aldolase also occurs.

GLYCOGEN BIOSYNTHESIS

Glycogen synthesis (Figure 1.3) requires the presence of the substrate G-1-P, uridine triphosphate (UTP), as well as certain synthetic enzymes. The synthesis of glycogen from uridine diphosphoglucose (UDP-glucose) is dependent on the enzyme glycogen synthetase. The enzyme phosphorylase is involved in the degradation of glycogen. Glycogen synthetase (uridine diphosphoglucose glycogen glucosyltransferase) has been isolated from muscle in partially purified form. It has a high affinity for glycogen and, in the liver, it is firmly bound to glycogen particles. This enzyme catalyzes

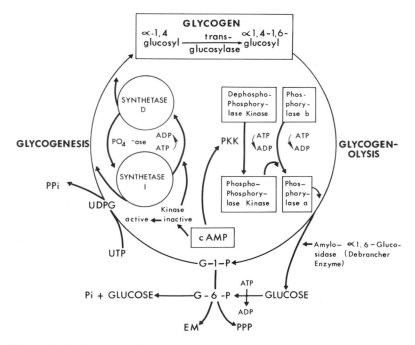

Figure 1.3. Pathways of glycogen synthesis and degradation. The role of cAMP in both glycogenesis and glycogenolysis is evident. *EM*, Embden-Meyerhof pathway; *PPP*, pentose phosphate pathway; *PKK*, phosphorylase kinase kinase.

the transfer of glucose from UDP-glucose to the growing chain of the glycogen molecule in an α-1,4-glucosidic linkage. Glycogen is the preferred acceptor, but a 4-residue maltotetrose will also serve as a minimum receptor. The enzyme glycogen synthetase exists in two forms: independent (I) is the dephosphorylated enzyme and dependent (D) is the phosphorylated enzyme which depends on the transfer of $\sim$ P from ATP by a glycogen synthetase kinase. The existence of the synthetase in two forms permits certain control mechanisms which are discussed below. The synthetase is responsible for the formation of α-1,4-glucosyl bonds. An amylo-(1,4→1,6)-transglucosylase is responsible for the branching of the glycogen molecule, i.e., the branching enzyme.

Control Mechanisms in Glycogen Synthesis

The phosphorylated enzyme (glycogen synthetase D) is activated by G-6-P, and this constitutes a major control mechanism whereby the synthesis of glycogen is stimulated as the level of G-6-P increases. For example, in classic glycogenosis I (von Gierke's), G-6-P phosphatase is missing; hence, the resultant accumulation of G-6-P stimulates increased glycogen synthesis via increased activity of the D-synthetase. The dephosphoenzyme (glycogen synthetase I) is inhibited by free UDP as would be expected when the supply of glucose and ATP is low, thus providing a mechanism for decreased glycogen synthesis. The formation of the active form of glycogen synthetase kinase depends on certain levels of cyclic adenosine 3′:5′-monophosphate (cAMP) formed from ATP by adenylate cyclase. This adenylate cyclase is activated by catecholamines; hence, in stress, there is a conversion of glycogen synthetase I to glycogen synthetase D so that glycogen synthesis is responsive to the level of G-6-P. Glycogen synthesis, therefore, occurs only in the presence of adequate sources of glucose and G-6-P. Glycogen itself inhibits glycogen synthetase phosphatase (hence, less of the dephospho (I) form). Therefore, when the amount of glycogen is high, the synthesis is more responsive to G-6-P, but when glycogen is low, the dephospho form becomes dominant.

GLYCOGEN BREAKDOWN

The breakdown of glycogen (Figure 1.3) is catalyzed by the enzyme glycogen phosphorylase. This enzyme has been isolated from muscle tissue and the active form has a molecular weight of approximately 500,000. There are certain common features of the amino peptide sequence of synthetase and phosphorlyase. Glycogen phosphorylase exists in a phospho as well as a dephospho form, the conversion from dephospho to phospho enzyme being dependent on a phosphorylase kinase, using ATP as phosphorylating agent. The only active form of the phosphorylase is the phospho form. Phosphorylase kinase itself is a complex enzyme existing in an active phosphorylated form and an inactive dephosphorylated form. The phosphorylated form of phosphorylase kinase is dependent on a phosphorylase kinase kinase using ATP as donor. Phosphorylase kinase kinase is activated by cAMP. Hence, in addition to making synthetase sensitive to G-6-P, epinephrine (via adenylate cyclase) also stimulates the breakdown of glycogen by activation of the kinase, and, hence, activation of the phosphorylated phosphorylase.

The phosphorylase is specific for the 1,4-glucosyl bonds; therefore, an additional enzyme (debranching enzyme) is required to hydrolyze the 1,6-bonds. It should be noted that the phosphorylase removes the 1,4-residues only to within 4 residues of a branch point. Hence, the glycogen remaining after phosphorylase action alone is limit dextrin. The enzyme glucan transferase transfers the remaining 3 residues before the branch point, and the debranching enzyme then removes the single α-1,6-glucosyl residue releasing free glucose. This glucose then must be rephosphorylated before further metabolism. Muscle phosphorylase is stimulated by epinephrine only, whereas liver phosphorylase is stimulated by both epinephrine and glucagon.

POLYOL PATHWAY

Certain tissues (e.g., lens of the eye, the liver, and the nervous system) are not dependent on insulin for the transmembrane transfer of glucose. Under conditions of ambient hyperglycemia, the freely diffusible glucose enters these cells in excessive amounts. If phosphorylation occurs then, G-6-P is formed; this intermediate has several fates available as discussed previously. Some of these tissues contain an aldose reductase which is capable of converting glucose for the polyhydroxyl (polyol) compound sorbitol. A similar mechanism results in the conversion of galactose to galactitol. Fructose may be formed from sorbitol via the L-iditol dehydrogenase enzyme.

D-Glucose   Sorbitol   D-Fructose

The polyols cross cell membranes very slowly and, consequently, oncotic forces result in an increase of water content of the cells containing increased polyols. Concurrent biochemical events may occur in these cells with excess polyols. For example, cataract formation due to polyol accumulation in the lens is associated with the following events: alterations of protein synthesis, amino acid transport, ion fluxes, inositol content, carbohydrate enzymes, and glutathione reductase. The decrease in glutathione reductase appears first after the increased fluid uptake; there is a resulting significant decrease in lens glutathione.

The polyol pathway in the cerebrospinal fluid (CSF) is regulated by ambient glucose concentration and has major implications in the genesis of both the acute and chronic aspects of diabetes mellitus. It has been suggested that in patients with diabetic ketoacidosis there is an increase of the polyol pathway in brain cells. Before therapy, dehydration and plasma hypertonicity are presumed to alleviate the consequences of the increased polyols in the brain, but an abrupt fall in blood glucose and osmolality causes a sudden shift of water to the brain, with increased CSF pressure as a result. It is, therefore, important, in the management of ketosis and hyperosmolar coma, that induction of hypotonicity is avoided.

Recent experimental studies have shown that an aldose reductase inhibitor, tetramethylene glutarate (TMG), prevents galactitol-induced cataracts in animals. The possible application of this study to clinical problems is under investigation.

GLYCOLYSIS AND GLUCONEOGENESIS

The pathways of glycolysis and gluconeogenesis (Figure 1.4) share several common, reversible reactions. There are also key enzymes in both sequences which are irreversible. The irreversible steps unique to the glycolytic pathway are mediated by the enzymes phosphofructokinase and pyruvate kinase. Phosphofructokinase is inhibited by ATP and citrate; therefore, in the face of adequate levels of ATP or of decrease in demand for the tricarboxylic acid cycle, a decrease in glycolysis results. This enzyme is also activated by cAMP. Pyruvate kinase is activated by fructose 1,6-diphosphate and is inhibited by ATP.

The irreversible steps unique to gluconeogenesis are mediated by the enzymes pyruvate carboxylase, phosphoenolpyruvate carboxykinase, and fructose-1,6-diphosphate phosphatase. Acetyl-CoA is an obligatory activator of the enzyme pyruvate carboxylase; therefore, this step in gluconeogenesis is activated only in the presence of adequate acetyl-CoA. Malonyl-CoA inhibits gluconeogenesis at this level and serves as a possible mechanism for enhancing lipogenesis from malonyl-CoA and acetyl-CoA. Phosphoenolpyruvate carboxykinase decarboxylates oxalacetate and phos-

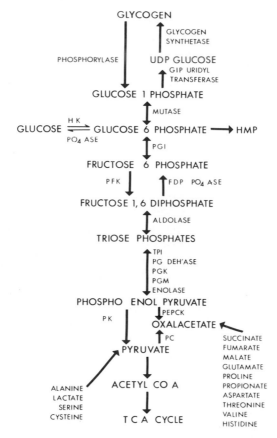

Figure 1.4. Glycolysis and gluconeogenesis. Steps common to both pathways and those unique to each are presented. Controlling mechanisms for the unique steps are described in the text. *PK,* pyruvate kinase; *PFK,* phosphofructokinase; *PC,* pyruvate carboxylase; *PEPCK,* phosphoenolpyruvate carboxykinase; *TCA,* tricarboxylic acid; *HK,* hexokinase; *TPI,* triosephosphate isomerase; *PGK,* phosphoglycerate kinase; *PGM,* phosphoglucomutase.

phorylates phosphoenolpyruvate. The synthesis of this enzyme is stimulated by cortisol, representing part of the mechanism of stimulation of gluconeogenesis by cortisol.

The various factors affecting these enzymes provide an efficient system of control of these reactions. Data are now available on the catalytic capacities of the enzymes unique to both cycles. The overall rate of glycolysis in liver, kidney, muscle, heart, and brain proceeds at 1 order of magnitude slower than the maximal capacity of phosphofructokinase. Liver and kidneys are almost exclusively active in the enzymes unique to gluconeogenesis.

While glycolysis provides each cell with a continuous supply of inter-mediates, the process of gluconeogenesis is not required for such con-tinuous supply. Nevertheless, there is a continuous hepatic and kidney gluconeogenic flux that maintains blood sugar and muscle glycogen even in the basal state. During muscular exercise the rate of gluconeogenesis increases as a result of the accumulation of lactate supplied to the liver and kidneys as substrate. In carbohydrate starvation, the increased availability of gluconeogenic amino acids and glycerol may stimulate gluconeogenesis. In addition, large amounts of acetyl-CoA from fatty acid will also stimu-late gluconeogenesis since acetyl-CoA is an obligatory activator of py-ruvate carboxylase. The process of gluconeogenesis is under hormonal control, e.g., glucocorticoids are known to increase the synthesis of phos-phoenolpyruvate carboxykinase and other gluconeogenic enzymes.

The role of alanine as a major controlling mechanism of gluconeogene-sis has been studied in considerable detail. In the fasting, as well as postabsorptive states, alanine is quantitatively the primary amino acid released by muscle. Hepatic conversion of alanine to glucose is con-siderable and exceeds that of all other amino acids. In prolonged fasting, the decreased gluconeogenesis is largely the result of diminished alanine release from muscle. In diabetes mellitus, the hepatic uptake of alanine is increased, and insulin depresses this hepatic alanine uptake. The "glucose-alanine cycle" involves the formation of alanine by the transamination of pyruvate derived from the glycolysis cycle. The amino acid (alanine) is then transported to the liver to be reconverted to glucose via gluconeo-genesis.

Relationship of Erythrocyte
2,3-Diphosphoglycerate to Oxygen Delivery to Tissues

The intermediate 2,3-diphosphoglycerate (2,3-DPG) in erythrocyte gly-colysis cycle exerts powerful effects on the oxygen-delivering potential of the red blood cell. This effect is shared by other compounds such as 3-phosphoglycerate (3-PG), 2-phosphoglycerate (2-PG), and phosphoenol-pyruvate, but 2,3-DPG has a greater effect and is present in larger amounts than ATP is in the red blood cell. Increased pH and inorganic phosphate also share this action in oxygen delivery from the red cell. When oxyhemo-globin (Hb-O_2) dissociates, the Hb competes with 2,3-DPG. Therefore, 2,3-DPG tends to push the Hb-O_2 dissociation curve to the right, whereas, in the presence of decreased 2,3-DPG, the oxygen dissociation curve is pushed to the left.

There are important clinical implications of this relationship of the red cell 2,3-DPG and glycolysis to the oxygen delivery capacity of hemo-globin. Acidosis decreases, and alkalosis increases, red cell DPG levels; therefore, rapid correction of alkalosis may delay optimal oxygen delivery to tissues by 10 hr. Transfusion with stored whole blood containing low levels of DPG permits rapid oxygen uptake by the red cells, but delivery to tissues does not increase until 24 hr later. Certain enzyme deficiencies in the erythrocyte, e.g., pyruvate kinase deficiency, cause increased 2-PG and 3-PG levels with decreased red cell oxygen affinity and relatively greater relative delivery of oxygen to tissues.

KREBS CITRIC ACID CYCLE

After anaerobic glycolysis (Embden-Meyerhof pathway) metabolizes glucose to pyruvate, this 3-carbon compound is oxidatively decarboxylated by the pyruvate dehydrogenase system to acetate. Glucose and fatty acids are completely metabolized to CO_2 and water by participation of the Krebs citric acid cycle (or tricarboxylic acid cycle) (Figure 1.5). The enzymes involved in this cycle are located in the mitochondria and operate in close association with the respiratory enzymes (Figure 1.6). Early studies showed that dicarboxylic and tricarboxylic acids added to respiring tissues resulted in marked increases in respiration. The resultant oxygen uptake was greater than could be accounted for by oxidation of the added acids. On the basis of such results, it was concluded that these intermediates serve a catalytic function and are regenerated during the oxidation. The Krebs citric acid cycle proceeds as eight reactions that are indicated in Figure 1.5. The cycle serves in anabolic and catabolic functions. This progression of the cycle also results in significant energy production that is derived from the formation of water rather than CO_2 production. The energy is used partly for heat generation to maintain body temperature and partly as chemical energy in form of ATP gained from oxidative phosphorylation. The isocitrate dehydrogenase, α-ketoglutarate dehydrogenase, and malate dehydrogenase reactions provide 3 ATPs each along with the production of NADH. The succinic dehydrogenase and succinyl thiokinase reactions result in the formation of 2 and 1 ATPs, respectively. $FADH_2$ is formed in the succinic dehydrogenase reaction. The total energy derived from these reactions is 12 ATPs or 96,000 cal per mole of activated acetate, so that 45% of the theoretically available free energy is stored as high energy phosphate.

Control Mechanisms in Citric Acid Cycle

The citric acid cycle involves coupling oxidation to phosphorylation. The rate of uptake of molecular oxygen depends on how rapidly the electron transport chain shuttles electrons to cytochrome oxidase which then reacts with molecular oxygen. The rapidity of this oxidoreduction transport will indirectly affect the rate of the initial oxidations. The generation of ATP directly affects the rate of reoxidation of the reduced components of the

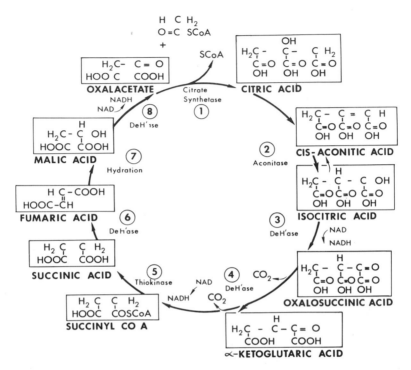

Figure 1.5. The Krebs citric acid cycle showing the metabolism of pyruvate and other intermediates to CO_2 and water with release of energy and reduced adenine nucleotides. Mitochondrial enzymatic steps are identified by numbers, namely: *(1)* citrate synthetase (inhibited by ATP); *(2)* aconitase catalyzes the dehydration of citrate to *cis*-aconitate and hydration of *cis*-aconitate to isocitric acid; *(3)* isocitric dehydrogenase catalyzes the oxidative decarboxylation of isocitric acid; *(4)* oxidative decarboxylation of oxalosuccinic acid by α-ketoglutarate dehydrogenase; *(5)* succinyl thiokinase reaction in which there is hydrolysis of the thioester link of succinyl-CoA (this is a substrate-linked phosphorylation in which GTP is produced); *(6)* succinic dehydrogenase reaction wherein succinic acid is dehydrogenated, with $FADH_2$ produced; *(7)* hydration of fumarate to malate; *(8)* malate dehydrogenase reaction resulting in production of oxalacetate and NADH.

respiratory chain (Figure 1.6). As ATP is cleaved to provide energy, the rate of respiration (and of cycle) increases rapidly, so that ADP and phosphorus will increase rapidly under such conditions, a type of feedback control. The initial reaction, the formation of citrate, is rate limiting. ATP is an inhibitor of citrate synthetase; hence, the initial entry of acetyl-CoA into the cycle is under control of availability of ATP. The ratios of AMP, ADP, and ATP undoubtedly determine the initial steps. For example, AMP stimulates glycogen phosphorylase, which would have the effect of eventually increasing acetyl-CoA. Similarly, AMP stimulates phosphofructokinase, another essential step in glycolysis.

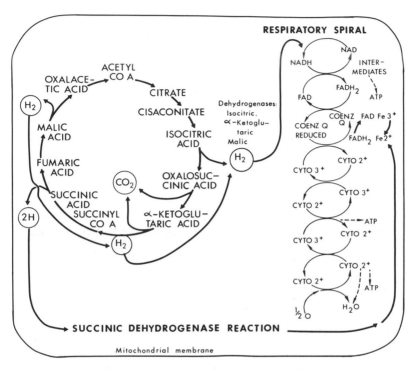

Figure 1.6. The Krebs citric acid cycle and the respiratory chain series of reactions. NADH is produced at three dehydrogenase reactions, viz., isocitrate, α-ketoglutarate, and malate. Reoxidation of each of these reduction equivalents by the respiratory chain produces 3 ATPs resulting in a total of 9 ATPs. Oxidation of succinate through reduced FADH yields 2 molecules of ATP, and the substrate-linked phosphorylation (succinyl-CoA thiokinase) yields 1 ATP. Hence, a total of 12 ATPs = 96,000 cal is released.

To summarize, citrate production is affected by activation of FDP production by AMP, inhibition of the same reaction by citrate, and inhibition of citrate synthetase by ATP. Citrate utilization is affected by the fact that AMP stimulates its oxidation and inhibits its utilization for synthetic reactions, and that citrate itself stimulates fatty acid synthesis. Thus, ATP production is kept in balance with the needs of synthetic reactions.

Catabolic functions of the Krebs tricarboxylic acid cycle are presented in Figure 1.7. These catabolic functions include entrance of carbohydrate and some amino acids via pyruvate in which alanine serves a unique function in gluconeogenesis by conversion to pyruvate after transamination. Similarly, various amino acids and fatty acids are transformed to succinyl-CoA, and urea cycle intermediates may enter the cycle through glutamate.

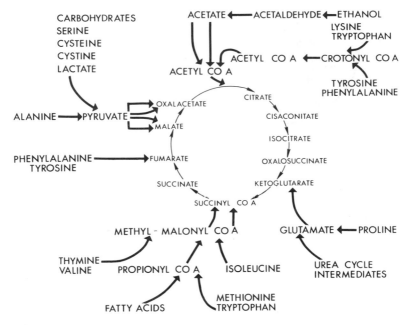

Figure 1.7. Catabolic functions of the Krebs citric acid cycle.

The anabolic functions of the tricarboxylic acid cycle are presented in Figure 1.8. The various biosynthetic functions includes the following processes: conversion of oxalacetate to phosphoenolpyruvate, an early step in gluconeogenesis; conversion of pyruvic acid to glycine to serine; acetyl-CoA conversion to malonyl-CoA, an early step in one of the lipogenic pathways; condensation of acetyl-CoA to form β-hydroxy-β-methyl-glutaryl-CoA (HMG-CoA), an essential step in the formation of cholesterol and steroids; entrance of citrate and α-ketoglutarate into the cytoplasm to form acetyl-CoA which may enter lipogenesis via the malonyl-CoA pathway; combination of succinyl-CoA with glycine to provide substrates for porphyrin synthesis; utilization of α-ketoglutarate for synthesis of glutamate which is involved in the generation of the urea cycle; and conversion of oxalacetate to aspartate in the pathway to synthesis of purine and pyrimidine nucleotides.

FAT METABOLISM

Fat metabolism has a relationship to the metabolism of carbohydrates not shared by that of proteins. The Embden-Meyerhof pathway supplies the major substrate acetyl-CoA for fatty acid synthesis. In a normal metabolic balance, the oxidation of glucose serves as a source of energy, the tri-

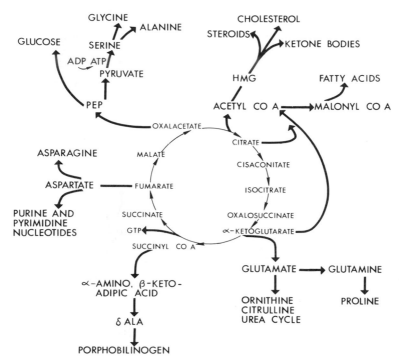

Figure 1.8. Anabolic functions of the Krebs citric acid cycle. *PEP*, phosphoenol-pyruvate.

carboxylic acid cycle intermediates are high, and this stimulates fatty acid biosynthesis by mechanisms involved in activation of acetyl-CoA carboxylase. Carbohydrate utilization prevents mobilization of fatty acids and promotes lipogenesis by favoring the synthesis of L-α-glycerophosphate in the fat cell.

Factors Controlling Fat Mobilization

Tissues differ markedly in their ability to generate energy requirements from glucose oxidation. For example, the brain utilizes glucose almost exclusively for energy; the glucose uptake by this tissue is independent of insulin. Fatty acids as such are not metabolized by the brain.

The adipose cell is made up of a large single droplet of triglyceride surrounded by a narrow cytoplasmic border containing the nucleus. Adipose tissue contains stored energy sufficient for energy requirements for 1 month. Formation of L-α-glycerophosphate is required for synthesis of triglyceride from free fatty acids (FFA); the glycerol released from triglyceride breakdown is unavailable for this purpose. Fat cells are unable to produce L-α-glycerophosphate from glycerol and ATP because of a lack of glycerokinase. There is continuous turnover of triglycerides in the fat cell caused by lipase action. The glycerol which is released readily diffuses into the circulating plasma to be metabolized in the liver. In the presence of glycerophosphate, resynthesis of triglyceride occurs. Triglyceride synthesis, therefore, requires carbohydrate utilization for generation of L-α-glycerophosphate. In fasting, where there is decreased availability of glucose, or in diabetes mellitus, where there is a failure of trans-membrane glucose transport, triglyceride breakdown exceeds resynthesis. FFA will be transported by plasma to liver, muscle, and extrahepatic tissues for utilization.

The biological half-life of depot lipids is 2–15 days, representing the rate of FFA release from triglyceride and not resynthesized to new depot fat. Circulating FFA level is normally about 500 μEq/liter, and the biological half-life is a few minutes. Thirty per cent of plasma FFA is cleared by one pass through the liver. FFA is transported bound to albumin, so that a marked decrease in serum albumin may influence FFA transport.

Triglyceride hydrolysis depends on the presence of "hormone-sensitive lipase." This enzyme is activated by catecholamine hormones, by adrenocorticotropic hormone (ACTH), thyroid-stimulating hormone (TSH), and glucagon, via participation of membrane adenylate cyclase. Insulin decreases this reaction by inhibiting the cellular level of cAMP.

Hormone-sensitive lipase activity is increased in the fasting state when the availability of glucose is markedly limited; hence, triglyceride synthesis is decreased. During the fasting state, there is a decrease in the insulin levels and, therefore, a rise in cAMP concentration. The decreased insulin level also decreases glycolysis, therefore, both events promote fatty acid mobilization. This latter effect (in fasting) is unrelated to changes in catecholamine levels.

Fatty Acid Synthesis

The major sites of fatty acid synthesis are the liver, gastrointestinal tract, and adipose tissue. Other sites of synthesis include the bone marrow and lungs. Fatty acid synthesis is not merely a reversal of the oxidation of fatty acids because: 1) the synthetic steps require NADPH, a coenzyme not required in the oxidation process; and 2) fatty acid synthesis occurs much more rapidly in non-mitochondrial areas than in the mitochondria.

The major site of fatty acid synthesis involves an aggregate of enzymes located in the cytosol of the cell. Secondary pathways for lengthening of fatty acids are located in microsomal and mitochondrial fashions. The fact that acetyl-CoA, the eventual substrate for fatty acid synthesis, is synthesized in the mitochondrial compartment posed questions as to the mechanism of generation of extramitochondrial acetyl-CoA. The following

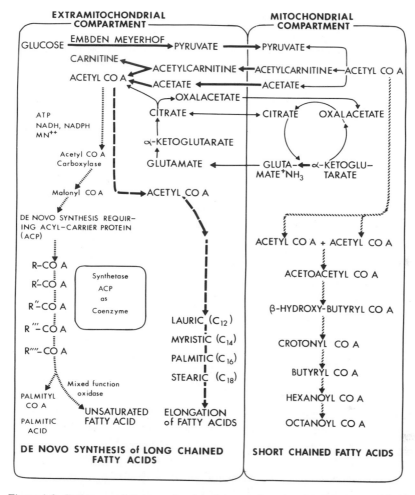

Figure 1.9. Pathways of lipogenesis, showing reactions in the extramitochondrial compartment leading to synthesis of long-chain fatty acids. The mitochondrial steps resulting in synthesis of short-chain fatty acids are also shown. NADPH is required in all three pathways of lipogenesis.

mechanism is proposed: viz., pyruvate, the end product of the Embden-Meyerhof pathway, diffuses into the mitochondrion where the pyruvate dehydrogenase complex converts it to acetyl-CoA. This end product does not penetrate the mitochondrial membrane. It has been suggested that the transport of acetyl-CoA across the mitochondrial membrane is due to the following (Figure 1.9):

1. Participation of carnitine, whereby the acetyl group is transferred to carnitine by an acetyl-CoA-carnitine transferase. This acetyl carnitine

penetrates the mitochondrial membrane and enters the cytosol. The acetyl group is then transferred to coenzyme A in the cytosol.

2. Acetyl-CoA may be deacylated in the mitochondrion, and the acetate diffuse through the membrane. The acetate is then recombined with CoA by acetate thiokinase in the cytoplasm.

3. Citrate, formed from condensation of acetate and oxalacetate, diffuses freely into the cytosol. The citrate cleaving enzyme in the cytosol then releases acetyl-CoA and oxalacetate in the extramitochondrial compartment.

Fatty acid synthesis is closely tied to the pathways of carbohydrate utilization (EM and HMP pathways) and to the tricarboxylic acid cycle.

In Figure 1.9, three pathways of fatty acid synthesis in the liver are described, the non-mitochondrial (malonyl-CoA system) which is the major pathway and two mitochondrial pathways. The overall reaction for synthesis of the fatty acid palmitic acid in the nonmitochondrial system (malonyl-CoA system) is:

$$8 \text{ Acetyl-CoA} + 16 \text{ NADPH} + 8 \text{ ATP} \rightarrow C_{15} H_{31} \text{ COOH} +$$
$$16 \text{ NADP} + 8 \text{ ADP} + 9 \text{ P}_i + 8 \text{ CoA}$$

It should be noted that NADPH is required in all three pathways.

Fatty Acid Oxidation (Figure 1.10)

Carbohydrate and protein each provide 4 cal/g whereas fat provides 9 cal/g. Fatty acids in the form of triglycerides are stored in an almost anhydrous form, whereas both proteins and carbohydrates are stored in an aqueous environment. Oxidation pathways of fatty acids involve β oxidation and deacylation reactions which result in the end products acetyl- or propionyl-CoA. These are finally oxidized to CO_2 and H_2O via the tricarboxylic acid cycle. The principal enzymes catalyzing β oxidation are located in the mitochondria. The tricarboxylic acid cycle and the respiratory chain couple the largest portion of the available energy to the generation of ATP. This energy is conserved in the reactive thioester intermediates.

The continuous operation of this cycle produces an acetyl-CoA pool. Oxidation of even numbered fatty acid (palmitic acid) is as follows:

$$CH_3 - (CH_2)_{14} - COOH + ATP + 8 \text{ CoA} + 7 \text{ NAD} + 7 \text{ Enz FAD} + 7 \text{ H}_2O \rightarrow$$

$$8 \text{ CH}_3 - \overset{\overset{\text{O}}{\|}}{\text{C}}\text{-SCoA} + AMP + PP_i + 7 \text{ NADH} + 7 \text{ H}^+ + 7 \text{ Enz FADH}_2$$

ATP is involved in activation of the substrate, but each reduced NAD coenzyme is associated with production of 3 ATPs. Therefore, a total of 7

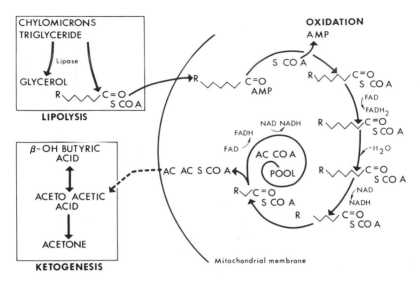

Figure 1.10. Fatty acid oxidation. Summary of release of triglycerides from chylomicrons, and the intramitochondrial steps.

X 3 or 21 ATPs is formed. Reduction of each flavin nucleotide provides 2 ATPs, so that the total net gain in this oxidation is 34 ATPs, i.e., 35 generated in the process minus the initial ATP involved in the initial activation.

Ketogenesis and Ketolysis (Figure 1.10)

If large amounts of fat are being mobilized and oxidized, the rate of oxidation of acetyl-CoA units may exceed the rate at which they condense with oxalacetate, as in diabetes mellitus and starvation. Alternative pathways for their utilization are ketogenesis and cholesterologenesis. The liver is very active in synthesis of ketone bodies, but their further metabolism via oxidative pathways takes place mainly in extrahepatic tissues. They diffuse into the circulation and are then metabolized. The ketone body β-hydroxybutyrate is oxidized back to acetoacetate in a reaction activated by thiokinase; succinyl-CoA can also be used for this purpose.

Factors Controlling Fatty Acid Synthesis

The main source of acetyl-CoA is pyruvate from the Embden-Meyerhof pathway. Pyruvate is converted to acetyl-CoA by the pyruvate dehydrogenase complex of enzymes. The rate-limiting step in fatty acid synthesis is the acetyl-CoA carboxylase reaction. This enzyme is decreased in fasting and in diabetes mellitus, and is increased with refeeding, as well as in hyperthyroidism. Fatty acid synthesis is stimulated by citrate, isocitrate, and by di- and tricarboxylic acids, but free fatty acids and acyl-CoA derivatives inhibit the acetyl-CoA carboxylase reaction. As NADPH is required in all three lipogenic pathways, the relative importance of the hexose monophosphate shunt, which provides this cofactor, is apparent.

Mobilization of Fatty Acids

Mobilization of fatty acids (Figure 1.11) from adipose tissue depends on the relative rates of the opposing processes of triglyceride lipolysis and fatty acid esterification back to triglyceride. The rate-limiting reaction in lipolysis is removal of the first long chain fatty acids from triglyceride to form a diglyceride. Removal of fatty acids thereafter is a rapid continuous process, but there is re-esterification which traps essentially all of fatty acids as triglyceride within adipocyte. The availability of glucose governs the rate of re-esterification and, hence, the rate of FFA production. Because adipose tissue cannot phosphorylate glycerol significantly, the α-glycerophosphate has to be made via the Embden-Meyerhof pathway from glucose, and it is, therefore, dependent on insulin. Transfer of glucose across adipose cell membrane is insulin dependent; hence, insulin is an effective regulator of FFA mobilization. The adipocyte is exquisitely sensitive to insulin and reduces its output of FFA in response to concentrations too low to affect blood sugar levels.

Effect of Fatty Acid Oxidation on Carbohydrate Metabolism

Fatty acid oxidation profoundly affects intermediary carbohydrate metabolism. In the liver, free fatty acids depress the action of pyruvate kinase,

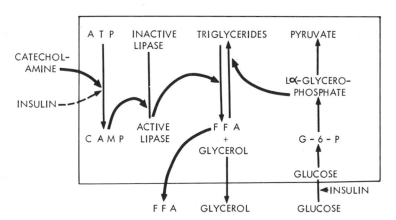

Figure 1.11. Mobilization of fatty acids and explanation of the roles of insulin, catecholamines, and cAMP in these processes. Note that insulin action (*broken line*) inhibits conversion of ATP to cAMP.

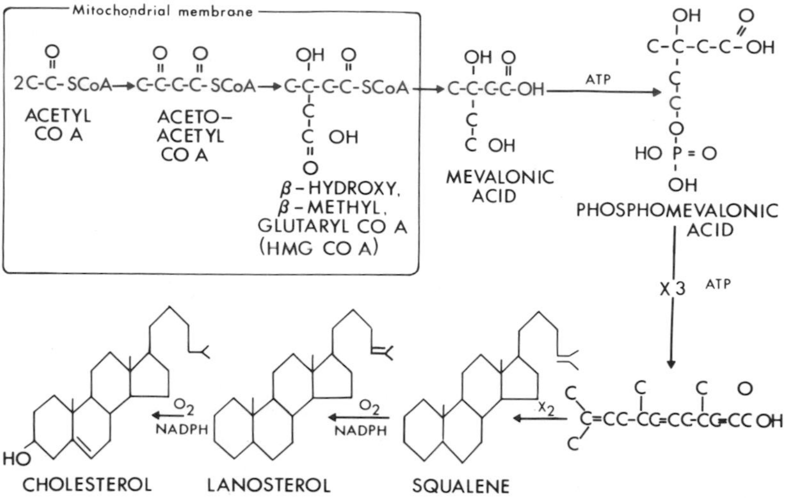

Figure 1.12. Cholesterol synthesis. Note that the steps to mevalonic acid are not necessarily confined to the mitochondrial compartment.

resulting in decreased glycolysis. Fatty acids increase hepatic glycogenesis via increased levels of G-6-P. Fatty acid oxidation induces increased gluconeogenesis by an increase in pyruvate carboxylase activity. In muscle tissue, free fatty acid oxidation increases the pool of acetyl-CoA which leads to increased levels of citrate via the tricarboxylic acid cycle. The high levels of citrate block phosphofructokinase activity, with resulting accumulation of F-6-P and G-6-P. The increased G-6-P increases the activity of dependent glycogen synthetase and decreases the hexokinase reaction. The net result is an increased glycogenesis. In addition, acetyl-CoA from fatty acid oxidation inhibits pyruvate dehydrogenase activity and, therefore, there is a decrease of pyruvate oxidation to acetyl-CoA.

Cholesterol Synthesis

Cholesterol is synthesized de novo in the mammalian cell from the substrate acetyl-CoA (Figure 1.12). The process is considered in five steps: 1) synthesis of β-hydroxy-β-methylglutaryl-CoA (HMG-CoA); 2) synthesis of mevalonic acid; 3) synthesis of the isoprenoid unit; 4) conversion of squaline to lanosterol; and 5) conversion of lanosterol to cholesterol.

The first step, synthesis of HMG-CoA, takes place in mitochondrial compartment. HMG-CoA, the precursor of mevalonate, can also be synthesized in extramitochondrial regions (similar to the steps involving acyl carrier protein derivatives in fatty acid synthesis). In steps 2 through 5, mevalonate formation and cholesterol synthesis occur primarily in the endoplasmic reticulum (ER) associated with microsomes.

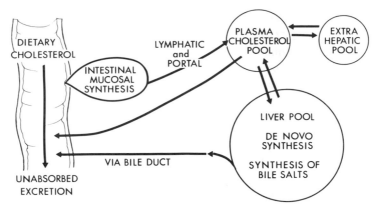

Figure 1.13. Cholesterol metabolism. Distribution of cholesterol among body pools.

Cholesterol Metabolism

Cholesterol (Figure 1.13) is involved in many biological processes, namely, substrate for steroid hormone, vitamin D, and bile salt synthesis. Highest concentrations are found in the adrenal cortex and the brain. Plasma and liver cholesterol are essentially a single pool with rapid turnover rate. There is virtually no exchange between plasma cholesterol and the central nervous system.

Cholesterol-degrading enzymes are most active in the liver. A significant amount of dietary cholesterol is excreted in the stools. Absorbed dietary cholesterol mixes with the plasma-liver pool and, in this form, is essentially indistinguishable from that synthesized de novo. There is an inverse relationship between absorbed cholesterol and synthesis. The major excretion pathway is via bile salts.

AMINO ACID METABOLISM

Amino acids are chemical compounds which contain amino groups and possess the prototype structure:

$$H_2N - \overset{\displaystyle R}{\underset{\displaystyle H}{\overset{|}{\underset{|}{C}}}} - COOH$$

They differ according to composition of the side chain and the presence of one or more NH_2 or COOH groups. They are classified as:

1. Aliphatic
    a. Neutral: 1 amino group, 1 COOH: glycine, alanine, α-amino-*n*-butyric, valine, isoleucine, leucine

  1 amino, 1 COOH; 1 OH groups; serine, threonine
  1 amino, 2 COOH: asparagine, glutamine
  Sulfur containing: cysteine, cystine, methionine
  β-amino compounds: taurine; β-alanine; β-aminoisobutyric
 b. Basic or cationic: 2 amino groups, 1 COOH: arginine, lysine;
    ornithine
 c. Acidic or anionic: 1 amino group, 2 COOH: aspartic, glutamic
2. Aromatic
 a. Neutral: phenylalanine, tyrosine
3. Heterocyclic
 a. Neutral: proline, hydroxyproline, tryptophan
 b. Basic: histidine

All biologically active amino acids are of the L-α-rotatory form. Relatively high content of protein in human diet supplies a large proportion of the amino acids needed for protein biosynthesis. In man, the eight essential amino acids are: 1) leucine, 2) isoleucine, 3) valine, 4) lysine, 5) methionine, 6) phenylalanine, 7) tryptophan, and 8) threonine. To provide sufficient amounts of these essential amino acids, the normal diet should contain 8–10% protein. Protein requirements vary according to age. At age 2 months, the requirement is 2.2 g/kg/24 hr; at age 6–12 months, 1.4 g/kg/24 hr; and, in the adult, 0.7 g/kg/24 hr. These requirements increase in the presence of infections, illness, menstruation, pregnancy, and lactation. Of the amino acids involved in protein synthesis, the 11 essential amino acids (Table 1.1) are synthesized in man. Others are obtained from plant and animal sources. Animals, therefore, need a source of complex nitrogen-containing compounds such as amino acids and proteins.

Table 1.1. Biosynthesis of Nonessential Amino Acids in Man

Amino acid	Origin of carbons and non-amino nitrogens
Alanine	All C from pyruvate
Aspartic acid	All C from oxalacetate
Cysteine	All C from serine S from methionine
Glutamic acid	All C from α-ketoglutarate
Glycine	Pyruvate via phosphoglycerate via serine
Histidine	Imidazole N-1, C-2 from adenylic acid, imidazol N-3 from glutamine
Proline and hydroxyproline	All C from glutamate
Serine	All C from pyruvate via phosphoglycerate
Tyrosine	Side chain from P-enolpyruvate; ring from erythrose 4-phosphate and P-enolpyruvate; in mammals from phenylalanine by hydroxylation

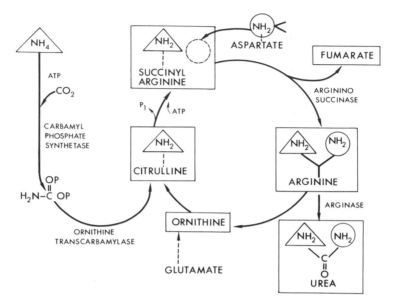

Figure 1.14. The urea cycle (Krebs-Henseleit cycle).

The conversion of inert N_2 to NH_3, the process of nitrogen fixation essential to all life, is limited to relatively few organisms. These include anaerobic azotobacter and anaerobic clostridium. The photosynthetic bacterium rhodospirillum rubrum and certain algae are also "nitrogen fixers." Leguminous plants like alfalfa in symbiosis with rhizobium located in root nodules also fix nitrogen. Although mammalian cells have three systems for catalyzing the incorporation of ammonia into various carbon skeletons, these are inadequate for total needs. Ammonia is essential to mammalian metabolism but, because of its toxicity, endogenous enzymatic methods for its disposition have evolved. These are the glutamine dehydrogenase reaction which interconverts the carbon skeletons of carbohydrates and amino acids, the ATP-dependent formation of glutamine, and the ATP-dependent formation of carbamylphosphate from CO_2 and NH_3.

The Krebs-Henseleit cycle is responsible for the synthesis of urea. The immediate sources of NH_2 groups are ammonia (ammonium ion) and the amino group of aspartate. Figure 1.14 presents the synthesis of carbamylphosphate, a reaction requiring the presence of ammonia, CO_2, 2 molecules of ATP, and a synthetase which is activated by N-acetylglutamate. The first ATP is utilized to form an enzyme bound "active carbonate" and the second ATP is involved in forming carbamylphosphate from NH_4 and "active carbonate." The ATP requirement is responsible for the essential reversibility of the reaction. Carbamylphosphate synthetase is associated with an active urea cycle, but is also present in tissues requiring pyrimidine synthesis.

The first step unique to the urea cycle is that catalyzed by ornithine transcarbamylase (carbamoylphosphate: L-aspartate carbamoyltransferase) which is found in the liver. The enzyme arginino-succinic synthetase is found in the liver and kidney and catalyzes the condensation of the amino group of aspartate with the C=O group of citrulline. Arginino-succinase catalyzes the cleavage of the N–C group of acyl guanidino group to form fumarate and arginine; the reaction is reversible and the equilibrium favors arginino-succinate.

Arginase is the unique enzyme of the urea cycle and is the hallmark enzyme of ureotelic animals. (This enzyme appears in the amphibian liver during metamorphosis, at which time the organism alters the nitrogen exertion mechanism from ammonotelic to ureotelic.) This enzyme is present in greatest amounts in the liver, accounting for the majority of urea synthesis. Low blood urea nitrogen (BUN) levels in liver disease are due to decreased arginase. The enzyme is also present in mammary gland, testes, kidney, and skin. (It is absent from liver of birds and reptiles.) Arginase levels are stimulated by adrenocortical hormones.

LITERATURE CITED

1. Coleman, J. E. 1974. Metabolic interrelationships between carbohydrates, lipids and proteins. *In* P. K. Bondy and L. E. Rosenberg (eds.), Diseases of Metabolism, pp. 107–220. W. B. Saunders Co., Philadelphia.
2. Krebs, H. A., and J. M. Lowenstein. 1960. The tricarboxylic acid cycle. *In* D. M. Greenberg (ed.), Metabolic Pathways, Vol. 1, pp. 129–203. Academic Press, New York.
3. Green, D. E., and D. M. Gibson. 1960. Fatty acid oxidation and synthesis. *In* D. M. Greenberg (ed.), Metabolic Pathways. Vol. 1, pp. 301–340. Academic Press, New York.

2

Clinical Disorders of Carbohydrate Metabolism

Circulating blood glucose is derived from two major sources—dietary carbohydrates and the process of gluconeogenesis. Glycogenolysis of stored carbohydrate contributes a quantitatively smaller portion of circulating glucose. Dietary carbohydrate may be considered nonessential in view of the production of glucose from other sources through gluconeogenesis. Nevertheless, considerable amounts of carbohydrate are included in the American diet in the form of vegetables, grain foods, and purified sugars (e.g., sucrose). The absorption of glucose from the gastrointestinal tract takes place after intraluminal processes, involving breakdown of starches and other glucose polymers by amylases and disaccharidases to release glucose. Certain foodstuffs also provide fructose and galactose so that the major hexose components for digestion include the three sugars listed above. Transmucosal transfer of these hexoses into the blood stream involves passive diffusion through the intestinal mucosal cells as well as intramucosal active processes involving phosphorylation (1).

Most ingested carbohydrate is converted to glucose. The resulting raised postabsorptive blood glucose level stimulates the release of insulin by the β islets of the pancreas. This process is mediated by mechanisms involving glucose itself, glucagon, as well as vagus impulses. An intricate system of checks and balances is responsible for maintenance of blood levels of glucose between 60 and 110 mg/100 ml (Figure 2.1). Pituitary growth hormone (GH), cortisol, and insulin, with participation or modulation by glucagon, normally exert a fine control of blood glucose levels (Figures 2.1 and 2.2). Glucose is the major energy source for the central nervous system, the red blood cells, the renal medulla, and bone marrow,

28   Habeeb Bacchus

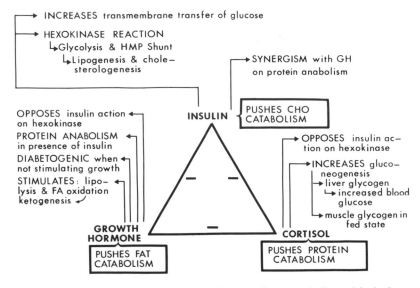

Figure 2.1. Endocrine factors in control of intermediary metabolism with the inter-relationships among the growth hormone, cortisol, and insulin. The *minus signs* indicate opposing actions on the metabolic parameters. Synergistic actions are also depicted in the scheme.

and, undoubtedly, the fine control of glucose levels is designed to serve these functions.

In conditions of lowered blood glucose, the levels are replenished by the processes of glycogenolysis (via catecholamines and glucagon), gluconeogenesis (via cortisol), lipolysis (via GH), decreased glucose utilization, and increased fatty acid oxidation. Hypoglycemia induces decreased insulin secretion, and this is followed by decreases in carbohydrate utilization, lipogenesis, and glycolysis. Increased oxidation of fatty acids leads to decreased generation of the tricarboxylic acid cycle and increased gluconeogenesis (see controlling factors, Chapter 1). The above processes provide sufficient carbohydrate for central nervous system metabolism and serve to promote utilization of other sources of energy for other tissues.

When the blood glucose is at the normoglycemic level of 100 mg/100 ml, the total glucose in circulating plasma, red blood cells, and extracellular fluids amounts to only 24 g, equivalent to 96 kcal. Tissue carbohydrate exists in the phosphorylated form and release of such forms into the blood stream requires the action of phosphatases from tissues such as the liver, muscle, and the intestinal mucosal cell. Stored carbohydrate in the amount of 200 g exists mainly in muscles and the liver, the component in the liver accounting for 60 g. The liver may release up to 3 mg/kg/min, equivalent to 10–12 g/hr or 40–48 kcal/hr in an average sized individual. Hepatic

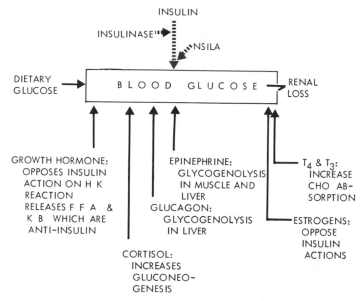

Figure 2.2. Control of blood glucose levels, including participation of dietary renal and endocrine factors. *Solid lines* refer to actions tending to increase blood glucose levels. *Broken lines* refer to inhibitory actions, e.g., insulin lowers blood glucose, but insulinase opposes insulin action. *NSILA,* nonsuppressible insulin-like activity.

glycogenesis is stimulated mainly by glucagon and muscle glycogenesis principally by catecholamines.

GLUCONEOGENESIS

This process whereby carbohydrate is formed from non-carbohydrate substrates occurs mainly in the liver (90%) and the kidneys (10%) in normal human subjects. A normal man fasting 2–3 days releases 180 g of glucose/24 hr via the splanchnic bed. Of this amount, the requirement by the central nervous system is 140 g, and by the formed elements of blood, 10 g. In addition, the renal medulla is glucose dependent. These sources account for only 560 kcal/24 hr, and, therefore, the major energy needs of the body are obtained from other processes. One process, that of lipolysis stimulated by catecholamines, cortisol, growth hormone, and glucagon, involves the release of triglycerides into free fatty acids (FFA) and glycerol. The FFA are utilized by muscle, and the glycerol provides substrate for the process of gluconeogenesis. Ketone bodies derived from oxidation of the fatty acids, as well as FFA, decrease glucose uptake by muscle. The human body is capable of utilizing up to 1500 kcal of ketone bodies daily.

ROLE OF KIDNEY IN GLUCOSE HOMEOSTASIS

The kidneys utilize glucose, but also function as an auxiliary glucose-producing organ. Renal gluconeogenesis is important during acidosis and prolonged starvation. In the obese patient starved for 35–40 days, the kidney may contribute around 45% of the glucose secreted into the blood stream. The kidney is also involved in carbohydrate metabolism through its production of the enzyme insulinase. This enzyme, also produced by the liver, plays a major role in the degradation of circulating insulin. In severe renal disease, the half-life of insulin in the plasma is prolonged. Electrolyte disturbances, which may be related to renal function, may affect carbohydrate metabolism also. Hypokalemia results in decreased insulin secretory capacity by the islet cells, whereas the opposite is found in the hyperkalemia.

ROLE OF CENTRAL NERVOUS SYSTEM IN GLUCOSE HOMEOSTASIS

The brain does not possess any storage form of carbohydrate. At rest, two-thirds of the total hepatic glucose is utilized by the brain, and indeed it has been suggested that "it is as if the production of glucose by liver glycogenolysis and gluconeogenesis were primarily directed by the brain" (1). In man, after 4–6 weeks of fasting, the central nervous system adapts by enzyme induction to the use of the ketone bodies acetoacetate and β-hydroxybutyrate as fuel to supplement the low amounts of glucose.

ROLE OF RED CELL MASS IN GLUCOSE HOMEOSTASIS

Red blood cells are dependent on glucose as the sole fuel, and the end product of glucose oxidation, lactate, constitutes a major part of the Cori cycle (lactate → pyruvate → gluconeogenesis). It is estimated that, in the 70-kg man with 3 liters of red blood cells, glycolysis in these cells accounts for 26 g of glucose/day (1).

ENDOCRINE FACTORS IN CONTROL OF CARBOHYDRATE HOMEOSTASIS

Endocrine factors in the control of carbohydrate homeostasis have been discussed previously (see Figures 2.1 and 2.2). Undoubtedly, the interplay between GH and factors facilitating its action, glucagon, and insulin deserve continued and closer research attention.

Growth hormone participates with insulin favoring protein anabolism

(2, 3) (Figure 2.1). This hormone also favors lipolysis, an activity supported by glucocorticoids, but this activity is suppressed by insulin. The output of pituitary growth hormone is increased by hypoglycemia, fasting, exercise, and certain stresses. The action of GH on glucose utilization is antagonistic to insulin action perhaps through a change in the sensitivity of the cellular glucose transport system. The participation of GH in glucose kinetics is also exemplified by the increased lipolysis which occurs in chronic diabetes mellitus and in chronic starvation. In these situations, the phosphorylating capacity is decreased (because of a block at the phosphofructokinase level) (see Chapter 1). This results in a rise in FFA which is responsible for a contrainsulin action, so that there is an abnormal glucose tolerance test in "starvation diabetes." Chronic excess of GH produces an insulin-resistant diabetic state accompanied by high insulin levels (3). Pancreatectomy largely abolishes the resistance induced by GH administration. Since adult-onset diabetes at isoglucose levels produces more insulin than normal, it is, therefore, likely that contrainsulin factors do play a role in this disorder.

INSULIN AND INTERMEDIARY METABOLISM

Insulin participates in several aspects of intermediary metabolism in the liver, adipose tissues, and muscles. These processes will be described later in this section. The hormone insulin is a peptide hormone consisting of 51 amino acids distributed in two chains, an A chain with 21 amino acids, and a B chain with 30 amino acids, linked by intrachain disulfide bridges. The synthesis (4–6) involves the following steps: 1) amino acids and peptides are synthesized on four membranes associated with ribosomes of the endoplasmic reticulum, and, thus, are transferred to the cisternae of the endoplasmic reticulum (ER); 2) these precursors are then transferred to the Golgi complex via "transition elements," and concentrated into granular material in the cisternae of the Golgi apparatus; 3) the secretory granules in the Golgi complex are made up of proinsulin which is an 85 amino acid peptide, a precursor of insulin; 4) conversion of proinsulin to insulin probably takes place in the maturing part of the Golgi apparatus through actions of pancreatic acinar trypsins and carboxypeptidase B. Cleavage of peptide 31–63 of the A chain releases insulin (consisting of A (1–21), and B (1–30) linked by disulfide bridges), and the C peptide (peptide 31–63). The C peptide probably plays a role in determining the fold of insulin, and considerable interspecies variation is noted in this fragment.

Release or destruction of insulin and proinsulin in the islet cells is mediated by the following processes: emiocytosis of mature secretory granules, emiocytosis of immature granules, microvesicular release, release through increased membrane permeability, or release by emiocytosis of physicochemically altered peptides (6).

Insulin Action on Hepatic Carbohydrate Metabolism

Insulin stimulates the three key enzymes for hepatic glycolysis: the hexokinase, phosphofructokinase, and pyruvate kinase reactions. The key hepatic gluconeogenic enzymes, pyruvate carboxylase, phosphoenolpyruvate carboxykinase, and fructose-1,6-diphosphate phosphatase, are depressed by insulin. The transport of amino acids into the hepatic cell is stimulated by insulin, which also independently catalyzes the incorporation of amino acids into protein. The incorporation of pyruvate and lactate into protein anabolism is also accelerated by insulin, and the energy for mitochondrial protein synthesis is provided by the process of oxidative phosphorylation which is stimulated by insulin. In insulin lack, hepatic glucose uptake is decreased, fatty acid uptake, ketogenesis, and ketone body release are increased, uptake of amino acids is increased, and gluconeogenesis is enhanced. This results in increased hepatic glucose release.

Actions of Insulin on Muscle Metabolism

The major function of insulin in muscle tissue is the stimulation of energy utilization. This process is initiated by the transfer of glucose across the cell membrane, the rate of this process being dependent on the concentration gradient. In insulin lack, glucose uptake and utilization are decreased, utilization of fatty acids and ketones is increased, and the release of amino acids is increased.

Actions of Insulin on Adipose Tissue Metabolism

The main action of insulin on the adipose cell is the stimulation of synthesis and storage of fat. The action involves the transfer of glucose across the cell membrane, as well as stimulation of the hexose monophosphate shunt. This pathway provides substrates and cofactors for the three pathways of lipogenesis. In the absence of insulin, the uptake of glucose by the adipocyte and the process of lipogenesis are decreased while lipolysis is increased.

Mechanism of Stimulation of Secretion of Insulin

Because of the time relationships of formation of intermediate metabolites, it seemed probable that the glucose molecule exerts the insulin-releasing action by stimulating glucoreceptors in the cell membrane. New studies on the mode of action of insulin once released reveal that insulin attaches itself to a specific receptor (probably glycoprotein) at the membrane. This event causes specific changes in the molecular structure of certain parts of the membrane (4). The changes activate transport carriers for certain sugars, amino acids, and electrolytes, and, at the same time, a second messenger (probably a sialopeptide) is released into the cell. The second messenger acts upon a reaction shared at some point by the processes of anabolism—glycogen synthesis, protein, fat, and nucleic acid synthesis.

GLUCAGON AND INTERMEDIARY METABOLISM

Glucagon is a polypeptide consisting of 29 amino acid residues which is secreted by α cells of the islets of Langerhans. Intestinal glucagon, presumably identical with that from the α cells, has been isolated from extracts of the colon, jejunum, duodenum, stomach, and, occasionally, from lymph nodes, skin, spleen, and tongue. Plasma glucagon levels are increased during fasting. The normal nonfasting level may approach 100 pg/ml. This substance is metabolized rapidly, with a biological half-life 25–50% that of insulin. In hypoglycemia and fasting, there may be a 2- to 3-fold increase in plasma glucagon. Glucagon stimulates phosphorylase activity and the breakdown of glycogen to glucose 1-phosphate. Blood glucose levels are thereby increased in the presence of pyruvate and intact adrenocortical function. The process of gluconeogenesis is stimulated by glucagon by an activation of the steps between pyruvate to phosphoenolpyruvate via oxalacetate. The release of membrane adenylate cyclase by glucagon mediates the process. Glucagon may also reduce the incorporation of amino acids into muscle protein.

HORMONAL CONTROL OF CARBOHYDRATE METABOLISM

Considerations of the hormonal interplay in control of carbohydrate metabolism are presented in part in Figures 2.1 and 2.2. The intricate process is also demonstrated by the events following the ingestion of a mixed meal. Three successive stages of response are noted after this stimulus: 1) insulin release; 2) insulin release coupled with GH release; and 3) GH effect alone.

1. With absorption of glucose and amino acids, there occurs an increase in the release of insulin. Initial release comes from a rapid pool in the β cell of preformed insulin. The later "continuous release" from a larger pool is derived from new synthesis of insulin in response to the challenge. In diabetes mellitus, the rapid pool is resistant to normal stimuli such as rises in blood glucose. The insulin released at this stage in normal subjects serves to dispose of the glucose, inhibit fat mobilization (via insulin action on lipoprotein lipase), and initiate labile protein synthesis.

2. In the second stage, i.e., release of insulin and GH, the insulin-induced drop in glucose stimulates release of GH which serves to limit glucose uptake through the antagonism to insulin actions on transport and phosphorylation mechanisms, as well as to promote protein synthesis.
3. In the stage of GH effect alone, which is the beginning of the postprandial fasting period, there is maintenance of protein stores, beginning of fat mobilization, and sparing of glucose.

TESTS OF CARBOHYDRATE METABOLISM

Tests of carbohydrate turnover range from estimation of fasting blood glucose levels to measurement of glucose levels after various challenges. The fasting blood glucose ranges between 60 mg/100 ml and 100 mg/100 ml. The value for plasma glucose is somewhat higher and may be calculated as follows:

(Blood glucose $\times$ 1.15) + 6 mg/100 ml = plasma glucose (mg/100 ml).

The postprandial blood glucose levels should return to fasting levels within 2–3 hr after meals. Abnormal values in this test are similar to those in the oral glucose tolerance test discussed below. Random blood glucose levels may be helpful in assessing carbohydrate metabolism provided that the conditions and the time the sample was obtained are known.

Glucose Tolerance Tests

In the oral glucose tolerance test (GTT), the subject is given a measured amount of glucose (50–100 g) solution by mouth. A prototype oral GTT is presented in Figure 2.3, which also presents the factors affecting the phases in the curve. The normal subject absorbs enough glucose during the first 30 min to raise the blood glucose by 30–50 mg/100 ml. After this, the rate of fall exceeds the absorption rate. By 120 min, the blood glucose should fall to within 10 mg/100 ml of the fasting level. In adrenocortical or pituitary insufficiency, the blood glucose drops to below 50 mg/100 ml and may induce clinical symptoms of hypoglycemia, although recent data indicate that even lower blood glucose levels may be tolerated without symptoms. The terminal rise in blood glucose levels during the GTT is ascribable to the processes of gluconeogenesis and glycogenolysis and is absent when gluconeogenesis is defective, as in adrenocortical insufficiency. The upper limits of the normal GTT are discussed below under analysis of the GTT. In diabetes mellitus, the fasting blood glucose may be elevated and the entire curve is displaced upward.

A flat GTT curve is seen in the presence of intestinal malabsorption, in adrenal insufficiency, and in pituitary insufficiency. Patients who are hyperactive, whether due to neuroses or other psychiatric problems, often

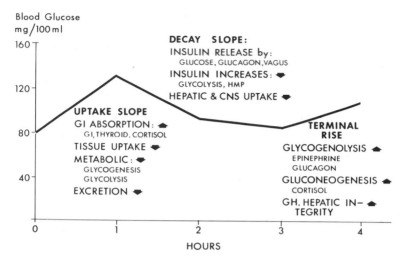

Figure 2.3. Metabolic processes in the normal glucose tolerance test. Processes involved in the different phases of the curve are presented. *Thick arrows* indicate directions of changes in blood glucose levels.

display a flat glucose tolerance curve. While this has been termed a normal variant, examination of the dynamics of the test from Figure 2.3 would suggest that rapid uptake and utilization due to hypermobility may be responsible for the shape of the curve in such conditions. In severe hyperthyroidism with hypermotility, the uptake may be decreased, but in most hyperthyroid patients there is a rapid absorption followed by a rapid fall-off of blood glucose.

Intravenous Glucose Tolerance Test

This procedure is most useful to avoid problems with gastrointestinal absorption. Fifty milliliters of 50% glucose is infused intravenously over a period of 2 min. Blood glucose levels are obtained at zero time and at 5, 10, 30, 60, and 90 min after the infusion. The peak level is observed at 5 min, after which an exponential fall-off occurs. The value k is a mathematical indication of the rate of glucose utilization. It is easily obtained by plotting the blood glucose levels on a logarithmic scale and time on a linear scale. The half-time is determined from the straight portion of the curve. Average normal subjects have a k value of 0.02 or a utilization rate of 2%/min, while diabetic patients have significantly lower k values. Patients with hypermetabolic states and hyperactivity associated with neuroses, as well as patients in certain degrees of malnutrition, may exhibit relatively flat intravenous GTT curves, reflecting increased muscle uptake of the infused glucose.

Insulin levels may be quantitated in the plasma samples obtained during the oral or intravenous GTT. A normal and appropriate rise in plasma insulin observed during the test is not noted in juvenile-onset diabetes and in small proportion of adult-onset diabetics. These constitute the insulinopenic diabetic group. Most maturity-onset obese diabetics show an exaggerated insulin response to the glucose challenge, reflecting the insulinoplethoric type of diabetes mellitus.

Cortisone-Glucose Tolerance Test

A challenge with a glucocorticoid hormone before an oral GTT unmasks the diabetic state in susceptible individuals. The patient is given 50 mg of cortisone acetate (or 12.5 mg of prednisone) 8 hr and again 2 hr before performance of the oral GTT. Blood glucose values exceeding the limits of the standard GTT reflect glucose intolerance.

Sodium Tolbutamide Response Test

This challenge with the hypoglycemic agent tolbutamide is useful to determine the presence of diabetes mellitus, to determine effectiveness of the drug, and as a test for insulin-producing tumors. In the test, the patient is given 1 g of sodium tolbutamide intravenously and blood is drawn at zero time, and at 30, 60, 90, 120, and 180 min or longer after the infusion. Alternatively, the patient may take 2 g of tolbutamide with 2 g of $NaHCO_3$ orally. In normal subjects, the blood glucose level drops to below 60% of the pretest value in the intravenous challenge. Normal subjects exhibit a blood glucose level at 30 min of below 78% of the baseline. Diabetic subjects exhibit values significantly in excess of those described above. In patients with insulinoma, there is a drop of glucose greater than 34% of the fasting level lasting 2 hr or longer.

Standardization of Oral Glucose Tolerance Test

The Committee on Statistics of the American Diabetes Association presented recommendations for the standardized oral GTT (7). The recommendations include adequate dietary preparation of around 150 g of carbohydrate daily for 3 days prior to the test. The test should not be performed within 2 weeks after an illness; drugs which may influence the GTT (e.g., diuretics or hormones) should be discontinued for at least 3 days; unusual activity should be avoided 8 hr prior to the test; and the patient should not be bedridden. There should be an 8-hr fast before the test.

Analysis of Glucose Tolerance Test

Analysis of the GTT requires careful consideration of all factors known to influence the turnover of carbohydrate. These factors include nutritional status, disease states, states of physical activity, and administration of drugs.

In the Wilkerson system, the diagnosis of diabetes mellitus based on the oral GTT requires the total of two or more points with use of the following criteria. One point each is given for blood glucose (mg/100 ml) >110 at 0 and 3 hr, and one-half point each for >170 at 1 hr, and >120 at 2 hr. This method is essentially the basis of the United States Public Health Service system. On the basis of the World Health Organization criteria, the diagnosis of diabetes mellitus is made if the 3-hr blood glucose level is 130 mg/100 ml or greater.

The Fajans-Conn system is widely used in this country and is highly recommended. In this system, the diagnosis of diabetes mellitus is made if any of the following criteria are met: blood glucose at 1 hr of 160 mg/100 ml or greater, blood glucose at 90 min of 140 mg/100 ml or greater, and blood glucose at 120 min of 120 mg/100 ml or greater. An alternative procedure is the summation of blood glucose values at 0-, 1-, 2-, and 3-hr intervals during the GTT. The diagnosis of diabetes mellitus is made if the sum of blood glucose levels at those intervals equals or exceeds 500 mg/100 ml; if plasma glucose values are employed, the critical figure is 600 mg/100 ml.

In view of the several factors which influence the GTT, it is recommended that a repeat GTT should be done after a reasonable interval if the initial test provided equivocal data. A GTT is valid only if it is performed in the patient adequately prepared by diet, who is not bedridden or on drugs such as hormones, kaliuretic, and hypoglycemic agents. It is also important that the test is not done within 2 weeks after an acute illness.

Advancing age may alter the GTT very slightly. The k value in the intravenous GTT is lowered by age. In renal failure, the oral GTT is of a diabetic type, a reflection of several abnormal mechanisms. Hypokalemia, whether spontaneous or induced by diuretics, is associated with a diabetic type GTT; this is corrected by potassium supplementation. Hypothyroidism is associated with a flat GTT, a reflection of decreased absorption. In hyperthyroidism, both the absorption and the falloff are increased. Impaired GTT is noted in acromegaly, hypocalcemia, the malignant neoplastic state, in myotonic dystrophy, as well as in certain hyperlipoproteinemias. In patients with hepatocellular disease, the GTT shows a diabetic pattern, and simultaneous insulin levels may be indistinguishable from the levels in maturity-onset diabetes mellitus.

DIABETES MELLITUS

Diabetes mellitus is ascribed to a relative or absolute deficiency of insulin and is characterized by impaired intermediary metabolism. The disorder in

Table 2.1. Classification of Diabetes Mellitus[a]

	Insulinoplethoric	Insulinopenic
7% of all diabetics	85–90%	10–15%
Age of onset	Adult (especially > 40)	< 15 years
Family history	+ −	+++
Body size	> 50% overweight	Normal or thin
Rate of onset	Slow	Rapid
Severity	Mild	Severe
Occurrence of ketoacidosis	Infrequent	Common
Stability	Stable	Unstable
Insulin therapy	None to very few	All
Insulin sensitivity	Decreased	Very sensitive
Response to sulfonylurea	50%	Very few to none
"Concomitants"	Less common; slower	> 90% in 20 years

[a]In addition to the above, the entity lipoatrophic diabetes, a diencephalic disorder characterized by absent or diminished adipose tissue, insulin insensitivity, without ketosis-proneness, is considered in classification of adults. It is recommended that the terms maturity-onset diabetes mellitus and juvenile-onset diabetes, hitherto referring to the insulinoplethoric and insulinopenic forms respectively, be dropped.

metabolism is characterized by appearance of hyperglycemia, glycosuria, and, if sufficiently severe, osmotic diuresis and ketonemia. Although there are familial clusters of diabetes mellitus especially among the insulinopenic group, the etiology of the disorder is unknown. Bilateral inheritance patterns are known in insulinopenic diabetics. The preponderant evidence, however, is that the inheritance pattern in most diabetics is multifactorial. Several experimental studies have implicated GH, cortisol, glucagon, catecholamines, insulin antagonists, viruses, islet cell exhaustion, insulin antibodies, as well as abnormal molecular species of insulin in pathogenesis of this disorder.

The classification of diabetes mellitus into three types is presented in Table 2.1. Of special significance is the fact that the insulinopenic diabetics fail to show an appropriate elevation of plasma insulin in response to a glucose challenge. In the insulinoplethoric group, on the other hand, there is a good response to the challenge, albeit occurring after the glucose peak, i.e., a delay in the insulin response.

Natural History and Course of Diabetes Mellitus

The evolution of the two major forms of diabetes mellitus, unless rigorously treated, is through an inexorably progressive course. Insulinopenic diabetics are subject to frequent episodes of diabetic ketoacidosis and other acute complications. Table 2.2 presents a staging classification of diabetes mellitus. Pathological changes in various organ systems due to

Table 2.2. Stages of Diabetes Mellitus

Stage		FBG[a]	GTT[a]	GC[a]-GTT	IRI[a] in GTT	Symptoms	Angiopathy
I	Prediabetes	Normal	Normal	Normal	+	0	+
II	Latent chemical	Normal	Normal	Abnormal	+	0	+
III	Chemical	Normal	Abnormal	Abnormal	+	+	++
IV	Overt	Abnormal	Abnormal	Abnormal	±	Usual	+++

[a] FBG, fasting blood glucose; GTT, glucose tolerance test; GC, glucocorticoid; IRI, immunoreactive insulin.

diabetes mellitus have been considered as complications, but are more appropriately considered as diabetic concomitants. These include the various comas in diabetes, diabetic nephropathy, diabetic retinopathy, diabetic neuropathy, and diabetic dermopathy. These are discussed in detail below.

Comas in Patients with Diabetes Mellitus

Although diabetic patients are subject to all of the possible causes of coma in the general population, there are special types of coma to which diabetics are especially prone. These are: 1) diabetic ketoacidotic coma; 2) hyperosmolar non-ketotic coma; 3) lactic acidosis; and 4) hypoglycemic coma. To facilitate understanding of the pathophysiology in these states, the patterns of intermediary metabolism of carbohydrates, lipids, and proteins are presented in Figure 2.4 representing the normal subject and Figure 2.5 representing the normal individual under the condition of starvation.

Diabetic Ketoacidosis   The fundamental derangement in diabetic ketoacidosis is a relative or absolute deficiency of insulin action. With decreased insulin effects, large amounts of glucose are produced by the liver (glycogenolysis and gluconeogenesis) and released into the circulation. Glucose freely enters the cells of the central nervous system and of the

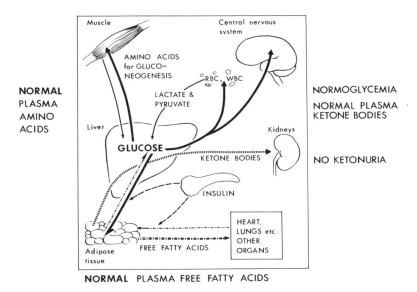

Figure 2.4. Carbohydrate, amino acid, and fatty acid metabolism in a normal individual under stable physiological conditions. The processes of gluconeogenesis, lipogenesis, lipolysis, and ketogenesis are depicted.

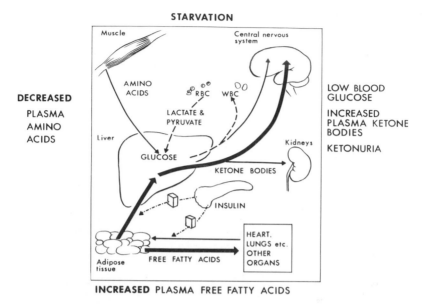

Figure 2.5. Carbohydrate, amino acid, and fatty acid metabolism in starvation. Pertinent laboratory data and mechanisms of the abnormalities are depicted. Note decreased insulin actions on lipogenesis, ascribable to decreased insulin caused by lower blood glucose as well as to anti-insulin actions of free fatty acids and ketone bodies.

renal tubules. The entrance of glucose into muscle cells, adipose tissue, and other cells is insulin dependent, and, in the insulin insufficiency state, a hyperglycemia results. Osmotic diuresis carries large amounts of water as well as extracellular and intracellular electrolytes into the urine. Limited fluid volume prevents further glucose loss; hence, there is an exacerbation of the hyperglycemic state.

In most patients in this state, the diagnosis of diabetes mellitus had been made previously, but there are exceptions, especially among juveniles whose first indication of diabetes mellitus is often an episode of keto-acidosis. The common precipitating events include decreased insulin treatment, increased glucose intake, or a combination of the two, acute or chronic infections, acute or chronic stress, surgery, thyrotoxicosis, pregnancy, hypercortisolemia, acromegaly, febrile illnesses leading to lipolysis and insulin resistance, insulin antibodies, and emotional trauma.

Symptoms and signs of diabetic ketoacidosis include polyuria and polydipsia occurring early, until the polyuria becomes limited by dehydration. The patient may also complain of anorexia with nausea and vomiting, weakness, malaise, and muscle aches, and abdominal pain, especially in children. On physical examination, the patient exhibits dry mucous mem-

42   Habeeb Bacchus

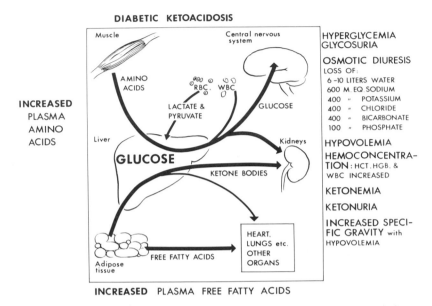

Figure 2.6. Carbohydrate, amino acid, and fatty acid metabolism in diabetic keto-acidosis. Pertinent laboratory data are presented outside the rectangle. Note the absence of significant insulin actions as well as increased gluconeogenesis and lipolysis.

branes (conjunctival, oral, and nasopharyngeal), acetone smell to breath, dry skin with decreased skin turgor, soft and sunken eyeballs, tachycardia, hypotension, weak, rapid pulse, and hypotension. The pattern of Kussmaul respirations (hyperpnea and dyspnea) and central nervous system depression, including headache, drowsiness, stupor, and confusion, may evolve into coma. Diabetic ketoacidosis should be differentiated from the hypoglycemic coma, lactic acidosis, hyperosmolar non-ketotic coma, salicylate poisoning, head trauma, cerebrovascular accident, septicemia or hypovolemic shock, and severe dehydration. The laboratory findings are presented in Figure 2.6 which also presents some data on mechanisms in this disorder.

   Treatment of Diabetic Ketoacidosis The goals of therapy in the management of diabetic ketoacidosis are to reverse hypovolemia, block lipolysis and reinstitute lipogenesis, restore the electrolytes lost, and to reinstitute carbohydrate utilization in the muscles, liver, adipose, and other tissues.

   The fluid deficit is replaced by the intravenous infusion of 2–4 liters of saline solution within the first 2 hr. The choice between 0.45% and 0.9% saline solution is often controversial, but, in view of the marked fluid deficit, it is desirable to employ 0.45% saline initially. If the patient is severely hypotensive, then it is prudent to administer normal saline instead of hypotonic saline. After the initial 2 hr, the intravenous saline is given at the rate of 1 liter/hr. It should be noted that full replacement of the fluid deficit with around 6–8 liters of saline will provide a total of 924–1232 mEq of sodium, considerably in excess of the sodium deficit ascribed to osmotic diuresis. The use of sufficient 0.45% saline to avoid the sodium excess is therefore recommended. Fluid replacement alone is followed by a measurable decrease of the hyperglycemia (presumably as a result of dilution), increased excretion, and reduced osmolality which is a strong anti-insulin factor.

Insulin therapy is instituted immediately after initiation of fluid replacement. Several protocols for insulin replacement have evolved, but greatest success is achieved with the use of intramuscular regular insulin or with intravenous regular insulin.

Therapy with Intramuscular Insulin   After institution of fluid replacement, regular (crystalline zinc) insulin is given initially at the dose range of 0.1 unit/kg body weight. In some regimens the patient is given a loading dose of 10–20 units of insulin (8). Subsequent management requires the administration of 5–10 units of insulin at hourly intervals until the blood glucose levels decrease to around 250 mg/100 ml. By this method of management, peak insulin levels in the serum are achieved within 3–4 hr of therapy, although improvement in the various metabolic parameters (glucose, ketones, and electrolytes) is noted within the first hour.

Therapy with Intravenous Insulin   Two methods of administration of insulin intravenously have been employed. In one regimen (9), the regular insulin is given as an intravenous bolus at intervals of 1–2 hr depending on the levels of hyperglycemia and ketoacidosis. If the blood glucose exceeds 300 mg/100 ml and the plasma ketone test is strongly positive, crystalline zinc insulin (150–200 units) is infused as a bolus. A similar dose is used if the blood glucose is greater than 750 mg/100 ml with weak to moderate plasma ketone test. Blood is obtained at hourly intervals for estimation of blood glucose, ketone bodies, and electrolytes. If, at the end of 1 hr, there is no decrease of the plasma ketones or of blood glucose, the initial dose is repeated. A drop in either measurement is followed by giving one-half of the initial dose in the succeeding hour. A drop in blood glucose without a decrease in plasma ketones is treated by repeating the initial dose of insulin. This is necessary because, despite the lowering of glucose levels, it is essential to correct the excess lipolysis. It is, therefore, occasionally necessary to infuse intravenous glucose to prevent insulin-induced hypoglycemia.

An alternative method employing intravenous insulin requires the constant infusion of insulin at the rate of 0.5–1.0 unit of regular insulin/kg/hr. This is infused with aid of a perfusion pump. Since insulin is adsorbed by glass and plastic in variable amounts, it is useful to add a protein-containing solution, such as serum albumin, to avoid this phenomenon. By this method, circulating levels of insulin of between 20 and 200 microunits of insulin/ml are readily achieved. This circulating level is known to be optimal for glucose transport. The major drawback of this method is the requirement for an infusion pump. Comparative studies have suggested a slightly greater tendency to hypoglycemia when the intravenous insulin regimen is employed.

Control of Electrolytes   As soon as it is clear that there is production of urine by the patient following the rehydration, potassium chloride is added to the intravenous infusions at the rate of 20–30 mEq every hour for the remainder of the acute treatment period (6–8 hr). This supplement is necessary in view of the potassium deficit associated with diabetic ketoacidosis (see Figure 2.6) and because of an impending exacerbation of hypokalemia on correction of intracellular acidosis, as well as by insulin action on cellular uptake of glucose and potassium levels drawn at the intervals indicated above. The infusion of sodium bicarbonate is reserved for marked acidosis with the blood pH at 7.0 or below. The recommended dosage is 44 mEq added to each liter of saline, to be continued until significant improvement in the pH is achieved. This therapy is not required very often. When the blood glucose levels are reduced to less than 250 mg/100 ml, and plasma ketones are not detectable, the patient may be treated with small subcutaneous doses of insulin. With careful management, the patient should recover from the emergency state within 8–10 hr. It is essential during this treatment period to ascertain the precipitating cause of the acute episode.

The differences in insulin requirements between the intravenous and intramuscular methods relate to the relative durations of insulin actions when insulin is given by the different routes. The plasma half-life of intravenously administered insulin is between 1 and 2 min, with peak hypoglycemic action at 20 min. In view of the short half-life by this route, large doses of insulin are required. Intramuscularly administered insulin, on the other hand, reaches the circulating plasma more slowly, but the duration of action is somewhat longer because of the "constant" release from the intramuscular site over a longer period.

Hyperosmolar Non-Ketotic Coma   Hyperosmolar non-ketotic coma is more commonly seen in older diabetics, and is relatively rare in insulin-openic diabetics. It is not infrequently the presenting problem in insulinoplethoric diabetics. The mortality rate in this disorder approaches 40%. These patients produce sufficient amounts of insulin to block excessive lipolysis, but insufficient amounts to assure glucose utilization. The hyperglycemia induces significant osmotic diuresis. This induces increased ingestion of fluids, often including sweetened beverages. Defects in the sensorium occurring in these patients subsequently lead to decreased fluid intake. This pattern of events culminates in the hyperosmolar state. Several observations indicate that the level of the sensorium correlates well with the plasma osmolality. Drowsiness is seen when the plasma osmolality is around 320 mOsm/liter, whereas stupor and coma occur at levels above 360 mOsm/liter. It is possible that the comatose state in diabetic keto-acidosis may also be at least partly due to increased osmolality.

Precipitating causes in hyperosmolar non-ketotic state may include renal disease, cerebrovascular accidents, other cardiovascular disorders, infections, sepsis, and other stresses. Many of these patients will have been taking diuretics.

The significant symptomatology includes, in addition to the early polydipsia and polyuria, lack of Kussmaul respirations, the presence of mental confusion, severe dehydration, stupor, coma, and seizures. It is important to distinguish this disorder from diabetic ketoacidosis (in which marked ketonemia is present) and other causes of hyperglycemia. The diagnostic laboratory data are presented in Figure 2.7. In addition to determination of blood glucose, urea nitrogen, and electrolytes, it is useful to ascertain the plasma osmolality. A calculated osmolality based on the observed serum Na and K (as mEq/liter), glucose, and urea nitrogen (BUN) (as mg/100 ml) and with the formula:

$$2(Na + K) + \frac{glucose}{18} + \frac{BUN}{2.8} = mOsm/liter$$

is reasonably accurate and is close to the value determined by an osmometer. Hyperglycemia may falsely lower the observed (determined) serum sodium levels. Electrolyte solutions exert 1 mOsm for 1 mEq; for nonelectrolyte solutions such as glucose, 1 mmole is equivalent to 1 mOsm in osmotic behavior. In osmotic equilibrium, 1 mOsm of glucose depresses the observed (determined) serum sodium by 1 mOsm (equivalent to 1 mEq). But, because a depression of sodium would require an equal amount of chloride, a depression of 1 mEq/liter of sodium represents a glucose increase of 2 mOsm/liter or 36 mg/100 ml. Based on these considerations it is possible to calculate the extent of depression of observed serum sodium on the basis of a formula which employs the excess of glucose over a normal of 100 mg/100 ml (i.e., blood glucose (mg/100 ml) − 100 mg/100 ml).

$$\frac{Glucose\ excess}{36} = depression\ of\ sodium\ (mEq/liter)$$

Therefore, the actual serum sodium is the sum of the observed (determined) sodium plus the "depression" value calculated above.

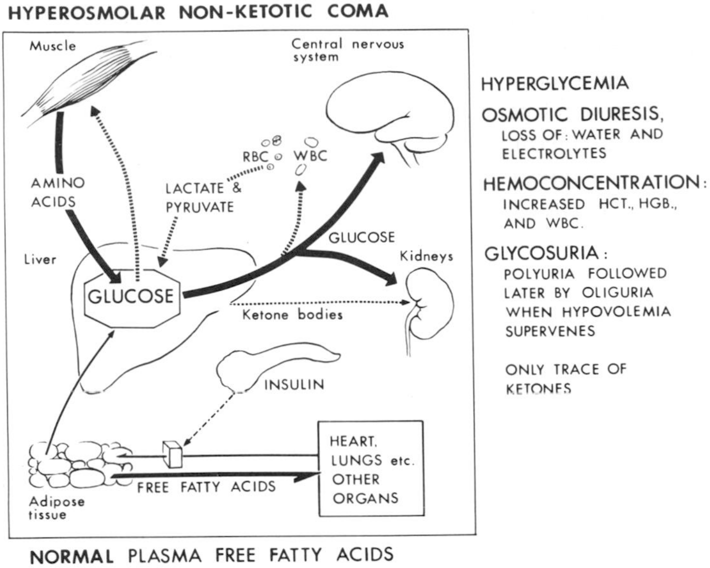

HYPEROSMOLAR NON-KETOTIC COMA

NORMAL PLASMA FREE FATTY ACIDS

Figure 2.7. Carbohydrate, amino acid, and fatty acid metabolism in hyperosmolar non-ketotic coma. Pertinent laboratory data are also presented. Sufficient insulin effects to prevent lipolysis are present.

Management of Hyperosmolar Non-Ketotic State   The goals of therapy are replacement of fluid volume and restoration of carbohydrate utilization by the use of insulin. Fluid therapy consists of the intravenous infusion of 0.45% saline as the first replacement (about 3–4 liters). In cases of hypovolemic shock, it is prudent to infuse 0.85% saline solution. It is important to avoid the induction of a hypo-osmolar state in the course of management so as not to precipitate osmolar disequilibrium with the central nervous system. This complication is discussed below.

Patients with hyperosmolar non-ketotic state, despite the hyperosmolality, lack several of the more powerful contrainsulin factors, such as elevated levels of free fatty acids and ketone bodies. Therefore, the insulin requirement is often less than in the ketoacidotic state. Accordingly, small doses of insulin are given intravenously (or preferably by intramuscular injection), the dosage being monitored by hourly determinations of blood glucose and serum electrolytes. Potassium replacement is started as soon as output of urine is assured. There is no need for bicarbonate therapy in this disorder.

Complications during Management of Diabetic Ketoacidosis and Non-Ketotic Hyperosmolar State   The therapeutic regimens for both diabetic ketoacidosis and hyperosmolar non-ketotic state may be complicated by aspects of vigorous management. Hypokalemia is a concomitant of the osmotic diuresis in both states, and it is exacerbated by the correction of glucose metabolism, and, in the case of ketoacidosis, of the acidosis. Potassium replacement is, therefore, essential in all patients except anephric patients and patients with severe renal insufficiency. In the latter groups, serum potassium values are higher than those observed in the absence of renal disease.

An osmotic disequilibrium may complicate management of both ketoacidosis and hyperosmolar state. The pathogenesis of this complication is of interest. During hyperglycemia, there is free entrance of glucose into the central nervous system. Aldoreductases convert the glucose to polyols, including sorbitol (see Chapter 1), which are less freely diffusible. On correction of the hyperosmolar state, and perhaps with creation of a hypo-osmolar state in the circulation, fluid is drawn by the osmotically active polyols in the central nervous system, resulting in increased cerebrospinal pressure, cerebral edema, seizures, and death. It is, therefore, prudent to avoid the induction of hyposmolality in the intravascular compartment.

A cerebrospinal fluid acidosis may complicate the management of diabetic ketoacidosis if significant amounts of bicarbonate are used. When bicarbonate is infused to ketoacidotic patients, the intravascular pH is corrected with a rise in bicarbonate. With lessening of the acidosis, the hyperventilation associated with ketoacidosis ceases, and the blood pCO_2 increases. Because CO_2 diffuses rapidly and bicarbonate diffuses slowly, across the blood-brain barrier, a severe acidosis in the CSF compartment may supervene. This mechanism has been cited as a basis of decreased brain function in patients receiving bicarbonate, but a similar disorder has been found occasionally in patients not receiving the alkalinizing solution.

Lactic Acidosis Lactic acidosis is a highly fatal disorder ascribed to increased anaerobic glycolysis complicated by intracellular hypoxia, resulting in a failure to convert lactate to pyruvate (10). Diabetic patients on phenformin therapy, or with associated hypoxemic states, may be subject to this disorder. The conversion of pyruvic acid to lactic acid requires the presence of a high NADH:NAD ratio and is increased in hypoxic states. The normal level of plasma lactate is around 1.0 mEq/liter, and of pyruvate, 0.1 mEq/liter, a lactate to pyruvate ratio (L:P) of 10. Increased levels of lactate are evaluated in terms of the L:P ratio so that, in conditions such as infusion of glucose, pyruvate, or bicarbonate, and in glycogenoses, an absolute increase of lactate is observed, but with a concomitant increase of pyruvate so that the L:P ratio remains essentially normal. A similar ratio is seen in hyperventilation. An excess of lactate and an elevated L:P ratio are seen after muscular exercise, in cardiovascular insufficiency, shock, cardiopulmonary bypass, acute hypoxia, leukemia, diabetes mellitus, renal insufficiency, ethanol ingestion, and in patients receiving epinephrine or phenformin. An idiopathic form is also recognized (10).

The clinical manifestations of lactic acidosis are usually those of the underlying and precipitating disorders. An acute onset with rapid progression to Kussmaul respirations, stupor, and coma is seen frequently. There is no acetone odor on the patient's breath, and hypotension and anoxemia are evident. The laboratory findings include those of the underlying disorder along with an elevated plasma lactate and L:P ratio and a decreased pH. The presence of an unexplained anion gap (over 16 mEq/liter) is invariably noted. Plasma ketone may be slightly elevated, but, since lactic acidosis depresses ketogenesis, a ketonemia is often absent.

In the management of lactic acidosis, special measures, along with treatment of the underlying disorder, are instituted. Fluid replacement is provided if the patient is in shock, treatment of diabetes mellitus is undertaken, and all medications known to precipitate or contribute to this state are discontinued. Bicarbonate is administered in large doses, essentially by the intravenous route. The bicarbonate deficit is estimated by the following formula:

$$(\text{Normal HCO}_3 - \text{patient's HCO}_3) \times \text{½ body weight (kg)} = \text{deficit of bicarbonate (mEq)}$$

It is recommended that 60–100% of this deficit should be replaced within 6–8 hr. In patients with fluid overload, the buffer tris(hydroxymethyl)aminomethane has been employed instead of bicarbonate. Methylene blue, which functions as a hydrogen acceptor, may be administered at a dose range of 1–5 mg/kg body weight. Even vigorous management by the above methods is frequently unsuccessful in lactic acidosis, and the prognosis of this disorder remains poor. The use of hemodialysis does not alter the prognosis significantly.

Hypoglycemic Coma   Although there are several etiologies of hypoglycemia (see discussion of hypoglycemic syndromes), the major etiologies of hypoglycemic coma in diabetics are usually excess insulin or sulfonylurea compounds and excess exercise. The common precipitating causes of hypoglycemic coma in diabetics include decreased glucose intake despite continued insulin or oral antidiabetic therapy, overtreatment with insulin or sulfonylureas, increased exercise, hepatocellular disease (with decreased gluconeogenesis), and decreased insulin requirement occurring late in pregnancy.

The clinical manifestations include those due to hyperepinephrinemia, such as weakness, tingling in the fingers or in the circumoral areas, sweating, tachycardia, "internal tremors," and nervousness. The cerebral hypoglycemic manifestations include headaches, diplopia, fainting, disorientation and mental confusion, and hysterical behavior. Persistence of severe hypoglycemia may lead to convulsions and permanent central nervous system impairment, as well as myocardial damage. Laboratory findings include the finding of blood glucose levels below 40 mg/100 ml; it should be emphasized, however, that many patients may be completely asymptomatic at this range of blood glucose values.

Because hypoglycemia of significant severity may be immediately life threatening, it is imperative that treatment be instituted immediately. A blood sample is obtained (to be sent for baseline study) and 50% glucose is infused intravenously without awaiting the results of the laboratory tests. Glucose (5–10%) infusion should be continued until it is ascertained that the blood glucose is stable at a normoglycemic level. It is prudent to observe the patient over the course of several hours or days depending on the antecedent dietary and drug therapy. Patients on long-acting insulin or especially those on chlorpropamide may have recurrent episodes of hypoglycemia despite the vigorous initial therapy. In some patients, intramuscular glucagon is often helpful. But, in all cases, it is essential that the cause of the hypoglycemia be identified. This definition might extend to definitive work-up of pituitary, adrenal, and hepatocellular functions, as well as ascertain whether the episode is due to drug therapy. (See also section on hypoglycemic syndromes.)

Diabetic Nephropathy

Renal disorders are frequently found in diabetes mellitus, especially in the insulinopenic variety (11). All insulinopenic diabetics have been observed to acquire nephropathy within 16 years of onset of the diabetes, and, according to one survey, all of the patients died within the succeeding 5 years. In other series, over 50% of all diabetic patients with diabetes for 10–20 years were found to be in renal failure.

Blood vessel disorders are prominent in diabetic nephropathy, and these include arteriolosclerosis, arteriosclerosis, glomerulosclerosis (glomerular capillaries), and capillary aneurysms (11). Infections in the kidneys are basis of pyelitis, pyelonephritis, and papillary necrosis.

Arteriosclerosis, although not unique to diabetes mellitus, is more severe in diabetic patients, especially when the main renal arteries and their branches are involved. Arteriolosclerosis in the kidneys (arteriolonephrosclerosis) is more common and more severe in diabetic patients. Hyaline deposits occur initially between intimal cells and elastic fibers, and this process is followed by hyaline invasion of the media, replacing the muscle cells. Thickening of the basement membrane is also noted. The increased incidence of hypertension in diabetes is ascribed to the above changes.

Diabetic glomerulosclerosis evolves in three forms: diffuse, nodular, and exudative. Diffuse glomerulosclerosis describes a characteristic thickening of variable degrees in the walls of glomerular capillaries, axially, as well as peripherally. The capillary lumens are reduced and become occluded. Periodic acid-Schiff (PAS)-positive (mucopolysaccharide) deposits form along the basement membrane to the endothelial cells, eventually with extensive deposits of polysaccharides, lipids, and hemoglobin. In contrast to the changes in membranous glomerulonephritis and nephrosclerosis, there is no splitting of the basement membrane, and it does not contain collagen.

Nodular glomerulosclerosis develops in glomeruli with the diffuse changes described above. Nodular sclerosis is the original Kimmelstiel-Wilson lesion which eventually occurs in 25% of all diabetics. Spherical nodules 20–100 μm in diameter are located at the periphery of the glomerular tufts, appear laminated, and exhibit one or more layers of nuclei near the periphery. Reticulin fibers, as well as PAS-positive glycoproteins and lipids, are deposited. This lesion is virtually specific for diabetes mellitus, with considerably higher incidence in the insulinopenic form.

Exudative glomerulosclerosis consists of the occurrence of a crescentic mass of deeply eosinophilic hyaline or refractile material usually attached to the inner side of the parental layer of Bowman's capsule, or, in the capillary lumen, surrounded by endothelial cells. This lesion contains mucopolysaccharide, protein, hemoglobin, and lipid. These exudative changes are not specific for diabetes mellitus as they are also found in chronic pyelonephritis with glomerular ischemic.

Capillary aneurysms occur in kidneys of diabetics and may antedate the other characteristic changes. Other renal changes in diabetes mellitus include thickening of the renal tubule basement membranes occurring in association with the glomerular changes described above. A fairly common finding in the tubular epithelium in patients dying of diabetes in a period of poor control is the Armanni-Ebstein lesion due to glycogen deposition in the tubule cells; vacuolization of cells is also seen. The Armanni-Ebstein lesion is reversible. In severe acidosis and hypokalemia, tubular vacuolization may occur.

Clinical Considerations in Diabetic Nephropathy   The initial clinical manifestation of diabetic nephropathy is a mild and intermittent proteinuria (20–100 mg/100 ml) accentuated by episodes of pyelonephritis, other infections, and diabetic ketoacidosis. Later in the course, proteinuria becomes permanent and may reach 5–10 g/24 hr. Edema, hypoproteinemia, and hypercholesterolemia complete the picture of the nephrotic syndrome. The urinary sediment contains bacteria, pus cells, doubly refractile fat droplets, and red blood cells. Increased $\alpha 2$ and β-globulin are seen on serum protein electrophoresis. Renal function is impaired so that azotemia, hypertension, and uremia and its complications (neuropathy, anemia, bleeding diathesis, circulatory failure, pericarditis, electrolyte problems, abnormal calcium metabolism, and renal osteodystrophy) complete the evolution of the disorder. Uremia is a major cause of death in these patients, and this tendency is increased by concurrent infections. It is estimated that it takes 10–20 years of known diabetes before clinical manifestations of nephropathy appear. While the severity of the diabetic disorder does not appear to be directly related to the occurrence or severity of nephropathy, the control of diabetes undoubtedly influences the outcome. Poorer controlled patients show a higher incidence of nephropathy.

There are several associated clinical problems of the urinary tract in diabetic patients. Cellular defense mechanisms (e.g., abnormal leukocyte behavior) predispose to the occurrence of pyelonephritis and urinary tract infections, perinephric abscess, cystitis, neuropathic bladder, cystitis emphysematosa, and pneumaturia. Treatment of these conditions is also more difficult in diabetic patients than in non-diabetics. Renal medullary necrosis (renal papillary necrosis) is quite rare in the general population, but is considerably more frequent in diabetics. The disorder is manifested by a severe septic illness, often associated with shock, flank pain, fever, dysuria, hematuria, pyuria, sloughing of the renal papillary tips, and ureteral colic. The disorder rapidly progresses to renal insufficiency, anuria, and death. The pathology in this disorder consists of necrosis of two-thirds of the renal pyramid, including the papillary tips; a majority of the pyramids are involved. The pathology may be unilateral or bilateral. Passage of papillary tips in the urine is a diagnostic finding of this disorder. Renal cortical necrosis may occur in diabetics after infections or poisoning and in diabetic pregnancy. Hematuria, oliguria, and uremia are the usual clinical findings.

Diabetic Retinopathy

The incidence of retinopathy ascribed to diabetes mellitus is quite high, with most of this group having simple (nonproliferative) retinopathy, and a smaller number showing proliferative changes. It is likely that the duration of diabetes mellitus is important in the pathogenesis since, after 20 years of diabetes mellitus, about 80% of patients may have some form of retinopathy. Slower progression and less severe types of retinopathy are seen in patients under good diabetic therapy. In patients with simple retinopathy and good vision, approximately 3% become blind after 5 years. In patients with proliferative retinopathy, about 50% become blind after 5 years. After the occurrence of vitreous hemorrhage, approximately one-third of the patients become blind after 4 years, and one-third have impaired vision.

There is a general correlation between the occurrence of diabetic retinopathy and that of generalized vascular disease so that the prognosis

Table 2.3. Diabetic Retinopathy

Classification	Appearance	History	Biochemical features	Treatment
Diffuse capillary retinopathy (diffuse irregular dilatation of retina)	Central retinal edema, microaneurysm and hemorrhage; neovascularization; vitreous hemorrhage; retinitis proliferans; retinal detachment, fibrosis, and atrophy; few hard exudates are found	Uncommon; age 30; on insulin for 10–20 years; lives about 6 years after becoming blind; progresses by stages to blindness in 2–4 years; unique to diabetes	↗ HGH[a] response; ↗↗ free fatty acids; insulin insensitivity; only mild degree of proteinuria and renal dysfunction by time blindness occurs	Control diabetes; suppress HGH with medroxyprogesterone; if progressive, total pituitary ablation; light coagulation of retinal vessels
Diabetic lipid retinopathy (progressive accumulation of hard exudates)	No major neovascularization; hard exudates, few microaneurysms and hemorrhage; slow progression, lipid formation and reabsorption	Overweight patients over 40 years of age and not insulin-dependent, often with large vessel disease; slow visual deterioration	Decreased HGH response to hypoglycemia; free fatty acids low for diabetics; may resemble type IV lipoproteinemia	Weight reduction; atromid S; pituitary ablation not indicated as it decreases lipolysis; photocoagulation not needed

Diabetic obstructive retinopathy (obstruction of retinal circulation)	Arteriolar disease; arteriolar obstruction, cotton wool spots, and cytoid bodies; venous obstruction and dilated veins may be present; flame and dot hemorrhages, vitreous hemorrhage, neovascularization, and retinitis proliferans may occur	Patients <30 years, on variable diet and insulin therapy; many have renal disease and hypertension; usually slowly progressive course	50% have type II hyperlipoproteinemia; hyperviscosity of plasma and α_2 macroglobulin often present; elevated ESR[a] and increased fibrinolysis	Measures to decrease intraocular pressure; treatment of the lipid abnormality, control of hypertension
Minimal diabetic retinopathy ("normal" retina in patient with diabetes >25 years)	Microaneurysms (<20), few hard exudates, no hemorrhages, no neovascularization	On rigorous insulin and diet control; may have peripheral neuropathy and cataracts	Moderately increased HGH response; normal free fatty acids, and blood glucose <150 mg/100 ml; no hyperlipoproteinemia	Encouragement and reassurance and continued close control of diabetes

[a]HGH, human growth hormone; ESR, erythrocyte sedimentation rate.

for life is guarded in patients with diabetic retinopathy. It is estimated that the mean duration of life after the development of blindness in diabetes is around 5 years. In the United States, diabetic retinopathy is the leading cause of blindness.

Table 2.3 presents a useful classification (12) of diabetic retinopathy which includes the pathogenetic mechanisms, clinical manifestations, prognosis, and treatment (12).

Diabetic Neuropathy

Diabetic neuropathy refers to a heterogeneous group of mononeuropathies, polyneuropathies, myelopathies, and encephalopathies, varying in type, nature of onset, severity, relationship to diabetes prognosis, and treatability. These is probably no specific diabetic neurological syndrome. A useful classification of neurological disorders found in diabetics is that of Locke (13) which is the basis of the data in Table 2.4. In all of the disorders listed, the keystone of management is control of the diabetes, but special procedures may aid in some of the disorders.

Diabetic Dermopathy

At least 30% of diabetic patients manifest cutaneous complications during the course of the illness. These disorders may be due to superimposed infection or to vascular, metabolic, or nutritional problems. Perineal moniliasis is frequently found, especially in the presence of glycosuria.

Shin spots, red-brown papules over the pretibral areas, may be scaly and hyperpigmented. Despite their appearance and location, they are not due to trauma. Necrobiosis lipoidica diabeticorum occurs in about 3% of diabetics, more commonly in women, and usually develops in the 3rd and 4th decades. It consists of a demarcated plaque with shiny atrophic surface; the plaque may start out as smaller lesions which later coalesce. It is due to an obliterative endarteritis followed by necrobiotic changes.

Management of Diabetes Mellitus

The long-term goals of diabetic management are to prevent the acute complications of the disorder (e.g., ketoacidosis, hyperosmolar coma, etc.) and to control or prevent the "concomitants" of diabetes mellitus. The maintenance of normoglycemia in association with ideal body weight is considered as tantamount to maintenance of efficient intermediary metabolism in diabetes. The major modalities in diabetic management include dietary control and insulin therapy. There is perhaps a limited role for oral hypoglycemic agents in certain insulinoplethoric diabetics.

Diet Therapy in Diabetes Mellitus Dietary management is directed to the achievement and maintenance of ideal body weight. Several height-weight curves and tables are available for use. A useful method for

Table 2.4. Neuropathies in Diabetes Mellitus

Disorder and structure	Etiology	Signs and symptoms	Major involvement
Radiculopathy (nerve root)	Probably vascular	Pain and sensory loss in distribution of a dermatome; clears spontaneously	Usually a single dermatome
Mononeuropathy (mixed spinal or cranial nerve)	Probably vascular	Pain, weakness, reflex changes, sensory loss in distribution of mixed spinal or cranial nerve; spontaneous recovery usually	Peroneal, femoral, sciatic, ulnar, radial, median nerves may mimic carpal tunnel syndrome; oculomotor, facial, auditory nerves
Polyneuropathy (nerve terminals)	Metabolic?	Glove and stocking sensory loss: mild peripheral weakness, absent reflex	Longest nerves affected first; hence, earliest symptoms in feet; perforating ulcers or charcot joints
Diabetic amyotrophy	Unknown	Anterior thigh pain: proximal weakness of legs; fasciculation and Babinski, self-limited	Quadriceps, hamstring proximal leg muscle groups
Autonomic neuropathy (sympathetic ganglion)	Unknown	Postural hypotension, anhydrosis, impotence, gastropathy, vesical atony, nocturnal diarrhea, retrograde ejaculation; pupillary changes: sluggish pupils or Argyll-Robertson pupils	

calculating ideal weight in male subjects is based on the assignment of 106 lb for the first 60 inches of height, and 6 lb for each additional inch, so that a 68-inch male should have ideal body weight of 154 lb (70 kg). In female patients, 105 lb are assigned to the first 60 inches, and 5 lb for each additional inch of height. Variations beyond data from these formulas depend on body frame size and muscular development. For weight maintenance, the total caloric requirement is 25–35 kcal/kg/24 hr distributed as 40% carbohydrate, 40% fat, and 20% protein. Therefore, weight maintenance in a patient of ideal body weight of 60 kg requires around 1,800 kcal, consisting of 720 kcal of carbohydrate (180 g), 720 kcal of fat (80 g), and 360 kcal of protein (90 g). To achieve weight loss, a caloric intake of 20 kcal/kg ideal body weight/24 hr or less is recommended. For weight gain, as is often required in insulinopenic diabetics, 35–45 kcal/kg ideal body weight/24 hr or more may be needed. The requirements given above apply to patients engaged in sedentary activities. Vigorous activity will necessitate increments in caloric intake estimated from the degree of physical activity.

Insulin Therapy in Diabetes Mellitus Insulin therapy is required in insulinopenic diabetics. These patients are usually at or below ideal body weights. The recommended insulin regimen is instituted to simulate the postprandial spurts in insulin secretion which are seen in normal subjects. As described previously, dietary challenge (carbohydrate and amino acids) stimulates the release of insulin in two pools. This postprandial spurt is absent or decreased in insulinopenic diabetics. In the above context, ideal insulin therapy requires three or four injections of crystalline zinc insulin daily, each 20 min before meals. There are several isolated reports attesting to the superior results with this method of insulin therapy. An alternative method, with an equal degree of success, requires the administration of split dosages of NPH (or lente) insulin along with crystalline zinc (regular) insulin given before breakfast and the evening meal. It is recommended that two-thirds of the total insulin dosage should be given in the morning and one-third prior to the evening meal. The schedule of insulin therapy simulates the postprandial spurts of insulin.

There is no indication for the longer acting forms of insulin (protamine zinc insulin or ultralente insulin) since they do not provide levels of insulin appropriate to needs as in the method described above.

The hypothalamic hormone somatostatin is now known to affect the pathogenesis and progression of diabetes mellitus (14). Somatostatin is known to inhibit the secretion of insulin and glucagon, the latter being strongly implicated in the progression of the concomitants of diabetes mellitus. Recent studies have shown that the precipitation of diabetic ketoacidosis in insulin-dependent diabetics by temporary withdrawal of insulin is prevented by somatostatin therapy (15). This effect is ascribed to the suppression by somatostatin of the secretion of glucagon which, through its actions on gluconeogenesis, ketogenesis, and lipolysis, is a prerequisite to precipitation of ketoacidosis. In view of these data, it is anticipated that the split dose insulin regimen should be supplemented with the simultaneous administration of somatostatin. It is likely that analogues of somatostatin with somewhat prolonged biological activity will serve this purpose well.

Maintenance of normoglycemia refers to achievement of blood glucose levels essentially with normal ranges at the various intervals after dietary challenge, similar to the normal ranges of the glucose tolerance curve. These values may be modified somewhat in other individuals. The amounts of subcutaneous insulin given at each interval are monitored by blood glucose levels initially two to four times daily, e.g., fasting blood glucose, 11:30 a.m. blood glucose, 4:00 p.m. blood glucose, and 8:00 p.m. blood glucose. The dosages of insulin are regulated according to the blood glucose levels. For example, hyperglycemia at 11:30 a.m. necessitates an increase of the morning component of regular insulin. If the 4:00 p.m. blood glucose is too low, then it is likely that the a.m. NPH insulin dosage should be reduced. The dosages of insulin may also be monitored by fractional urine tests for glycosuria four times daily, using second voided specimens to provide information on blood glucose levels at specific times. This indirect criterion is not applicable in patients who may have renal threshold problems (as in renal disease and pregnancy). The actual combination of NPH (or lente) and regular insulins employed depends on the glucose levels; NPH and regular insulin may be mixed in any proportion without alteration of their individual activities. But whenever lente and regular insulin are mixed at ratios approaching 1:1, there is alteration of activity to an indeterminate duration. The ratio of NPH to regular insulin is usually 2–5 NPH:1 regular, but this may be modified to suit the specific situations.

The preparations of insulin which are now widely used are of the "single peak" variety, whether of lente, NPH, or regular, and these are packaged as U-100, i.e., 100 units/ml. This single peak insulin is superior to previous forms of insulin which were mixed with variable amounts of proinsulin and insulin dimers, some of which are responsible for allergenicity of insulin preparations. The lipodystrophy occasionally found at insulin injection sites does not occur when "single peak" insulin is used.

Oral Hypoglycemic Agents   Oral hypoglycemic agents are of limited usefulness in the long-term management of diabetes mellitus. Two groups of agents are now available: the sulfonylureas and the biguanides. The mechanism of action of the former group involves enhancement of insulin secretion by the β islet cells; therefore, these agents have no place in the management of insulinopenic diabetes. Some data suggest that the sulfonylureas support the postprandial spurt in insulin secretion so that the insulin response corresponds more closely to the dietary challenge. Observations of severe and long-standing hypoglycemia in chlorpropamide-treated patients who have undergone a period of decreased food intake suggest, however, that the enhanced postprandial spurt is not the major mode of action. Decreased gluconeogenesis and glycogenolysis are minor actions of these drugs also.

All sulfonylurea drugs contain the benzene ring, a sulfonyl group, and urea. The available drugs in this group are: tolbutamide (1-butyl-3-p-tolylsulfonylurea),tolazamide(1-(hexahydro-1-azepinyl)-3-p-tolylusulfonyl-urea), chlorpropamide (1-propyl-3-p-chlorbenzene sulfonylurea), and acetoheximide (N-(p-acetylbenzylsulfonyl)-N'-cyclohexylurea). These agents also exert some extrapancreatic actions including an antithyroid effect, a possible hypertriglyceridemic effect, an increase in stomach emptying, a blush reaction after ingestion of alcohol, and an effect on platelet adhesiveness. A potentially useful action of these agents is the inhibition of phosphodiesterase activity in the renal tubule, thus exerting an antidiuretic action. The metabolism, exertion rate, and duration of action of these agents are given in Table 2.5.

The biguanides do not directly affect the secretion of insulin and, in normal subjects, do not lower the blood glucose levels. The mechanism of action of these drugs is not fully known. A malabsorption of glucose has been found in patients on biguanides and this action may well be the major effect of these agents in diabetic management. Other data indicate that they may induce a state of cellular hypoxia by altered tricarboxylic acid cycle electron transfer, as well as decrease gluconeogenesis.

The use of oral hypoglycemic agents is contraindicated in the management of insulinopenic diabetes mellitus. Brittle diabetes, ketosis-proneness, the presence of severe infections, and surgical procedures are also contraindications to the use of these agents in diabetic management. The diabetics to whom these agents are given are usually insulinoplethoric diabetics who are overweight and whose diabetes can be controlled by restoration of ideal body weight. It is, therefore, prudent to institute a strict diet in preference to the use of the oral agents. If, on achievement of ideal body weight, hyperglycemia remains a problem, then the patient should be re-evaluated for the probability of insulinopenic diabetes. In such patients, insulin levels are found to be inappropriately low for the blood glucose levels.

Some diabetologists institute oral hypoglycemic therapy only after proof of their effectiveness. Accordingly, the patient is submitted to the oral or intravenous tolbutamide test, and the blood glucose levels are monitored. Failure of a response is good indication for alternative methods of diabetic control.

Table 2.5. Pathways of Metabolism and Excretion of Oral Hypoglycemic Sulfonylureas

Drug	Metabolism	Excretion in 24 hr; residual	Duration of effect (hr)
Tolbutamide	Hepatic; rapid	As carboxytolbutamide; nearly all	6–8
Chlorpropamide	<1% metabolized; strongly protein-bound	60% in 24 hr; remainder unchanged	20–60
Acetoheximide	Reduced in liver to hydroxyheximide, which is more active	60% excreted in 24 hr	10–16
Tolazamide	Rapid hepatic metabolism	85% excreted in 24 hr	10–16

In cases where there is evidence of some action, the maintenance dose given should be the smallest effective dose. The recommended maximal dose of tolbutamide is 2–3 g/day; of chlorpropamide, 750 mg/day; of acetoheximide, 1.5 g/day; and of tolazamide, 1.0 g/day. Toxic effects of these agents include skin eruptions, dizziness, lethargy, gastrointestinal upsets, toxic hepatitis, agranulocytosis, and, possibly, cardiovascular disease. As pointed out above, a high incidence of refractory hypoglycemia is frequently observed in older patients on these drugs, especially those of long duration of action.

Indications for use of biguanides are quite limited but, perhaps, similar to those for sulfonylureas. The dose range is 50–100 mg daily. Lactic acidosis may follow the use of this type of medication, especially in patients who may have hypoxemic states.

Management of Diabetes Mellitus in Surgical Patients The diabetic patient who is scheduled to undergo elective surgery is restricted from oral feedings overnight. On the morning of surgery, an intravenous infusion of 5% glucose in normal saline is started, and, at the same time, one-half of the maintenance dose of insulin (NPH or lente) is given by subcutaneous injection. Following surgery, while the patient is in the recovery room, blood is drawn for glucose determination. The remainder of the maintenance dosage of insulin is given in two one-fourth amounts as crystalline zinc insulin 4–6 hr apart, depending on the blood glucose levels. In the patient previously maintained on oral agents, it is assumed that the insulin requirement is less than 40 units/day. One-half of an arbitrary 20–30 units, i.e., 10–15 units of NPH (or lente) insulin are given in the morning, and the rest of the estimated total made up in one-fourth amounts (regular insulin) for two doses as described above. In all cases, the dosage of insulin is monitored by blood glucose levels.

Diabetes Mellitus in Pregnancy

The mutual interaction of diabetes mellitus and pregnancy may alter the course of both clinical states. Diabetes mellitus significantly influences the course and outcome of pregnancy, and there is a significantly increased fetal death rate in diabetic mothers because of glycogen deposition in the placenta, as well as the occurrence of renal vein thrombosis. There is a distinct tendency for larger babies in diabetic pregnancy, and this feature may antedate the discovery of the diabetic state. The large size of the babies is due to increased deposition of glycogen due to the actions of growth hormone, genetic factors, and maternal hyperglycemia, resulting in fetal β islet cell hyperplasia. Infant morbidity as a result of diabetes in the mother may include hypoglycemia and hyperbilirubinemia. The most frequent complications of diabetic pregnant women are hydramnios, toxemia, and ketoacidosis.

The incidence of diabetes in pregnancy has been estimated to be between 1 in 350 and 1 in 1000. The course and natural history of the diabetic state are altered by pregnancy through diabetogenic factors. These alterations are manifested by the appearance of: 1) gestational diabetes (diabetic state of any degree appearing during pregnancy, with remission after delivery, and recurrence in a subsequent pregnancy); 2) latent chemical diabetes revealed by pregnancy; 3) intensification of subtotal diabetes to a degree in which total diabetes is simulated; and 4) precipitation of a permanent form of diabetes appearing as severe ketoacidosis.

Diabetogenic Factors in Pregnancy Normal pregnancy is characterized by several diabetogenic influences, the placenta producing several factors which may affect carbohydrate metabolism. These include somatomammotropin (HCS) or human placental lactogenic hormone (HPL) which exerts a growth hormone-like activity and placental thyrotropin which may possibly increase maternal thyroid function and induce glucose intolerance. There is some evidence to suggest the occurrence of increased growth hormone in pregnancy with its attendant anti-insulin effects. An increased level of plasma cortisol in pregnancy is largely due to increased levels of cortisol-binding globulin; competition for this binding substance later in pregnancy by progesterone may displace cortisol with resulting increased free cortisol levels. This could potentially exert anti-insulin effects and increase maternal gluconeogenesis. The increased estrogen production in pregnancy may also oppose insulin action. Quantitatively more important is the production of placental insulinase which destroys insulin. But the most important diabetogenic influence in pregnancy is the "fasting metabolism state" stimulated by somatomammotropin in the maternal compartment. In this state, there are moderately increased levels of free fatty acids and ketone bodies which exert marked anti-insulin effects, leading to decreased glucose utilization. This action presumably suppresses glucose utilization in the maternal compartment and permits carbohydrate utilization in the fetal compartment. There is a decrease in the renal threshold for glucose in pregnancy, but the degree of this change is often variable.

In the non-diabetic pregnant patient, the glucose tolerance test is normal despite an evident hyperinsulinism. The diabetic pregnant patient shows poorer glucose tolerance despite this hyperinsulinism. Carbohydrate intolerance is progressive into the third trimester, at which time the patient may become more ketosis-prone and may require increasing amounts of insulin except in the last week of pregnancy. Labor is characterized by a tendency to hypoglycemia and a decreased insulin requirement.

Pregnancy adversely affects the concomitants of diabetes so that there is an increased susceptibility to neuropathy as well as cardiovascular lesions. Latent nephropathy and retinopathy may become overt, some features of which may be partly reversible. There is also an increased susceptibility to skin and urinary tract infections in pregnant diabetics.

Diagnosis of Diabetes Mellitus in Pregnancy   In the first trimester, the standards for diagnosis of diabetes mellitus are essentially those employed in non-pregnant individuals. The Fajans-Conn criteria indicate that the diabetic state is present if the blood glucose levels at 60, 90, and 120 min exceed 160, 140, and 120 mg/100 ml, respectively. In the second and third trimesters, the diagnosis of diabetes is made if the blood glucose is greater than 170 mg/100 ml at 1 hr and greater than 120 mg/100 ml at 3 hr after the glucose challenge.

Management of Pregnancy in Diabetes   Obstetricians classify pregnant diabetics on the basis of age of onset, duration, and "concomitants" of diabetes, ranging from class A, essentially chemical diabetes, with 100% fetal salvage, to class R with severe diabetes with repeated fetal loss. Individualization of management is imperative in all cases. Careful calculation of the date of delivery is necessary because early delivery is often warranted. Delivery at 36 weeks is the earliest stage with a reasonable chance of fetal survival. Determinations of urinary estriol sulfate and pregnanediol, preferably serially, are employed to monitor health of the fetus and placenta respectively (see Chapter 18). An acute drop of estriol levels to below 5 mg/24 hr from previously higher values, without a drop in pregnanediol, usually reflects defects in the fetal compartment.

Management of Diabetes in Pregnancy   The keystone of therapy is diet and, when necessary, supplemented with insulin. Some workers have employed oral antidiabetic agents in pregnant patients successfully, but, because of possible teratogenicity and other toxicity, it is probably better to use insulin if the diabetes is not controllable by diet alone (see also section on oral agents). The American Diabetes Association diet appropriate to the ideal body weight is given to the patient (see section on diet therapy in diabetes). Ideal body weight in pregnancy is calculated as the ideal non-pregnant weight (based on height-weight curves) plus an increment appropriate for the pregnancy. The allowable weight gain throughout the pregnancy is 25 lb, with the greatest increase in the latter half of the second trimester and in the third trimester. If, despite maintenance of ideal body weight, there is significant hyperglycemia, then insulin should be added to the management. The therapeutic goal is the maintenance of normoglycemia (appropriate to the stage of pregnancy; see diagnostic standards) in the presence of ideal body weight (appropriate to the stage of pregnancy). In the above context, in the second and third trimesters, the desired blood glucose levels should be below 170 mg/100 ml and 130 mg/100 ml at 1 and 3 hr, respectively, after meals. It is occasionally prudent to permit somewhat higher levels in order to protect the fetus from the effects of maternal hypoglycemia. Glycosuria is a crude guide only and should not be the basis for determining the dosage of insulin. A decrease of insulin requirement occurs just before delivery, and it is, therefore, essential that blood glucose and glycosuria should be carefully monitored.

Management of Diabetic Ketoacidosis in Pregnancy   The management of diabetic ketoacidosis in pregnant patients is essentially similar to that in non-pregnant patients except for the contribution of the "fasting metabolism state" to insulin requirement. Doses of insulin required to control ketonemia may precipitate hypoglycemia. It is, therefore, often necessary to give the patients supplemental glucose while trying to control the ketonemia. On the day of elective delivery, the patient should be restricted from oral feedings overnight or be allowed only oral liquids. An intravenous infusion of glucose (5% in water) is started, and the patient is given a subcutaneous injection of insulin. The dosage schedule of insulin is as follows: 1) one-half of the prepregnancy dosage of NPH (or lente) insulin is given before the glucose infusion; 2) at the end of delivery, the remaining one-half of the prepregnancy dose is given as regular insulin in equal (one-fourth plus one-fourth) portions at 4- to 6-hr intervals depending on the blood glucose levels. It is well to note that the insulin requirement decreases markedly on removal of the placenta (i.e., removal of placental insulinase, somatomammotropin, and other anti-insulin factors in pregnancy).

HYPOGLYCEMIC SYNDROMES

Hypoglycemia is a reflection of several possible derangements in intermediary carbohydrate utilization with a resultant depression in the blood glucose to abnormally low levels (16). Symptoms of hypoglycemia are noted in most patients when the blood glucose level in the adult reaches 40 mg/100 ml or below, but there are data indicating that the ability of patients to tolerate hypoglycemia varies among individuals, some being completely asymptomatic at even lower blood glucose levels. It is also known that infants may also tolerate glucose levels somewhat lower than 40 mg/100 ml. There is some evidence that, in addition to the level of blood glucose, the rate of fall of glucose may also precipitate symptoms. It is of importance that the diagnosis of a hypoglycemic syndrome requires the presence of symptoms during the time of low blood glucose levels as well as reversal of symptoms on restoring the glucose levels to normal.

Clinical manifestations in the hypoglycemic syndromes evolve in two phases, the hyperepinephrinemia phase and the cerebral phase. Occasionally the symptoms of the two phases may overlap. The clinical manifestations of the hyperinephrinemic phase are related to the release of epinephrine which is a compensatory reaction designed to increase blood glucose levels by increased hepatic glycogenolysis. The findings noted during this phase include diaphoresis, weakness, hunger, internal tremors, and tachycardia. When the drop in blood glucose takes place more slowly and over a period of several hours, the cerebral hypoglycemic manifestations occur. These include diplopia, headache, blurred vision, mental confusion, incoherent speech, bizarre behavior, coma, and convulsions. Sensory and motor deficits may also be noted.

Etiology of Hypoglycemic Syndromes

The various causes of these syndromes are presented in Table 2.6 in which they are classified into fasting and non-fasting types. This grouping is justified as the most useful information to be obtained from the patient pertains to the times of occurrence of the symptoms and their relationship to meals. On the basis of this historical information, confirmatory laboratory studies may be conducted.

Laboratory Studies in Hypoglycemic Syndromes

In the diagnostic work-up of the hypoglycemic syndrome associated with fasting, blood glucose levels are measured during a prolonged fast or after a challenge with tolbutamide. Insulin levels are obtained simultaneously in the above studies. In the prolonged fast regimen, the patient is committed to a fast of 72 hr during which periodic blood glucose levels are measured. In event of a significant hypoglycemia associated with symptoms, the test is discontinued. The plasma insulin levels in the samples with significantly low blood glucose levels are quantitated. Elevated insulin levels in the presence of low blood glucose would be compatible with excessive insulin production.

In the tolbutamide challenge, the patient is given 1 g of sodium tolbutamide intravenously. Glucose levels are measured in blood samples obtained at zero time, 30, 60, 120, and 180 min after the infusion. A marked drop in blood glucose by 30 mm after tolbutamide, without a significant return to normoglycemic levels, is found in insulinoma. Insulin levels done with this test also show elevated values inappropriate to the blood glucose levels. A challenge with glucagon to induce insulin release from an insulinoma is another useful diagnostic test.

In the diagnostic work-up of non-fasting hypoglycemia, the most useful test is the glucose tolerance (oral or intravenous). The standard 4-hr oral glucose tolerance test may be prolonged if there is no discernible terminal rise in the blood glucose curve. Representative types of glucose tolerance curves in hypoglycemic syndromes are presented in Figure 2.8. Two types of "reactive" hypoglycemia curves are shown. In the reactive "functional" hypoglycemia, a nadir of blood glucose occurs at 90- to 120-min intervals.

Table 2.6. Hypoglycemic Syndromes

I. Fasting hypoglycemia
  A. Pancreatic islet cell tumor (insulinogenic betacytoma); adenoma, single or multiple; carcinoma with metastases; associated with adenomas of other endocrine glands (MEA)
  B. Epithelioid tumor from foregut anlage: pancreatic tumor in islets producing insulin and other peptide hormones; carcinoid tumor producing insulin
  C. Massive extrapancreatic neoplasm: mesothelioma, adrenocortical carcinoma, hepatocellular carcinoma, gastrointestinal carcinoma
  D. Diffuse liver disease
  E. Anterior pituitary hypofunction
  F. Adrenocortical hypofunction: primary failure; secondary to hypothalamic pituitary failure, biosynthetic defects
  G. Glycogenoses I (von Gierke's), III (Cori's), and VI (Hers')
  H. Ethanol and poor nutrition

I. Fasting hypoglycemia *continued*
  I. Ketotic hypoglycemia of childhood
  J. Leucine hypersensitivity
  K. Neonatal hypoglycemia (transient) in infants of diabetic mothers
  L. Erythroblastosis fetalis
  M. Idiopathic hypoglycemia of childhood
  N. Drug induced: insulin administration; oral hypoglycemic drugs

II. Non-fasting hypoglycemia
  A. Alimentary hyperinsulinism
  B. "Reactive" hypoglycemia of early diabetes mellitus
  C. "Functional" (reactive) hypoglycemia
  D. Hereditary fructose intolerance (fructose-1-P aldolase deficiency)
  E. Galactosemia (galactose-1-P uridyltransferase deficiency)
  F. Maple syrup urine disease (BCKA) (deficiency of branched-chain α-keto acid decarboxylase)
  G. Familial fructose and galactose intolerance

The diagnosis is made with certainty if the glucose levels drop to 40 mg/100 ml or below and are associated with symptoms described previously. This disorder is most commonly seen in young individuals, often the high-strung types. Characteristically, this group of patients do not exhibit seizures or convulsions. In the reactive hypoglycemia of early diabetes mellitus, the nadir of blood glucose occurs at the 4-hr interval in the glucose tolerance test. This is a reflection of the late peak in insulin release following a carbohydrate challenge in insulinoplethoric diabetes. Such pattern is not found in insulinopenic diabetics.

Flat glucose tolerance curves are found in carbohydrate malabsorption and in pituitary and adrenocortical insufficiency. The lack of a terminal

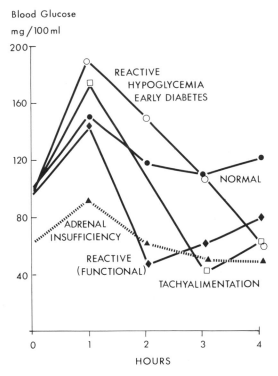

Figure 2.8. Oral glucose tolerance curves in hypoglycemic syndromes. A representative normal curve is presented for comparison. Note that in reactive (functional) hypoglycemia the 1-hr glucose level is lower than in the curves of tachyalimentation and in early diabetes.

rise in the curve is a reflection of decreased glycogen stores and gluconeogenesis as occur in adrenal insufficiency. Flat glucose tolerance curves are also seen frequently in nervous individuals, a reflection, probably, of increased neuromuscular uptake and utilization of carbohydrate. It is of interest that, in this group of patients, the curve reverts to normal with management of the underlying nervous disorder.

Treatment of Hypoglycemic Syndromes

Surgical therapy, if feasible, is recommended for betacytomas. Quite frequently islet cell carcinoma may be palliated with medical therapy with the use of diazoxide (17) or streptozotocin (18). For pituitary or adrenocortical insufficiency, the appropriate hormone replacements are undertaken (see Chapters 14 and 15). For reactive hypoglycemia of the insulinoplethoric diabetics, appropriate dietary management is instituted, essentially as recommended in the section on therapy for diabetes mellitus. For the reactive "functional" hypoglycemia, a high protein, low carbohydrate diet (120–140 g of protein, 75–100 g of carbohydrate, plus maintenance calories as fat) is recommended (16). The diet is distributed on a three to four meals per day schedule. Frequent feedings are not necessary in this disorder. For alimentary hypoglycemia (tachyalimentation), small feedings restricted in carbohydrate and with low fluid intake are given four to six times daily. This regimen is designed to prevent rapid absorption of carbohydrate characteristic of this disorder.

The diagnosis of hypoglycemic syndromes has been subject to considerable faddism in recent years. Indeed, some groups ascribe almost all ailments known to man to hypoglycemia. Such groups also recommend the use of adrenocortical extract (in amounts equivalent to around 1 mg of cortisol daily) for management of hypoglycemia. This practice is not justified in the light of valid scientific knowledge and is to be strongly criticized. Attention is directed to editorials on this topic in the major medical journals (19).

INSULIN RESISTANCE PHENOMENA IN DIABETIC PATIENTS

Insulin resistance phenomena are occasionally seen in diabetic patients treated with insulin. Severe resistance is relatively rare, however. The major clinical manifestations are increasing requirement to maintain normoglycemia or complete failure to control blood glucose despite large

Table 2.7. Factors in Insulin Resistance Phenomena

Hormonal	Growth hormone
	Cortisol
	Glucagon
	Placental lactogen
	Aldosterone (via hypokalemia)
	Catecholamines
Intermediary metabolites	Free fatty acids
	Ketone bodies
Humoral factors	"Bound" versus "free" insulin
	Synalbumin insulin antagonist
	"Atypical" versus "typical" insulin
	Insulin antibodies
Mechanical and biophysical	Microangiopathy
	Tissue resistance
	Hyperosmolality

amounts of insulin. Some authorities suggest that insulin resistance should not be considered unless the requirement for insulin is greater than 200 units/day. On the other hand, insulin resistance has been confirmed in patients taking considerably less insulin. The diabetic state is characterized by several factors which support insulin resistance. The various factors involved in insulin resistance phenomena are classified and listed in Table 2.7. Several of these factors have been considered in previous sections.

Insulin Antibodies as Cause of Resistance

Species differences in insulin reside in amino acids 8 and 10 in the A chain and amino acid 30 in the B chain. In position 8 (A chain), the amino acid in human, pig, and rabbit insulins is threonine, while alanine occupies this position in beef insulin. In position 10 (A chain), isoleucine is the amino acid in human, pig, and rabbit insulin, whereas, in beef insulin, it is valine. In position 30 (B chain), threonine is the amino acid in human insulin, alanine in pig and beef insulins, and serine in rabbit insulin. The antigenicity of insulin is more dependent on the structure of the A chain. It is now known that antibody production in man varies with the species of origin of the insulins used. Antibody production to beef and sheep insulins is greatest, followed by pork and horse insulin, with the least antibody production against fish insulin.

In patients with insulin antibodies (labeled) [131] I-insulin migrates in the γ-globulin serum fraction, whereas normally it migrates with the α-globulin fraction. The insulin-antibody complexes are biologically inactive and are usually degraded slowly. But spontaneous separation of the complex may release insulin and precipitate hypoglycemia. Of patients who develop insulin resistance due to antibody production, 75% are over 40 years of age, 50% develop the problem within 5 years of starting insulin, and 30% may show cutaneous or systemic allergies. Diagnosis of insulin resistance due to antibodies requires the presence of increased antibody levels. It is important to recognize that insulin antibodies are not usually found in patients who never received exogenous insulin; it is also probable that all patients receiving exogenous insulin may have detectable antibody levels. High titers are consistent with significant resistance. An alternative procedure is to determine the migration of labeled insulin on serum protein electrophoresis as indicated above.

Treatment of Insulin Resistance Caused by Antibodies

In the management of this disorder, it is useful to stop all insulin while the patient is under supervision and blood glucose and other parameters may be assessed. A different species of insulin, e.g., dealaninated insulin, may be tried—initially as a challenge with crystalline zinc insulin. The use of oral agents is not strongly indicated since these patients are insulinopenic diabetics. Glucocorticoid therapy may be instituted to stop further anti-gen-antibody complexing and to enhance degradation of existing complexes. This therapy may also influence some of the "tissue resistance" factors. The steroid is usually started in the form of prednisone 60–80 mg daily. Blood glucose levels are monitored closely, as, typically, a hypoglycemia may supervene within 2–3 days. After a therapeutic response, the dosage of glucocorticoid is reduced stepwise to 10 mg/day. The patient is then weaned off the steroid while a new species of insulin is tried. With the use of the "single peak" insulins, the likelihood of insulin antibody formation is considerably less.

CARBOHYDRATE METABOLISM IN ERYTHROCYTES

Several hemolytic anemias associated with erythrocyte enzyme deficiencies are due to inborn metabolic errors. These are characterized as: 1) deficiencies of enzymes of the Embden-Meyerhof pathway; 2) deficiencies in the hexose monophosphate shunt pathway; and 3) deficiencies in certain non-glycolytic enzymes.

The developing erythrocyte possesses the full machinery for replication, differentiation, and self-sustenance. The reticulocyte, despite the absence of a nucleus, has a limited capacity for lipid and protein synthesis and incorporation of hemoglobin iron. Beyond this stage, the mature, non-nucleated erythrocyte lacks the DNA, RNA mitochondria, and other intracellular organelles, and has only vestiges of the tricarboxylic acid cycle. Therefore, the erythrocyte is incapable of synthesizing new proteins; hence, no new enzymes. Its complement of enzyme proteins decay at various biological half-times. The erythrocyte is uniquely dependent on the pathway and hexose monophosphate shunt for its small energy needs. The EM pathway is responsible for ATP production as well as for recycling NAD → NADH. The HMP shunt is responsible for the conversion of NADP to NADPH which is required for maintenance of reduced glutathione (GSH), i.e.,

$$GS - SG \rightarrow 2 \ GSH$$
$$NADPH \rightarrow NADP$$

The erythrocyte lacks the ability to convert the energy of NADPH to high-energy phosphate bonds.

Two intermediates of intermediary glucose metabolism are especially high in the erythrocyte: 2,3-diphosphoglycerate (2,3-DPG) and glucose 1,6-diphosphate. The metabolic significance of this fact is only partly known. The intermediate 2,3-DPG is formed:

$$1,3\text{-DPG} \xrightarrow{\text{2,3-DPG mutase}} 2,3\text{-DPG}$$

and can be returned to the EM pathway via the Rapoport-Leubering shunt:

$$2,3\text{-DPG} \xrightarrow{\text{Phosphatase}} 3\text{-phosphoglycerate} + P_i$$

This shunt bypasses the ATP-producing step mediated by phosphoglycerate kinase:

$$1,3\text{-DPG} \xrightarrow{\text{Kinase}} 3\text{-PGA}$$

In the erythrocyte, 90% of glucose metabolism takes place via the EM pathway, but the contribution of the HMP shunt is greatly increased by any drug or agent which oxidizes GSH. Transaldolase and transketolase permit entry of intermediates of the HMP shunt to the EM pathway, so that it is calculated that the metabolism of 1 mole of glucose to lactate provides a net gain of 2 ATPs. However, this amount in energy is not fully realized because of the Rapoport-Leubering shunt, which is variable. Energy is required by the erythrocyte for maintenance of its shape, for pumping cations across its membrane against electrochemical gradients, for protecting its structure against oxidative stresses, and for resisting the conversion of oxyhemoglobin to methemoglobin. The ultimate lifespan of the erythrocyte is a result of slow denaturation of its irreplaceable enzymes and failure to maintain its relatively small energy production. In the presence of genetic enzymatic defects, this pattern is further disturbed.

Hemolytic Disorders of Embden-Meyerhof Pathway

Erythrocyte Pyruvate Kinase Deficiency (20) Over 100 cases of this autosomal recessive disorder have been described since 1961, mainly in the U. S. and Europe. A particularly high incidence has been reported among some Amish families. Patients with this disorder exhibit no distinguishing or pathognomonic stigmata of chronic hemolysis. They may have jaundice, slight to moderate splenomegaly, variable hepatomegaly, and an increased incidence of cholelithiasis. A neonatal anemia or compensated hemolytic process in adulthood may be seen. Exacerbation of hemolysis occurs in illnesses and surgery. Jaundice or anemia, or both, are noted in infancy or early childhood. Rarely, leg ulcers may occur. Survival to adulthood is common but a few gravely affected children may show growth retardation and prominent frontal bosses. Hematological manifestations include an anemia with hemoglobin usually ranging between 6–12 g/100 ml and hematocrit between 17–37 g/100 ml. Because of a moderate reticulocytosis, macrocytes may occur. Erythrocytes show normochromia, with slight anisocytosis and poikilocytosis. Bizarre cell forms, including irregularly contracted erythrocytes, cells with irregular borders, elongated forms, and, occasionally, nucleated forms as well as acanthocytes may be seen.

After splenectomy, Pappenheimer bodies, siderocytes, Howell-Jolly bodies, and target cells may appear.

Unconjugated serum bilirubin is slightly to moderately elevated, and fecal urobilinogen is increased. The plasma hemoglobin is normal, but haptoglobin is low or absent. Serum iron is normal or slightly increased, and the total iron-binding capacity (TIBC) is normal. Osmotic fragility of incubated cells is variable and there is autohemolysis on sterile incubation for 48 hr; this is correctible by ATP. No Heinz bodies are seen in this disorder. Associated findings include bone changes of hyperplastic bone marrow, with increased bone marrow hemosiderosis. Cholelithiasis may occur at an early age. Increased erythrocyte 2,3-DPG may permit oxygen delivery to tissues.

Ferrokinetic studies in this disorder reveal short plasma clearance time, and the erythrocyte lifespan is moderately to severely shortened. The spleen may "temper" PF-deficient cells, particularly the reticulocyte, so that their destruction by the liver is increased, and splenectomy usually permits longer cell lifespan. Definitive laboratory studies include assay of red blood cell hemolysate for pyruvate kinase. Patients with this disorder show about 5–25% of normal in most patients, whereas heterozygotes have 50% activity. Incubation of erythrocytes under sterile conditions shows increased hemolysis. Prevented by ATP and other compounds, this autohemolysis test is not specific, however. The following defects (21) are also presented in Table 2.8: erythrocyte hexokinase deficiency; erythrocyte glucose phosphate isomerase (GPI) deficiency; erythrocyte triosephosphate (TPI) deficiency; erythrocyte phosphoglycerate kinase (PGK) deficiency; erythrocyte 2,3-diphosphoglycerate mutase deficiency; and erythrocyte enolase deficiency.

Hexose Monophosphate Shunt in Erythrocyte Metabolism

The two early steps in this pathway, viz., G-6-P dehydrogenase and the phosphogluconate dehydrogenase reactions, provide for the generation of NADPH. Defective generation of this pathway is followed by GSH deficiency, especially if observations over several days are averaged. However, individual values may occasionally be normal. Decreased O_2 consumption and CO_2 production also result from this disorder. Occasionally, however, this is not evident, e.g., as in A type deficiency. In such patients, these decreased parameters become evident when NADPH oxidation is hastened, as with addition of methylene blue. The formation of methemoglobin in erythrocytes with G-6-P dehydrogenase deficiency is less than in normal cells when exposed to nitrosobenzol. The NADP:NADPH ratio is increased in G-6-P dehydrogenase deficiency, and increased activities of erythrocyte GSH-reductase, aldolase, hexokinase, and lactic dehydrogenase are noted. In G-6-P dehydrogenase deficiency (22), there is a decrease in NADPH

Table 2.8. Inherited Hemolytic Anemias in Erythrocyte Glycolytic Enzyme Deficiencies[a]

Enzyme defect	Occurrence	Features
Pyruvate kinase	Most common after G-6-P dehydrogenase	Described in text
Hexokinase	Rare	Hemolysis; reticulocytosis, enzyme defect in RBC[b] and WBC platelets; rare association with Fanconi syndrome
Glucose phosphate isomerase	Rare	Enzyme deficiency in RBC and WBC; some polymorphism in enzyme; splenectomy occasionally helpful
Triosephosphate isomerase	Rare	Enzyme deficiency in RBC, WBC, nerves, and muscles; spasticity is present; usually due before age of 5 years
Phosphoglycerate kinase	Rare	Enzyme deficient in RBC and WBC; X-linked inheritance; splenectomy decreases hemolysis
Phosphoglucomutase	Extremely rare	Probably autosomal recessive
Phosphofructokinase	Rare	50% decrease in enzyme in RBC; no splenomegaly or anemia; moderately reduced RBC lifespan; see glycogenosis VII
Enolase	Rare	95% decrease in RBC enzyme; inheritance unknown

[a] Autosomal recessive inheritance unless indicated otherwise.
[b] RBC, red blood cell; WBC, white blood cell.

diaphorase (NADP-linked methemoglobin reductase) and pyrophosphatase. Premature aging of erythrocytes and an abnormality of stromal elements have been observed in this disorder. In G-6-P dehydrogenase deficiency, the cells are normal when tested by Coombs' antiglobulin technique, the Ham acid hemolysis test, and the fragility tests, but cell lifespan is slightly shorter than normal.

Changes Induced in G-6-P Dehydrogenase-deficient Erythrocytes during Drug Administration   Primaquine, sulfa drugs, or fava bean ingestion are followed by a rapid fall in average erythrocyte GSH, resulting in major erythrocyte destruction. Thereafter, the GSH returns to normal. The hemolysis-inducing compounds cause changes in the erythrocytes through alterations in surface characteristics rendering them more sensitive to lysis by the reticuloendothelial system in vivo. Formation of Heinz bodies (hemoglobin denaturation products) and depletion of GSH precede the destruction of the erythrocytes.

Clinical Considerations in G-6-P Dehydrogenase Deficiency   G-6-P dehydrogenase deficiency is inherited as an X-linked trait. Female heterozygotes with this trait produce two populations of erythrocytes, one with normal G-6-P dehydrogenase and the other with decreased enzyme content. Many mutant forms of this enzyme are known. The A type of G-6-P dehydrogenase deficiency is found in 35% of American Blacks. In this form, the enzyme moves rapidly on starch-gel electrophoresis. The B type, in which the enzyme moves more slowly on electrophoresis, is found in 65% of Blacks and in nearly all Caucasians with G-6-P dehydrogenase deficiency. Beutler classifies the clinical types as A−, A+, and Mediterranean types. Patients with the A− type are essentially asymptomatic except when challenged by drug administration or infection. Two or three days after ingestion of the drug noxious in these patients, there occurs dark urine, this being the only manifestation in mild cases. In more severe cases, the patient may suffer back and abdominal pain associated with weakness, the urine becomes black, and icterus develops. Many erythrocytes then show presence of Heinz bodies, and hemoglobin, hematocrit, and erythrocyte values fall rapidly, while the reticulcyte count increases. The "acute hemolytic phase" subsides in 5−7 days, and even if drug administration continues, there is a recovery phase where the above parameters return to normal. It is suggested that the refractory state which develops is due to an alteration in reactivity of the erythrocyte population. There are studies which reveal that sensitivity to the hemolytic action of drugs such as primaquine is a function of cell age. The A− type of G-6-P dehydrogenase deficiency is a more severe clinical disorder. The erythrocyte G-6-P dehydrogenase activity is considerably lower than in A+ type. Congenital non-spherocytic hemolytic anemia associated with G-6-P dehydrogenase deficiency has been described in some patients with variant

G-6-P dehydrogenase. These patients may have varying degrees of hemolysis despite absence of drug ingestion.

Tests designed to detect G-6-P dehydrogenase deficiency include Heinz body formation, GSH stability, and dye screening tests which depend on NADP reduction. The methemoglobin reduction test is based on the principle that methemoglobin reduction by methylene blue is HMP shunt dependent. Fresh blood is required for the test, and abnormal results are also associated with NADPH diaphorase deficiency. The methylene blue absorption test requires the measurement of methylene blue bound to fresh erythrocytes. The ascorbate cyanide test may be positive also in GSSG deficiency, GSSG reductase deficiency, pyruvate kinase deficiency, and in certain hemoglobinopathies. The fluorescent spot test has high specificity. The test is based on the principle that reduced pyridine nucleotides fluoresce while oxidized forms do not. The test is done on filter paper and ultraviolet fluorescence is determined.

It has been suggested that the gene for G-6-P dehydrogenase deficiency confers some protection against falciparum malaria as the malaria parasites require the HMP shunt and GSH for optimal growth. There is a remarkable similarity in geographic distribution of G-6-P dehydrogenase deficiency and falciparum malaria.

Phosphogluconate dehydrogenase deficiency in erythrocytes is suggested to cause a syndrome of hemolysis similar to G-6-P dehydrogenase deficiency.

Deficiencies of Non-Glycolytic Enzymes

These include the following: 1) glutathione reductase deficiency, which has been shown to be responsible for a hereditary hemolytic disorder; 2) ATPase deficiency, which, as a basis of a hemolytic disorder, has been suggested but not definitely proved; 3) glutathione peroxidase deficiency (GSH Px), which is described as causing a rare hemolytic reaction following transfusion; 4) glutathione deficiency (GSH; GSSG), which is caused by decreased synthetase activity (inability to incorporate glycine into GSH; the cells are primaquine sensitive); and 5) several high ATP syndromes have been described, two associated with hemolysis.

GLYCOGEN STORAGE DISEASES

The glycogen storage diseases or glycogenoses are usually due to defects in enzyme reactions in the degradation of glycogen to glucose. Several disorders have been described; at least types I through VIII are established as specific entities. A scheme of glycogenesis and glycogenolysis was presented in Figure 1.3.

Type I glycogenosis, or classic von Gierke's, is inherited as an autosomal recessive characteristic. The clinical features include short stature with proportional growth, poor muscular development, the presence of xanthomas, increased capillary fragility, and osteoporosis. The patients may have convulsions secondary to hypoglycemia. A chronic acidosis leads to negative calcium balance. At birth, the liver is found to be enlarged, but the spleen is of normal size. The kidneys are enlarged, and glycogen accumulation in the kidneys may lead to Fanconi syndrome. The patients also exhibit a hyperlipidemia secondary to increased lipid synthesis. Hyperuricemia may lead to uric acid nephropathy and tophaceous gout. The biochemical defect responsible for this disorder is a deficiency of glucose-6-phosphate phosphatase. As a result of intracellular accumulation of G-6-P, the dependent glycogen synthetase is activated, with resulting increased glycogen synthesis. Failure of glycogenolysis following epinephrine injection is reflected by a failure of a rise in blood glucose. Definitive diagnosis of this disorder is made by demonstration of decreased G-6-P phosphatase in a liver biopsy specimen. Treatment consists of frequent feedings to maintain blood glucose levels. Some studies suggest that diazoxide may be helpful in management of this disorder.

Type II glycogenosis, or Pompe's disease, or acid maltase deficiency, is inherited as an autosomal recessive characteristic. The patients exhibit marked hypotonia despite normal muscle mass and firmness. Symptoms may start by the age of 2 months. The patients are markedly dyspneic because of respiratory muscle weakness. Cardiomegaly and cyanosis are prominent findings in these patients. Blood glucose, lipids, and ketones are within normal limits, as are the responses to epinephrine or glucagon. These patients die by 5 months of age as a result of cardiorespiratory failure. The disorder is caused by a deficiency of lysosomal α-1,4-glucosidase in the tissues involved. Liver biopsy specimens reveal an accumulation of vacuoles loaded with glycogen. Urine and leukocyte α-1,4-glucosidase (acid maltase) levels are decreased or absent. There is no effective treatment of this disorder. As a preventive measure, amniocentesis and fibroblast culture in pregnant patients with a family history of this disorder and proof of the deficiency indicates therapeutic abortion.

Type III glycogen storage disease, or Cori's disease, or limit dextrinosis, is also inherited as an autosomal recessive characteristic. The clinical manifestations include a progressive myopathy in patients in whom the storage disorder affects the muscles. There is growth retardation, and the patients exhibit a hepatosplenomegaly as well as cardiomegaly due to glycogen infiltration. There is no renal involvement in this disorder, and the liver size has been observed to return to normal at puberty. Some patients may rarely show evidence of hepatic cirrhosis. The hypoglycemia is not as severe as in type I, and the levels of serum uric acid may be normal or elevated. The biochemical lesion in this disorder is a deficiency of the debrancher enzyme (amylo-1,6-glucosidase). Diagnosis is confirmed by finding of an abnormal form of glycogen in liver biopsy and a decreased level of debrancher enzyme activity. The prognosis in this disorder is good, and management requires a high protein diet.

Type IV glycogen storage disease, or amylopectinosis, is also known as Andersen's disease. The disorder is of autosomal recessive inheritance and is quite rare. The clinical pattern is of failure to thrive and hypotonia. The patients exhibit a hepatosplenomegaly and progressive cirrhosis which is fatal by the age of 2 years. Glucose tolerance test is normal and the response to epinephrine or glucogen is variable in these patients. The disorder is caused by a deficiency of the brancher enzyme in glycogen synthesis (1,4-1,6-transglucosylase), so that the tissues show abnormal outer chains of glycogen. Diagnosis is based on the finding of abnormally branched type of glycogen in liver biopsy and on a demonstration of decreased leukocyte brancher enzyme activity. Treatment consists of supportive management of the liver disease and the complicating ascites.

Type V glycogen storage disease, or McArdle's disease, is also called muscle phosphorylase deficiency and is inherited as an autosomal recessive characteristic. The disorder is characterized by the occurrence of severe muscle cramps, myoglobinuria, and creatinuria after vigorous exercise. These patients eventually have muscle wasting. Hypoglycemia is not a manifestation of this disorder. The biochemical defect in this disorder is a deficiency of muscle phosphorylase. Diagnosis is confirmed by the failure of venous lactate to increase after exercise and by the finding of decreased muscle phosphorylase in biopsy specimens.

Type VI glycogenosis, or Hers' disease, is inherited as a rare autosomal dominant characteristic. The patients exhibit growth retardation, hepatomegaly, hypoglycemia, hyperlipidemia, and lactic acidosis. The disorder is due to a deficiency of liver phosphorylase, and the diagnosis is confirmed by this finding.

Type VII glycogenosis is a rare disorder which is ascribed to a decrease in hepatic phosphofructokinase, an enzyme essential to the glycolytic pathway. This disorder may also occur in the muscle since myoglobinuria is also a feature.

Type VIII glycogenosis is an X-linked inherited disorder which is characterized by hepatomegaly caused by glycogen accumulation. The disorder is caused by a deficiency of hepatic phosphorylase.

Clinical Disorders of Galactose Metabolism

Galactose is derived from dietary lactose which is cleaved in the intestinal mucosa to release glucose and galactose. This monosaccharide has four major alternative facts, viz., the formation of galactolactone as the initial step to the pentose phosphate pathway, the formation of galactose 1-phosphate by the enzyme galactokinase, the formation of uridine diphospho-galactose from galactose-1-P, and the reduction to galactitol by an aldo-reductase (Figure 2.9).

Clinical disorders from errors in galactose utilization are caused by toxicity of large amounts of the monosaccharide itself and its reduction product, galactitol. Two major types of galactosemia are recognized. One type, caused by a defect in the enzyme phosphogalactose uridyltransferase, is characterized by severe systemic effects. The more recently discovered type of galactosemia caused by galactokinase deficiency is of lesser clinical severity.

Congenital galactosemia caused by transferase deficiency is an auto-somal recessive inherited disorder. The early clinical manifestations include anorexia, vomiting, diarrhea, abdominal distension, and hypoglycemia. Hepatocellular damage may result in jaundice and ascites. Renal involve-ment is manifested by proteinuria and aminoaciduria. Accumulation of galactose 1-phosphate and galactitol causes damage in erythrocytes, lens (cataracts), kidneys, and the cerebral cortex (retardation). Galactose 1-phosphate interferes with phosphoglucomutase in glycogen breakdown, and this is the basis of the hypoglycemia. Diagnosis is suggested by the

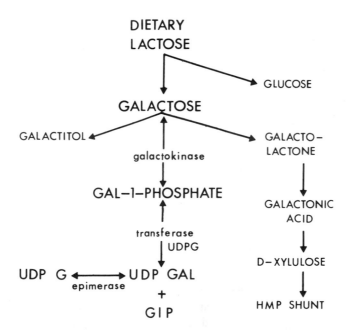

Figure 2.9. Biochemical defects in clinical disorders of galactose metabolism. En-zyme defects are described in text.

presence of increased amounts of nonglucose reducing substances in the urine. Definitive diagnosis may be made by finding of increased levels of galactose 1-phosphate and galactitol in erythrocytes. NAPDH fluorescence of erythrocytes has also been employed in detection of the disorder. Treatment requires exclusion of galactose from the diet and the removal of milk and milk sugars. Certain nutritional substitutes, such as nutramigen, have been helpful.

Galactosemia caused by galactokinase deficiency is an autosomal recessive disorder in which the only major clinical manifestation is the formation of cataracts late in the course of the disorder. There are no neurological or gastrointestinal problems associated with this type of galactosemia. An accumulation of galactose and galactitol is the basis of cataract formation in the lens. Diagnosis is suggested by the finding of nonglucose reducing substances in the urine and the finding of elevated galactose and galactitol. Erythrocyte galactokinase deficiency may be a diagnostic feature. Treatment consists of a diet low in galactose.

LITERATURE CITED

1. Levine, R., and D. E. Haft. 1970. Carbohydrate metabolism. N. Engl. J. Med. 283:174–183, 237–247.
2. Cahill, G. E. 1971. Physiology of insulin in man. Diabetes 20: 785–799.
3. Altszuler, N., I. Rathgeb, and B. Winkler. 1968. The effects of growth hormone on carbohydrate and lipid metabolism in the dog. Ann. N.Y. Acad. Sci. 148:441–458.
4. Levine, R. 1970. Mechanisms of insulin secretion. N. Engl. J. Med. 283:522–526.
5. Renold, A. E. 1972. The beta cell and its responses: Summarizing remarks and some contributions from Geneva. Diabetes 21 (Suppl. 2):619–631.
6. Sharp, G. W. G., C. Wollheim, W. A. Mullen, A. Gutzeit, P. A. Truehart, B. Blondel, L. Orci, and A. E. Renold. 1975. Studies on the mechanism of insulin release. Fed. Proc. 34:1537–1548.
7. Klimt, C. R., T. R. Prout, R. Bradley, H. Dolger, G. Fisher, C. F. Gastineau, H. Marks, C. L. Meinert, O. P. Schumacher, and invited contributors. 1969. Standardization of the oral glucose tolerance test. Diabetes 18:299–307.
8. Alberti, K. G. M. M., T. D. R. Hockaday, and K. C. Turner. 1973. Small doses of intramuscular insulin in the treatment of diabetic "coma." Lancet 2:515–522.
9. Kanter, Y., and A. N. Bessman. 1975. Small versus large doses of insulin in diabetic ketosis. Western J. Med. 122:509–513.
10. Oliva, P. 1970. Lactic acidosis. Am. J. Med. 48:209–225.
11. Solomon, M. A. 1965. Diabetic nephropathy: Clinicopathologic correlation. A study based on renal biopsies. Metabolism 12:687–698.
12. Beaumont, P., and F. C. Hollows. 1969. Classification of diabetic retinopathy, with therapeutic implications. Lancet 1:419–424.

13. Locke, S. 1964. The peripheral nervous system in diabetes mellitus. Diabetes 13:307–311.
14. Gerich, J. E., M. Lorenzi, V. Schneider, J. H. Karam, J. Rivier, R. Guillemin, and P. H. Forsham. 1974. Effects of somatostatin on plasma glucose and glucagon levels in human diabetes mellitus: Pathophysiologic and therapeutic implications. N. Engl. J. Med. 291:544–547.
15. Gerich, J. E., M. Lorenzi, D. M. Bier, V. Schneider, E. Tsalikian, J. H. Karam, and P. H. Forsham. 1975. Prevention of human diabetic ketoacidosis by somatostatin. N. Engl. J. Med. 292:985–989.
16. Conn, J. W., and H. S. Seltzer. 1955. Spontaneous hypoglycemia. Am. J. Med. 19:460–478.
17. Fajans, S., J. C. Floyd, C. A. Thiffault, R. F. Knopf, T. S. Harrison, and J. W. Conn. 1968. Further studies on diazoxide suppression of insulin release from abnormal and normal islet tissue in man. Ann. N.Y. Acad. Sci. 150:261–280.
18. Murray-Lyon, I. M., A. L. W. F. Eddleston, R. Williams, M. Brown, B. M. Hogbin, A. Bennett, J. C. Edwards, and K. W. Taylor. 1968. Treatment of multiple-hormone-producing-tumor with streptozotocin. Lancet 2:895–898.
19. Cahill, G. F. 1974. "A non-editorial on non-hypoglycemia." N. Engl. J. Med. 291:905–906.
20. Valentine, W. N. 1972. Pyruvate kinase deficiency and other enzyme deficiency hemolytic disorders. In J. B. Stanbury, J. B. Wyngaarden, and D. S. Fredrickson (eds.), The Metabolic Basis of Inherited Disease. 3rd Ed, pp. 1338–1357. McGraw-Hill Book Co., New York.
21. Valentine, W. N. 1968. Hereditary hemolytic anemias associated with specific erythrocyte enzymopathies. Calif. Med. 108:280–290.
22. Beutler, E. 1972. Glucose-6-dehydrogenase deficiency. In J. B. Stanbury, J. B. Wyngaarden, and D. S. Fredrickson (eds.), The Metabolic Basis of Inherited Disease. 3rd Ed., pp. 1358–1388. McGraw-Hill Book Co., New York.

3

Lipid
Metabolism

Lipids provide approximately 41% of the daily caloric intake in the American diet and serve as vehicles for delivery of the fat soluble vitamins A, D, E, and K in the gastrointestinal tract. The aromas and flavors of foods are also dependent on the lipid content. Dietary carbohydrate (roughly 47% of the American diet) and protein (approximately 12% of diet) may be converted to lipids in the body. U. S. Department of Agriculture statistics indicate the average daily diet in the U. S. A. contains 3,120 kcal, which is considerably in excess of requirements. A considerable portion of the excess calories is deposited as triglycerides in adipose tissues; these serve as a source of calories after release as free fatty acids. On the average, a 70-kg man, with 5% body weight as adipose tissue, has 31,500 kcal stored as lipid (i.e., 3,500 g). These lipid deposits maintain life in time of inanition or starvation.

In the American dietary, 34% of lipids are derived from vegetable sources and 66% from animal sources of which 45% is ingested as butter, margarine, oils, and shortening, 32% from meat, and 15% from dairy products other than butter. Approximately 98% of dietary lipid is in form of triglycerides, 700 mg in the form of cholesterol for which the main sources are eggs (1 egg contains 275 mg of cholesterol), brain, liver, butter, and to a small extent, meats. The remainder of dietary lipid is in form of phospholipids. Most of the calories derived from lipids come from the fatty acids in triglycerides, fatty acids constituting 95% of the triglyceride molecule. Fatty acids are distributed approximately as 40% monounsaturated oleic acid; 12% polyunsaturated linoleic acid, and 37% various saturated fatty acids, including palmitic and stearic acid.

Milk products and coconut oil contain mainly saturated fatty acids. Solid margarines prepared from soybean or cotton seed oil vary markedly in their fatty acid composition, containing 15–35% saturated, 40–60% monounsaturated, and 10–40% polyunsaturated fatty acids. The fatty acid composition of lipids from animals also varies considerably, largely reflecting the constitution of the animals' diets. It has been shown that the fat content of poultry feed affects the fatty acid composition of the eggs and, in man, chylomicrons in the serum closely approximate the composition of ingested lipid. Various modifications, largely oxidative, may take place during storage of dietary lipids.

The fatty acids arachidonic and linoleic which are not synthesized in man and other animal sources are termed essential fatty acids. Experimental essential FA deficiency in rats causes scaliness of the skin, alopecia, decreased reproductive capacity, and growth (effects which are ascribed to an increased basal metabolic rate and a decreased formation of high energy phosphate bonds). Essential fatty acid deficiency has not been observed in the adult man, but infants receiving low fat diets have dry, scaly, thickened skin, impaired utilization of calories, and decreased growth. It is recommended that the adult should consume at least 2% of the total dietary as essential fatty acids; infants require 3–4%. Dietary polyunsaturated fatty acids also serve an important function as prostaglandin precursors.

DIETARY LIPIDS

The dietary lipids include fatty acids (FA), triglycerides (TG), phospholipids (PL), and sterols. Fatty acids exist mainly as esters of naturally occurring alcohols such as glycerol, but small amounts may exist in amide linkage, or in the free form, FFA. FA from animal tissues are usually even-numbered, unbranched, and monocarboxylic, and are classified according to chain length and the numbers of double bonds in the molecule. A standard system (1) employs a numerical system in which the first numeral refers to the number of carbons; this is followed by a colon. The second numeral refers to the number of double bonds, and their locations are identified by superscripts, e.g., 2:0 refers to the 2-carbon acetic acid which lacks a double bond; $18:2^{9,12}$ refers to linoleic acid which contains 18 carbons, 2 unsaturated bonds located respectively at carbon atoms 9 and 12. FA solubility depends on the ratio of polar hydrophilic carboxyl group to the non-polar residue; for example, acetic acid is completely soluble in water, but, in other FA, increased numbers of methylene groups decrease the water solubility. Glycerides include mono-, di-, and triglycerides. The substituents on the glycerol molecule are identified by a stereospecific numbering system (*sn*), e.g.:

(1)

$$
\begin{array}{ll}
& \text{H} \\
& | \\
\text{H} - \text{C} - \text{OH} & 1 \\
& | \\
\text{HO} - \text{C} - \text{H} & 2 \\
& | \\
\text{H} - \text{C} - \text{OH} & 3 \\
& | \\
& \text{H} \\
\end{array}
$$

sn-glycerol

(2)
$$H_2 - C - O - C - R$$
$$HO - CH$$
$$H_2 - C\,O\,H$$

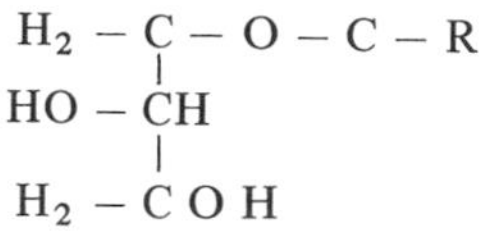

1-acyl-sn-glycerol
(a monoglyceride)

(3) $$CH_3(CH_2)_7CH-CH(CH_2)_7 \ - \ C-O-\underset{|}{\overset{C-O-\overset{O}{\overset{||}{C}}-(CH_2)_{14}-CH_3}{}}C-H \quad O$$
$$H_2C - O - \overset{O}{\overset{||}{C}} - (CH_2)_{16} - CH_3$$

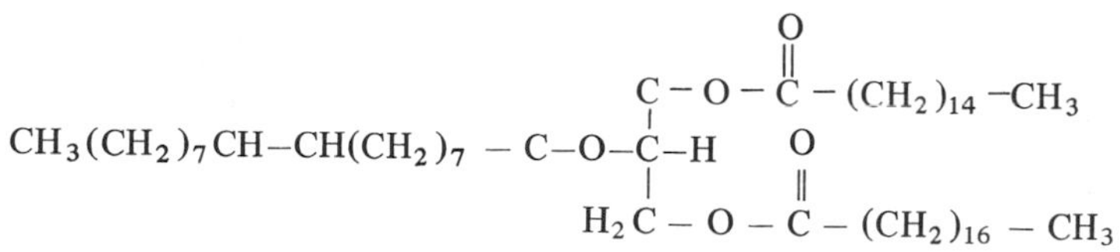

L-palmityl-2-oleyl-3-stearoyl-sn-glycerol
(a triglyceride)

Triglycerides (TG or neutral fat) constitute the most abundant lipid in animal tissues and serve as an important energy reservoir. TG are soluble only in non-polar solvents. TG which are liquid at room temperature are called oils; those which are solid are called fats. TG from animal sources usually contain 2 to 3 different FA in each molecule; the most common are oleic (18:1), palmitic (16:0), stearic (18:0), linoleic ($18:2^{9,12}$), and palmitoleic ($16:1^8$). In man, saturated FA occur mainly at positions 1 and 3. PL occur in all biological membranes. They also occur in serum as lipoproteins and in egg yolk. These compounds play an important role in electron transport, oxidative phosphorylation, and energy-linked transmembrane transfer of ions. PL are classed as 1) derivatives of sn-glycerol-3-P (L-α-glycerophosphate), 2) derivatives of sphingosine, and 3) carbohydrate-containing glycolipids. Examples of phospholipid structures are as follows:

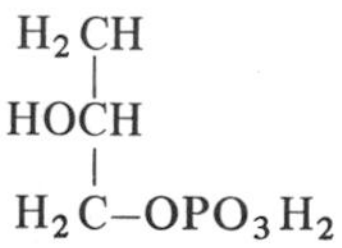

$$H_2\,CH$$
$$HOCH$$
$$H_2C-OPO_3H_2$$

sn-glycerol-3-P or L-glycerophosphate

and

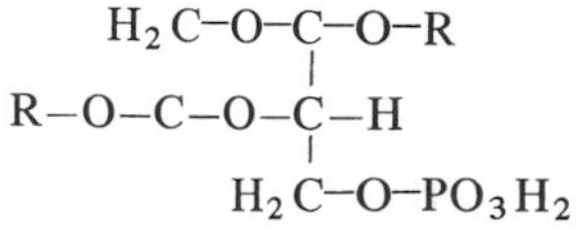

$$H_2C-O-C-O-R$$
$$R-O-C-O-C-H$$
$$H_2C-O-PO_3H_2$$

1,2-diacyl sn-glycerol 3-phosphate

Phosphatidyl derivatives are classified according to the moiety forming a diester with the phosphoric acid of phosphatidic acid.

$$H_2C-O-\overset{\overset{\displaystyle O}{\|}}{C}-R$$

$$HO-CH$$

$$H_2C-O-\overset{\overset{\displaystyle O}{|}}{\underset{\underset{\displaystyle O}{|}}{P}}-O-CH_2-N-(CH_3)_3$$

3-sn-phosphatidylcholine (lysophatidylcholine or lysolecithin)

The 3-sn-phosphatidylcholines are called lecithins, and they are dipolar compounds with isoelectric point near 6.5. They constitute the most abundant PL in serum. The 3-sn-phosphatidylinositols make up the cephalins which occur in high concentrations in the brain. These compounds have isoelectric point around 3.1. Sterols are derived from the cyclopentanophenanthrene skeleton and form the bulk of the nonsaponifiable fraction of lipid extracts. The principal sterol in man is cholesterol which serves as substrate for bile acids and steroid hormones.

Intestinal Lipid Metabolism

The events from the ingestion of lipids to their distribution to various tissues and organs are conveniently considered in four stages: 1) intraluminal processes; 2) absorption into intestinal mucosal cell; 3) intramucosal processes; and 4) transport from the mucosa to the liver and other organs (2–4) (Figure 3.1). The important intraluminal processes are emulsification, lipolysis, and micelle formation. Emulsification is the process whereby mastication followed by gastric contractions renders the ingested TG into an emulsion which is presented to the duodenum. Bile salts, phospholipids, lysolecithins, and monoglycerides aid in the emulsification process. Fat absorption does not occur in the stomach except in the rare condition of "intestinal metaplasia" which is found in pernicious anemia. Emulsification is disturbed in conditions causing rapid gastric emptying, bile salt deficiency, and in pancreatic insufficiency.

Lipolysis takes place in the duodenum where hydrolysis of 1- and 3-positions of triglyceride by pancreatic lipase (glycerol ester hydrolase) occurs at the oil-water interface of the emulsion. The pancreatic enzyme activity is increased by bile salts and Ca^{++}. This hydrolytic reaction is essentially irreversible and results in the release of free fatty acids (FFA), monoglycerides (MG), and diglycerides (DG). The released FA exist as soaps in the intestinal lumen as they are neutralized by the presence of bicarbonate. Similar processes involve phospholipids and cholesterol. Lipolysis is decreased when there is interference with release of pancreatic enzymes and the presence of decreased bicarbonate. Clinical disorders affecting intraluminal lipolysis include: pancreatitis; pancreatic insufficiency; mucoviscidosis (cystic fibrosis), in which conditions there are

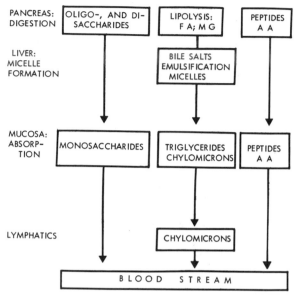

Figure 3.1. Processes in digestion of lipids and other foodstuffs. Note the dependence of lipid absorption on the processes of lipolysis, emulsification, and micelle formation.

decreased pancreatic enzymes; and the Zollinger-Ellison syndrome, in which increased gastric hydrochloric acid, decreased intestinal bicarbonate, and acid inactivation of lipase lead to malabsorption of lipid.

Micelle formation refers to the formation of polymolecular aggregates caused by the detergent action of bile salts. Bile salts account for 80% of cholesterol breakdown in the liver and the enterohepatic circulation of bile salts, which amounts to 20–30 g/day (2 cycles/meal), regulates hepatic cholesterol metabolism. The bulk of bile salt absorption takes place in the ileum. Micelle formation is dependent on conjugated bile salts and this process is enhanced by MG, FA, and PL, whereas diglycerides and TG lower micellar solubility. It is from micelles that the bulk of lipids are absorbed into the intestinal mucosal cell.

Clinical disorders affecting intestinal micelle formation which cause decreased formation or delivery of conjugated bile salts to the duodenum result in lipid malabsorption. These include biliary obstruction, interruption of enterohepatic circulation of bile salts, and drug effects. Biliary obstruction from several causes results in diminished bile salt delivery to the duodenum. In the absence of bile salts, absorption of FA and TG decreases 50% and that of cholesterol and fat soluble vitamins almost disappears. Interruption of the enterohepatic circulation of bile salts results in depletion of the bile salt pool. This problem may arise after resection of the distal bowel which is the site of absorption of these salts. After jejunal resection, the ileum can efficiently absorb lipids, but the jejunum is incapable of absorption of bile salts. Clinical disorders affecting this process include regional enteritis, ileal involvement in chronic ulcerative colitis, radiation enteritis, scleroderma, Whipple's disease, and enterocolic fistula. The malabsorption in the above conditions takes place because the critical micellar concentration is not reached in the duodenum and jejunum. Ingestion of cholestyramine binds bile salts in the intestinal lumen and results in interruption of their reabsorption. Large amounts of this drug may induce cholerrheic enteropathy because increased amounts of bile salts are thus permitted to reach the colon.

Absorption into Intestinal Mucosa   The absorptive surface of the intestinal mucosa is considerably enlarged by the formation of microvilli which are covered with mucopolysaccharide. Substances to be absorbed enter the microvillar cytoplasm and are transported to the lateral plasma membrane and, after certain intramucosal processes, are discharged into the blood vessels or lymphatic channels. Compounds released by lipolysis diffuse passively from the micellar oil-water interface into the brush border of the intestinal mucosa. This process is decreased in adult celiac disease (gluten enteropathy, characterized by villous atrophy), lymphoma, carcinoma, radiation enteritis, mesenteric vascular occlusion, amyloid infiltration, infestation with strongyloides stercoralis, giardiasis, bacterial and viral gastroenteritis, carcinoid, hyperthyroidism, disaccharidase deficiency, and in neomycin excess.

Intramucosal Processes   Within the intestinal mucosal cells, FA and MG are re-esterified to TG (Figure 3.2). With the participation of protein, phospholipids, and cholesterol, the TG is packaged into chylomicrons in which form the lipid is transported from the cell to the lymphatics. The primary pathway of intramucosal TG synthesis is via the monoglyceride shunt whereby the fatty acid CoA molecule condenses with MG to form a diglyceride. The addition of an acyl-CoA in presence of the appropriate transferase results in the formation of triglyceride. Alternative pathways include the condensation of acyl-CoA with L-α-glycerophosphate derived from the glycolytic pathway. The apoprotein and β-globulin required for chylomicron formation are synthesized by the intestinal mucosal cell. This synthesis is blocked by agents such as puromycin, cycloheximide, and ethionine. Clinical disorders which decrease the intramucosal synthesis of triglycerides are Addison's disease in which there are decreased levels of the enzymes thiokinase and mono- and diglycerate transacylase, congenital abetalipoproteinemia, and hypobetalipoproteinemia. In the latter conditions, the absence of the apoprotein precludes chylomicron formation.

Transport through Lymphatics to Liver and Other Tissues   After chylomicrons (CM) are packaged in the smooth endoplastic reticulum of the

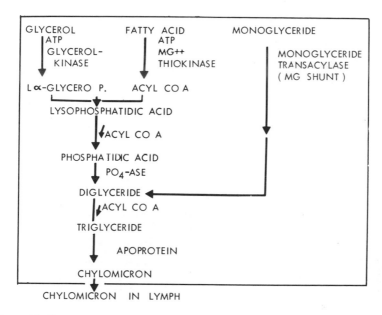

Figure 3.2. Intramucosal processes in lipid absorption by the intestinal mucosal cell.

intestinal mucosa, they are discharged into lacteals at the lateral border of the intestinal cell. The CM then flow through intestinal lymph vessels and nodes into the thoracic duct and eventually into the systemic circulation. In man, one-half of thoracic duct lymph flow is decreased during sleep and increased during and after meals. Dietary TG is detected in thoracic duct lymph within 10–20 min after a fatty meal. The rate of entry of CM is greater than the rate of removal, hence, the phenomenon of postprandial hyperlipemia. The half-life of the individual CM is 5–15 min. There is normally complete clearing of CM from the plasma within 6 hr, the clearance rate being directly proportional to particle size. The liver, adipose tissue, and RE system are the main sites of chylomicron removal. Disorders involving this process include Whipple's disease (intestinal lipodystrophy), which is a bacterial infection of the lamina propria so that lipid and other nutrients cannot be absorbed, and intestinal lymphangiectasia, in which there is obstruction in the lymphatic system.

BILE ACID METABOLISM

Bile acid synthesis occurs only in the liver, the formation of the primary bile acids requiring the presence of the substrate cholesterol as well as several enzymes and cofactors located in various geographic areas in the cell (Figure 3.3). The biochemical steps include: 1) the hydroxylation and

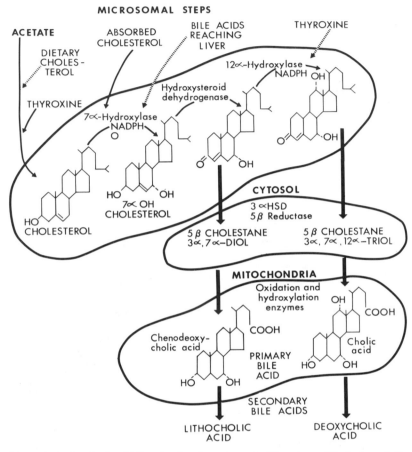

Figure 3.3. Synthesis of bile salts showing rate-controlling steps of 7α hydroxylation and 12α hydroxylation and factors influencing these reactions. Note the intracellular compartmentalization of the synthetic steps. *Broken arrows* indicate inhibitory influences.

dehydrogenation reactions which take place in the endoplasmic reticulum (microsomes); 2) the reduction steps which take place in the cytosol (cell sap); and 3) the shortening of the side chain which takes place in the mitochondria (5–7). Conversion of primary bile acids (cholic and cheno-deoxycholic acids) to secondary bile acids takes place in the colon and, occasionally, in the small intestine via action of bacterial enzymes, e.g., as in *Streptococcus fecalis, Bacteroides,* and *Clostridia.*

At least two feedback controlling mechanisms regulate bile acid synthesis. These are the amount of bile acids reaching the liver via the enterohepatic circulation (ileum (plus colon) to portal vein) and the amount of cholesterol absorbed from the diet. Both factors affect the essentially irreversible 7α hydroxylation reaction which takes place in the liver microsomes. It is worth noting that there are very few steroid metabolites outside of the bile acid series which are hydroxylated at C-7. Diversion of bile salt from the bile duct or sequestration of bile salts by cholestyramine activates the bile acid production rate markedly by inducing increased enzyme synthesis. Animal experiments have shown that, on total biliary drainage, the liver responds by a 10-fold increase in cholesterol degradation, the liver possibly degrading more cholesterol than is present in the total liver pool of cholesterol. As an increased rate of cholesterol synthesis occurs after disturbance of the enterohepatic circulation, the total body pool of cholesterol is unchanged. The sequestration of bile salts by cholestyramine is followed by decreased cholesterol levels in the serum, presumably because the rate of breakdown to the bile salts is greater than the elevation of cholesterol synthesis. Concomitant changes in lipoprotein metabolism may also contribute to this process. Increase in dietary cholesterol is followed by a severalfold increase in bile acid synthesis. Concomitantly, there is a decrease in bile endogenous synthesis of cholesterol in the liver.

Thyroid hormone administration, or hyperthyroidism, is followed by an increased cholesterol synthesis. The low cholesterol levels found in these states are caused by the activation of increased synthesis of the cholesterol side chain-oxidizing enzyme, a secondary regulatory factor. Thyroid hormone probably slows the 12α-hydroxylase system with resultant increase in chenodeoxycholic acid/cholic acid. Although there is a decrease in cholesterol synthesis in hypothyroidism, the decreased degradation of cholesterol to bile acids is largely responsible for the hypercholesterolemia found in this state. The bile acids, cholic acid (trihydroxy) and chenodeoxycholic acid (dihydroxy), are conjugated prior to discharge into the intestinal lumen. Glycine and taurine are the weak bases which are conjugated with these acids, essentially in the ratio of 3:1 (G:T ratio). The preferred substrate for bile salt conjugation is taurine, but often glycine is more available. The bile salts function to: 1) emulsify lipids and triglycerides and stabilize the emulsion by preventing the coalescence of the emulsion droplets, thus permitting the action of water-soluble pancreatic lipase on the water-insoluble triglyceride; 2) participate in the formation of micelles from which optimal intestinal absorption of FA, MG, and fat-soluble vitamins takes place; 3) serve as detergents and solubilize cholesterol in mixed micelles; and 4) serve as cofactors for cholesterol esterase which cleaves cholesterol esters. Cholic acid, glycocholic acid, and taurocholic acid are specific cofactors for extracellular cholesterol esterase.

Enterohepatic Circulation of Bile Salts

A specific sodium-dependent transport system for absorption of conjugated and unconjugated bile salts is located in the distal 100- to 150-cm

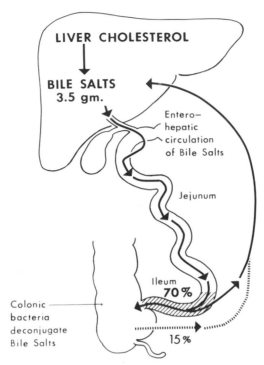

Figure 3.4. Enterohepatic circulation of bile salts depicting the quantitative importance of the process in bile salt economy.

segment of the ileum. In addition, there is passive absorption of unconjugated (deconjugated) bile salts, and glycine-conjugated bile salts in the small intestine and the colon (Figure 3.4). The active transport mechanism is relatively independent of the number of hydroxyl groups in the bile salt molecule. The most likely requirement for this transport system is the presence of a positive and a negative charge on the transport site which permits the movement of the bile salt against a concentration gradient. This ileal active transport system applies to all bile salts and is responsible for 70% of reabsorbed bile salts.

Passive Processes in Bile Salt Absorption

The complete mechanism of the passive processes in bile salt absorption is not known, but the factors involved possibly include osmotic water flow and sieving effect, passive ionic diffusion, or passive nonionic diffusion. These steps are responsible for approximately 15% of daily bile salt circulation and also involve the deconjugated bile salts which may occur in the colon (via bacterial deconjugases) and, to a small extent, in the ileum.

When there are deconjugating bacteria present in the small intestine, passive absorption may also take place in this location.

The total bile salt pool in man is 3.5 g, the bulk of which is reabsorbed twice during each meal, or approximately 21 g of bile salts is emptied into the small intestine daily. Based on these figures, approximately 14.7 g of conjugated bile salt and between 0.5 and 3.1 g of unconjugated bile salt are reabsorbed via colon and terminal ileum. It is suggested that colonic absorption continues throughout the day, regardless of time of meals.

In the process of reabsorption, these bile salts enter the portal system bound to albumin. The conjugated bile salts are re-excreted into the lumen, but the deconjugated bile salts are conjugated with the available glycine and taurine (usually a G:T ratio of 3:1) and re-excreted. The fecal loss of bile is about 0.52 g/day (0.2–0.8 g) and represents a major catabolic pathway for cholesterol excretion, approximately 50% of total steroid excretion. This amount of bile is replenished by new synthesis from cholesterol.

Clinical Disorders Related to Altered Bile Salt Kinetics in Ileal Diseases

Disturbance of the integrity of the ileum by surgery, neoplasm, infection, and by disease processes alters the reabsorption of the bile salts so that they are discharged into the colonic lumen where deconjugation processes caused by bacterial enzymes take place. Similar deconjugation may occur in the small intestine in the presence of an incompetent ileocecal valve. The deconjugated bile acids are absorbed in the colon and small intestine and carried via the portal system to the liver where reconjugation takes place. The amount of reconjugation and the type of conjugates depend on the availability of glycine and taurine. Because of greater availability of glycine, the G:T ratio of the reconjugated salts approaches 15:1 in comparison to the normal 3:1. The recirculation of deconjugated bile salts depletes the available stores of taurine. Experimental data have revealed that taurine feeding may normalize the G:T ratio in patients with ileal disorders. Although the above processes tend to conserve the pool of bile salts, the total pool is not maintained; hence, there is a compensatory synthesis of new bile acids from cholesterol. As was pointed out earlier, the feedback regulation of the 7α hydroxylation enzyme involves reabsorbed bile acids.

Clinical Entities that Result from Disturbances in Bile Salt Reabsorption

Cholerrheic enteropathy is a syndrome of watery diarrhea associated with loss of bile salt into the colonic lumen when ileal absorption is insufficient. The accumlation of dihydroxy bile salts in the colon is responsible for inhibition of colonic salt and water absorption. Cholestyramine is a useful agent in this disorder because it induces intraluminal sequestration of the dihydroxy bile salts. A secondary increase in the synthesis of trihydroxy bile acids, which aids in the processes of lipid absorption, aids in the amelioration of diarrhea associated with cholerrheic enteropathy.

Bacterial metabolism of increased amounts of bile acids reaching the colon in patients with diseases of the ileum is associated with an increased occurrence of renal calculi. The increased reconjugation of deconjugated bile salts and subsequent re-entry of these salts into the colon provide increased amounts of such salts for bacterial action. It has been proposed that glycine is released and is oxidized to glyoxylate which is reabsorbed and carried to the liver. Glyoxylate is metabolized to oxalate by the liver and excreted in the urine. The above explanation has been disputed recently. Hyperoxaluria and oxalate stone formation have been found in several patients with ileal resection. Oral treatment with taurine (4 g/day) corrects the ratio of reconjugation of the reabsorbed deconjugated bile acids in the liver; hence, a resultant decrease in the hyperoxaluria and oxalate stones.

Steatorrhea is often found in ileal disease and is due to a decrease of efficient postprandial recirculation of conjugated bile salts. Increased hepatic synthesis of bile salts is insufficient for adequate micellarization of lipid. Oral bile salts may be of therapeutic value, but often may contribute to a "cholerrheic enteropathy." As a result, the best treatment is the use of medium-chained triglycerides (MCT) which do not require bile salts for their absorption.

An increase in incidence of cholelithiasis is found in patients with ileal disorders. The mechanism is not clear; it is possible that because of decreased bile salts there are periods during food ingestion when cholesterol solubility is inadequate, leading to lithiasis.

Clinical Disorders Related to Altered
Bile Acid Kinetics in Duodenojejunal Diseases

Duodenojejunal disorders occasionally lead to decreased cholecystokinin, so that there is decreased gall bladder contraction following a meal. This leads to inadequate discharge of bile salts and decreased enterohepatic circulation with consequent insufficient exposure to bacterial flora, resulting in altered taurocholate kinetics in patients with nontropical sprue. A similar phenomenon is observed in Whipple's disease; in nontropical sprue, the process is corrected by a gluten-free diet.

Clinical Disorders Related to Altered Bile
Acid Kinetics in Conditions of Intestinal Bacterial Overgrowth

Abnormal bacterial flora is responsible for the malabsorption found in "blind loop" syndrome. This process is readily diagnosed by intubation, the detection of bacterial count $> 10^5$/g of small bowel content, and the presence of unconjugated bile salt at this level (since, under normal conditions, only conjugated bile salt is found in the upper small intestine).

Clinical Disorders of Intestinal Lipid Metabolism

Clinical disorders of the intestinal lipid metabolism are conveniently classified according to the nature of the processes involved in the defects (4). Accordingly, these disorders are discussed under the following headings: 1) clinical disorders of intraluminal lipid metabolism (including emulsification, lipolysis, and micelle formation); 2) clinical disorders caused by errors in absorption of lipid into intestinal mucosa; 3) clinical disorders of intramucosal metabolism; and 4) disorders of lipid transport from mucosal cell to liver and other tissues.

In the disorders to be considered, varying degrees of steatorrhea or excess fecal loss of fat are encountered. Steatorrhea is accompanied by weight loss and muscle wasting secondary to negative caloric balance, abdominal distension, crampy abdominal pain and borborygmi secondary to decreased transit time of intestinal contents, and hyperperistalsis caused by increased osmotically active content in the lumen.

Clinical Disorders of Intraluminal Lipid Metabolism These disorders are considered under the headings of the processes of emulsification, lipolysis, and micelle formation.

Emulsification The emulsification of lipids in the intestinal lumen is disturbed in the presence of impaired gastric motility and emptying, and, in gastrectomy, because of impaired mixing of intraluminal contents and pancreatic secretions. Intestinal bypass surgery is accompanied by an impaired acid-induced release of secretion and consequent decreased release of pancreatic enzymes, hence, decreasing the emulsification process. In addition, impaired emulsification occurs in the absence of bile salts.

Disorders of Intraluminal Lipolysis Disorders of the pancreas which result in the secretion of <10% of levels of lipolytic enzymes or in decreased bicarbonate in the intestinal lumen may result in malabsorption of lipids. In acute pancreatitis, pancreatic enzymes (lipase and trypsin) may escape from the cell and duct and cause lipolysis and fat necrosis in adjacent tissues and in mediastinal, pleural, pericardial, bone marrow, and subcutaneous areas. Pancreatic insufficiency usually results from tissue destruction and fibrosis following recurrent active pancreatitis. This condition is associated with significant diarrhea with attendant losses of sodium, potassium, calcium, magnesium, iron, copper, and water. The stools are soft, gray, oily, and foul, and may float because of high lipid content. Malabsorption of certain fat soluble vitamins may lead to hyperkeratosis follicularis due to malabsorption of vitamin A, abnormal bleeding (correctible by parental injection of vitamin K) secondary to vitamin K malabsorption, decreased calcium absorption due to inadequate absorption of vitamin D and malabsorption of calcium which is attributable to abnormal vitamin D absorption as well as to bile salt deficiency and formation of insoluble calcium soaps in the intestinal lumen. Tetany, osteomalacia, and pathological bone fractures may result from calcium malabsorption. Creatinuria, ceroid deposits in tissues, hemolysis, and a myopathy may result from decreased absorption of vitamin E in pancreatitis. Concretions in the duct system and tumor replacement may be causes of pancreatic insufficiency.

In fibrocystic disease of the pancreas (mucoviscidosis) in children, secretions block pancreatic ducts, resulting in progressive pancreatic fibrosis. Inspissated bile causing similar involvement of the bile ducts may lead to bile duct proliferation, periportal fibrosis, biliary cirrhosis, portal hypertension, and hepatic failure. Malabsorption results from decreased release of bile salts. In mucoviscidosis, there is an increase in sweat chloride (> 60 mEq/liter). In the Zollinger-Ellison syndrome (gastrin-secreting pancreatic adenomas), excessive HCl secretion from the stomach is the probable basis of multiple recurrent peptic ulcers. Inactivation of lipase and neutralization of bicarbonate by high levels of HCl result in steatorrhea. The pancreatic adenomas are frequently multiple with a high incidence of malignancy. As complete excision of the tumor is often impossible, the treatment of choice is total gastrectomy.

Micelle Formation Disorders of micelle formation have been described in detail under the discussion of bile salt metabolism.

Clinical Disorders Caused by Errors in Absorption of Lipid into Intestinal Mucosa Adult celiac disease (gluten-induced enteropathy, nontropical sprue, idiopathic steatorrhea) is clinically characterized by weight loss, crampy abdominal pain, and generalized malabsorption of food, vitamins, and water. At least 50% of patients had symptoms in childhood and there are strong indications that this is an inheritable disorder. The incidence of diabetes mellitus is quite high in these patients. The clinical manifestations are precipitated by ingestion of gluten from wheat, barley, buckwheat, rye, and malt; gluten is a water-insoluble peptide which is rich in proline and glutamine. It has been found that this peptide will exacerbate the clinical signs by causing a defect in the absorptive epithelium of the intestinal mucosa and possibly by altering certain aspects of intramucosal metabolism. In this disorder, there are characteristic alterations in the morphology of the wall of the small intestine, including short and blunt villi and a flattened villous tip covered by a pseudostratified cuboidal or squamous epithelium, only a narrow band of columnar epithelial cells being seen. The microvilli are shortened, fewer, and fused. These changes result in a marked decrease in the absorptive area. On histochemical studies, decreased levels of ATPase, esterases, acid phosphatase, and succinic dehydrogenase are found. There are also decreased goblet cells and impaired mucin secretion. Plasma cell and lymphocytic infiltration of the lamina propria are also characteristic.

In addition to malabsorption in this state, there is a massive diarrhea with loss of salt and water. Decreased xylose absorption reflects the mucosal defect. Hypoalbuminemia is caused by both malabsorption and protein-losing enteropathy. Postprandial levels of plasma amino acid (especially glutamine) are increased. Urinary excretion of 5-hydroxyindole acetic acid, indole-3-acetic acid, kynurenic acid, and xanthurenic acid are increased in untreated patients—all reflecting a deficiency of pyridoxin. Several patients also have a disaccharidase deficiency. Complete remission occurs after a few days to weeks on a gluten-free diet. Pyridoxin replacement is necessary, especially in the early treatment phase. A sine qua non for diagnosis of nontropical sprue is villous atrophy on a jejunal biopsy. These changes may also occur in tropical sprue, in congenital hypogammaglobulinemia, in some patients with acquired hypogammaglobulinemia, and in patients with specific deficiency of gamma A. Hypogammaglobulinemia and steatorrhea are found in the presence of nodular hyperplasia of the small intestine. Associated features are low levels of IgA, IgG, and usually IgM, and decreased antibody production with recurrent upper respiratory infections. In some patients with this disorder, splenomegaly, pernicious anemia, carcinoma of the stomach or colon, giardiasis, and pancreatitis may be seen. Villous atrophy with associated malabsorption may occasionally be found in the lymphomas. Occasionally a malabsorption syndrome and steatorrhea are associated with extensive skin diseases: exfoliative dermatitis, erythrodermic psoriasis, dermatitis herpetiformis, and widespread eczema. In these disorders, the gastrointestinal symptoms improve as the skin responds to therapy.

Radiation enteritis is caused by a defect in cell renewal in which the villi are flattened and crypts are shortened and for which there is no specific therapy. Other steatorrhea syndromes caused by defective lipid absorption into the intestinal mucosa include midgut ischemia secondary to mesenteric artery occlusion, amyloidosis, strongyloides stercoralis, hookworm, giardiasis, and neomycin excess. Rapid transit of contents through the small bowel may be associated with steatorrhea in viral and bacterial gastroenteritis, carcinoid, hyperthyroidism, and disaccharidase deficiency.

Clinical Disorders of Intramucosal Metabolism   In adrenocortical insufficiency (Addison's disease), glucocorticoid deficiency results in malabsorption as these hormones are required for the optimal activity of the enzymes involved in triglyceride synthesis in intestinal mucosal cells, viz., microsomal thiokinase, monoglyceride, and diglyceride transacylase. In congenital abetalipoprotenemia (abetalipoproteinemia, acanthocytosis), an autosomal recessive inherited disorder, there is an inability to manufacture the β-globulin (B-protein) of β-lipoprotein and chylomicrons. Clinical features of this disorder evolve within the first 2 years of life as failure to thrive, steatorrhea, diarrhea, and abdominal distension made especially worse by ingestion of lipids. Evidence of involvement of the nervous system becomes apparent at age 5 and above when the patients develop ataxia, intention tremors, athetoid movements, muscle weakness, mystagmus, and absent deep tendon reflexes. Intelligence may be unhindered, but emotional lability may be pronounced. The neurological signs are presumably secondary to extensive demyelimization of the posterior columns, spinocerebellar cortex. Late in the course of the disorder, retinitis pigmentosa may occur in some patients. The erythrocytes exhibit a thorny (spiny) shape (acanthocytosis) and may have an increased tendency to hemolysis, but no anemia. The most striking chemical abnormality is marked decrease of serum lipids, and the most useful screening test for this disorder is the serum cholesterol which is usually less than 90 mg/100 ml, a level seen only in Tangier disease, severe malnutrition, and in some anemias. Serum TG are the lowest reported for any disease, being less than 20 mg/100 ml. The intestinal mucosal cell and the liver are lipid infiltrated because of the inability to discharge the lipids. In these patients postprandial hyperlipemia, which normally follows a fatty meal, does not develop. Diets low in fat will decrease steatorrhea, diarrhea, and abdominal distension, but the resulting caloric deficit may lead to growth retardation. Therapy with MCT (which do not require chylomicron formation) is helpful, but there are as yet no long-term data on improvement of the hematological and neurological problems.

Hypobetalipoproteinemia is seen in severe debilitating illness and in certain malabsorption syndromes. This disorder may be seen in adults, and the basic defect may be similar to that in congenital abetalipoproteinemias.

Disorders of Lipid Transport from Mucosal Cell to Liver and Other Tissues Whipple's disease (intestinal lipodystrophy) is characterized by extreme debility, abdominal pain, diarrhea, steatorrhea, weight loss, arthralgia, increased skin pigmentation, lyphadenopathy, polyserositis, and arthritis. This disorder is most often observed in men between 40 and 60 years. The unique pathological finding in this disorder is presence of lipoprotein containing PAS-positive, sickle-form particles in histiocytes probably representing atypical form of bacteria. These bodies may be found in histiocytes of the intestinal mucosa, liver, pancreas, spleen, lymph nodes, bone marrow, subendocardium, epicardium, lungs, adrenals, and central nervous system. Diagnosis may be made by biopsy of any of these sites, but the most convenient sites are the small intestine and the colon. The histological appearance of the small intestine reveals extensive infiltration at the base of the lamina propria with distorted villi which appear wide and flat. Lipid and other nutrients cannot be transported across this diseased barrier, and a disturbance in fatty acid esterification may also be present. Treatment with 1,200,000 units of penicillin and 1 g of streptomycin daily for 14 days followed by 1 g of tetracyline daily for 1 year is highly successful in this disease. Intestinal lymphagiectasia represents a heterogeneous group of disorders in which there is an obstruction of lymphatic flow resulting in chylous effusion into small bowel. Lipids, iron, copper, and calcium are lost with the gastrointestinal lumen. Lymphopenia is a common feature as chyle contains lymphocytes. Biopsy of the intestinal wall reveals dilated intestinal lymphatics. Causes of lymphatic obstruction include pelvic and retroperitoneal nodes, atresia, hypoplasia, stenosis of the lymphatics, and acquired fibrosis of lymphatics occurring in regional enteritis, lymphoma, carcinoma, intestinal tuberculosis, trauma, and Whipple's disease. Lymphatic obstruction may cause chylous effusions into the pleural space, peritoneal cavity, and genitourinary tract. Hypoalbuminemia observed in this state may cause edema of the extremities. The best diagnostic procedures include peroral intestinal biopsy, the fecal excretion of ^{131}I-polyvinylpyrrolidone (PVP), ^{51}Cr albumin, or ^{131}I-albumin given intravenously, and treatment consists of low fat, high protein diet, and the use of medium-chain triglycerides.

Considerations in Diagnosis of Malabsorption of Lipids

Lipid malabsorption may occur as an isolated phenomenon as well as part of generalized malabsorption of other foodstuffs. For this reason it is essential to undertake procedures to establish the nature and extent of the defect in absorption. These purposes are served by tests ranging in simplicity of 72-hr stool collection for fat and nitrogen contents to the complexity of peroral intestinal biopsy and examination by light or electron microscopy. Tests may be designed to specifically measure the absorption of food constituents based on the unique processes involved in the absorption mechanisms (see Chapter 4, Figure 4.1).

In addition to the otherwise standard studies, such as gastrointestinal x-rays, endoscopy, and serum chemistry data, the following procedures are recommended (4) in the differential diagnosis of malabsorption syndromes: 1) fecal fat determination (72 hr); 2) fecal nitrogen determination (72 hr); 3) xylose absorption test; 4) B_{12} absorption test; and 5) peroral biopsy of small intestinal mucosa.

1. The fecal fat determination is most reliably done on a 72-hr collection. Normal fecal fat is approximately less than 7% of dietary intake. Accordingly, on a typical diet with fat intake of 60–100 g/day, the patient with malabsorption of fat will excrete more than 7 g/24 hr. It should be noted that, even on a fat-free diet, the normal individual excretes approximately

3 g/day because of sloughing of intestinal mucosal cells and a significant amount of bacterial lipids.

2. Fecal nitrogen determination done on a 72-hr collection from a normal subject on a balanced protein diet normally ranges from 2.0–2.5 g/24 hr. A component of this value is undoubtedly from endogenous processes. The test is not reliable in the presence of protein-losing enteropathy.

3. The xylose absorption test is a measure of integrity of the intestinal mucosa, as the carbohydrate substance is absorbed passively in the proximal small intestine. The fasting patient is given 25 g of xylose orally, and a 5-hr urine collection, made during good flow, is obtained. Normal subjects excrete in excess of 4.5 g during this period; patients over the age of 50 years may show a slight decrease in the excretion of this substance. Patients with defective intestinal mucosal cells excrete considerably decreased amounts of this substance during the test time.

Table 3.1. Summary of Clinical Disorders of Intestinal Lipid Metabolism

Cause	Diseases
Insufficient intraluminal pancreatic enzyme activity (malabsorption of fats, CHO, protein)	Chronic pancreatitis, pancreatic carcinoma, cystic fibrosis are characterized by severe steatorrhea with fecal fat >30–40% of intake and severe azotorrhea with >4.2–7.5 g of N/24 hr. Xylose and B_{12} absorption, and small intestinal biopsy normal
Insufficient intraluminal bile acid activity resulting in isolated steatorrhea	Intra- or extrahepatic biliary obstruction with or without jaundice, choledochocolonic fistula, intestinal stasis, multiple strictures, blind loops, diabetic neuropathy, and scleroderma
Intramural small intestinal disease	Gluten enteropathy, tropical sprue, dermatitis herpetiformis, nongranulomatous jejunitis, Whipple's disease, primary and secondary amyloidosis, multiple myeloma, eosinophilic gastroenteritis, food allergy, small bowel ischemia caused by atherosclerosis, polycythemia, vasculitis, Kohlmeier-Degos disease, small bowel resection, jejunectomy, massive resection, or bypass
Defective apoprotein	Abetalipoproteinemia
Lymphatic defects	Intestinal lymphangiectasia, lymphoma

Table 3.2. Major Histological Findings in Small Intestinal Biopsy

I. Biopsy essentially diagnostic of:
  A. Normal: fingerlike normal villous pattern, intact surface epithelium, normal crypts
  B. Gluten enteropathy: villous atrophy, changes in surface epithelium, hypertrophy of crypt epithelium, lamina propria infiltrated with chronic inflammatory cells
  C. Whipple's disease: loss of villous structure, mucosal flattening, infiltration of lamina propria with macrophages with PAS-positive cytoplasmic inclusions. Bacilli-like structures beneath basement membrane and between macrophages
  D. Abetalipoproteinemia: normal villous structure, cytoplasmic droplets positive to fat stains
  E. Amyloidosis: presence of amyloid deposits after staining with Congo red
  F. Mast cell disease: large number of mast cells in lamina propria, muscularis mucosa, and submucosal areas

II. Small intestinal biopsy compatible with:
  A. Radiation enteritis
    1. Acute changes: decreased mitosis in crypt cells, shortening of villi and crypts, and infiltration of lamina propria with plasma cells and neutrophils
    2. Chronic changes: connective tissue proliferation and thickening, loss of submucosal vascularity
  B. Lymphangiectasia: dilation of lacteals and lymphatics in lamina propria distortion of some villi. Villous and crypt epithelium essentially normal. Lymphatics contain lipid-filled macrophages
  C. Tropical sprue: villous atrophy, pleomorphic cells in lamina propria; pleomorphic lymphocytes infiltrate and destroy crypts. Mucosal lymphatics dilated
  D. Nongranulomatous jejunitis: loss and flattening of villi with crypt distortion; infiltration of lamina propria with mononuclear cells. No granulomas
  E. Scleroderma: collagen encapsulation of Brunner's gland; fibrosis and fragmentation of muscularis mucosa
  F. Eosinophilic gastroenteritis: villi and lamina propria diffusely infiltrated with eosinophils
  G. Dermatitis herpetiformis: villous atrophy and inflammatory cell infiltration of submucosa
  H. Hypogammaglobulinemia: absence or flattening of villi, decrease or absence of plasma cells in lamina propria; lymphocytic infiltration of submucosa
  I. Parasitism: varying degrees of attenuation and blunting of villi with cellular infiltration of lamina propria. Specific parasites may be seen in crypts or mucosa

4. The B_{12} - absorption test involves the binding of labeled vitamin B_{12} with intrinsic factor in the stomach, transport of the complex to the absorption sites in the ileum, absorption into the portal circulation, and flushing out of the labeled B_{12} with a parenteral injection of unlabeled B_{12}. Normal individuals excrete 10% or more of the labeled B_{12} in 24 hr. If, on addition of intrinsic factor, the excretion is less than 6%, then a diagnosis of B_{12} malabsorption is confirmed.

5. Peroral small intestinal biopsy is performed by the use of hydraulic and suction biopsy capsules which are inserted into the intestinal lumen through the mouth. The usual biopsy site is the jejunum. Diagnostic patterns may be obtained by microscopic examination of the specimens. Less useful tests in the differential diagnosis of malabsorption include the application of the oral and intravenous GTT, the serum carotene level, and tests for absorption of labeled triolein.

Clinical and laboratory features of several malabsorption disorders are summarized in Table 3.1. Tables 3.2, 3.3, and 3.4 summarize histological findings of intestinal biopsy specimens from several disorders. The clinical and laboratory features of malabsorption syndromes of uncertain etiology are presented in Table 3.5.

LIPID TRANSPORT IN SERUM

Because of their insolubility in plasma, various lipids, whether derived from dietary sources or synthesized endogenously, are transported in plasma bound to various protein (or glycoprotein) structures. These protein-bound lipids, lipoproteins, are complex macromolecules which are visualized as containing an inner core of lipid, primarily TG and cholesterol esters, and an outer coat of protein and PL. The lipid to protein binding is noncovalent, and the looseness permits exchange of lipid among various lipoproteins as well as between serum and tissues. The proteins which serve for lipid transport include albumin for FFA transport, A- and B-apoproteins which are present in lipoproteins, prebetalipoproteins, and β-lipoproteins which serve as the major transport system for specific groups of lipids (8, 9).

Lipids serve at least five biological functions: 1) They provide for energy production via oxidation of lipids. This is the source of at least one-half of the energy for basal metabolism. Lipids serve as a very efficient storage form of energy containing 9 cal/g. These stores are utilized during exercise and in fasting 2) as integral parts of all cellular membranes, 3) as thermal insulation, the heat conductivity of lipids being approximately one-third that of water, 4) as a protective cushion for various organs and the skeletal system, and 5) as important secondary characteristics by the distribution of secondary sexual features.

Lipids required for the above functions are synthesized by various tissues, either in tissues performing the functions, or in cases by other organs. For example, most fatty acids and triglyceride synthesis occur in the liver and adipose tissue, but they may be utilized by other tissues. These compounds are transported as lipoproteins or, in the case of fatty acids, as FA-albumin complexes. It is estimated that two-thirds of the lipids in lipoproteins are phospholipids and cholesterol and are, at least in part, structural. The most important function of serum lipoproteins is transport of cholesterol and TG. The liver supplies most of the endogenous TG, and adipose tissues supply all of the FFA.

Lipoprotein Fractions in Serum

Lipoproteins differ in several physicochemical characteristics and serve different functions. One major property separating these compounds is the relative density; other properties include electrophoretic mobility, flotation properties, and carbohydrate and protein contents. The following classes of lipoproteins are recognized:

1. Chylomicrons are the largest and lightest of the lipoproteins. This fraction contains, by weight, 80–95% TG which is derived from exogenous or dietary sources, 2–5% cholesterol, 3–6% PL, and 1–2% protein. The high content of TG in this form gives the plasma a turbid appearance. If serum or plasma is left standing at 4°C for 12–24 hr, all of the CM float to the top of the tube and form a creamy layer. CM are synthesized in the intestinal mucosal cell and serve as the transport medium for TG to plasma and to tissues of utilization. Normal individuals exhibit a transient chylomicronemia after a fatty meal, but the presence of CM 12–16 hr postprandially is abnormal and is indicative of a defect in the metabolism (degradation) of TG.

2. Very low density lipoproteins (VLDL; prebetalipoprotein) are made up of both A- and B-apoproteins, and function to transport endogenously synthesized glycerides. The metabolic turnover of endogenously synthesized TG is slower than that of exogenous TG (i.e., in CM). This VLDL or prebetalipoprotein fraction contains 55% TG, mainly of endogenous origin, 22% PL, 5% free cholesterol, 8% cholesterol esters, and 10% protein. The turbidity of this fraction remains uniformly distributed throughout the serum sample after storage in the cold. The exclusive source of VLDL is the endoplasmic reticulum of the liver. Ingestion of a high carbohydrate diet (including alcohol) or medium-chained triglycerides is followed by increased levels of VLDL, an example of "carbohydrate induction." The A- and B-apoproteins required for synthesis of this fraction are made from amino acids by the liver; the protein combines with TG to form lipoproteins. After delipidation of VLDL in peripheral tissues by lipoprotein lipase, the apoprotein is reused by the liver.

Table 3.4. Malabsorption Syndromes Secondary to Multiple Defects

Disease	Mechanism of malabsorption defects	Tests
Zollinger-Ellison	Excess gastric acid production denatures pancreatic enzymes, precipitates glycine conjugated bile acids, and causes nonspecific mucosal changes; hence, defects in lipolysis, micellarization, and absorption	Fecal fat $>$ 26% of intake; xylose absorption is slightly decreased; B_{12} absorption is normal
Scleroderma	Decreased intestinal motility with intestinal stasis. Also structural changes in mucosa-increased plasma cells within lamina propria. Other changes in submucosa and muscularis	Fecal fat $>$24% of intake; fecal N is normal; xylose absorption; B_{12} absorption
Ileal dysfunction	Decreased enterohepatic circulation of bile acid (Crohn's disease and ileal resection) leading to decreased jejunal fat absorption. Loss of ileal absorptive capacity also	Fecal fat $>$24% of intake; slight azotorrhea; xylose absorption normal; B_{12} absorption low
Postgastrectomy	Gastrectomy, especially Billroth II with loss of pyloric function and bypass of duodenum leading to decreased pancreatic secretory response to meals. Poor mixing and emulsification. Also rapid intestinal transit decreases absorption time. Also, often there is secondary villous atrophy of intestine	Fecal fat $>$18% of intake; little or no azotorrhea; low B_{12} absorption

| Radiation enteritis | Mucosal injury: villi and crypts shortened. Occasional ulceration, occasional thrombosis. Ileal damage leads to decreased enterohepatic circulation of bile salts | Fecal fat $>35\%$ of intake; azotorrhea >6.5 g/24 hr; xylose and B_{12} absorption decreased |

Malabsorption Syndromes of Uncertain Etiology

Disease	Mechanism of malabsorption defects	Tests
Mast cell disease	Rarely a cause of steatorrhea. Possible mechanisms include increased gastric secretion and increased intestinal motility secondary to histamine and other mast cell products	Fecal fat $>45\%$ of intake; xylose and B_{12} absorption are normal
Hypogammaglobulinemias	Primary form most often associated with steatorrhea. Other forms (dysgammaglobulinemia associated with nodular lymphoid hyperplasia, congenital hypogammaglobulinemia) rarely associated with malabsorption	Fecal fat $>19\%$ of intake; no azotorrhea; xylose absorption slightly low; B_{12} absorption low

Table 3.5. Malabsorption Syndromes of Uncertain Etiology

Disease	Mechanism of malabsorption defects	Tests
Carcinoid syndrome	Rarely a cause of steatorrhea. Perhaps related to actions of 5-OH tryptamine or similar amines. Perhaps also tumor masses or vessel involvement	Fecal fat variable; xylose absorption low; B_{12} absorption?
Diabetes mellitus	Possible causes are gluten enteropathy type changes, pancreatic insufficiency, and autonomic neuropathy; may have hyper- or hypomotility of intestinal tract. Also bacterial overgrowth may play a role. Usually found in insulin-dependent diabetics	Fecal fat >34% of intake; fecal N >5 g/24 hr; xylose and B_{12} absorption usually normal
Thyrotoxicosis	? Increased motility	Occasional steatorrhea
Addison's disease	Decrease in microsomal enzymes thiokinase, mono- and diglyceride transacylase	Occasional steatorrhea
Hypoparathyroidism	Mechanism unknown	Occasional steatorrhea

Parasitic infestations (Strongyloides, Schistosomiasis, Giardiasis, Coccidioidomycosis)	Morphological changes in mucosa, flattening of villi, disorganization of epithelial cells, inflammatory reaction	Moderate steatorrhea; xylose absorption is decreased
Drugs		
Cholestyramine	Binds bile acids, thus decreasing micellarization leading to steatorrhea in doses >12 g/day	Steatorrhea related to dosage
Colchicine	Disturbs epithelial cell function and renewal	Loss of fat, nitrogen, and electrolytes; decreased xylose absorption
Cathartic agents	Mucosal changes	
Neomycin	Changes in villi, ↓ lipolysis, precipitate bile salts	Steatorrhea; ↓xylose absorption

3. Low density lipoproteins (LDL; β-lipoproteins) have a mean density of 1.032 and appear to be derived, at least in part, from the intravascular breakdown of VLDL. This fraction carries about 75% of the cholesterol in serum, most of which is known to be structural, but some of the cholesterol is undoubtedly also transported. The average composition of this LDL fraction is 11% TG, 22% PL, 8% cholesterol, 37% cholesterol esters, 1% FAA, and 21% protein. LDL do not produce turbidity in plasma, even in increased amounts. Esterases, as well as some other enzymes, migrate with this fraction.

4. High density lipoproteins (HDL; α-lipoproteins) float in solutions with densities between 1.063 and 1.21 and will not precipitate with polyanions such as heparin or manganese chloride. The average composition of this HDL fraction is 6% TG, 26% PL, 3% cholesterol, 15% cholesterol esters, and 50% protein. The fatty acid patterns of the lipids carried by α- and β-lipoproteins are similar. This fraction is normal constituent of normal plasma and does not produce turbidity when present in excessive amounts.

5. Very high density lipoproteins (VHDL) with density >1.21 are of glycoprotein structure. The glycoproteins are capable of combining in the liver with lipids to form lipoproteins.

6. Free fatty acids constitute the greatest amount of lipids transported in the plasma; and these compounds are transported bound to albumin. Quantitative studies indicate that 25 g of FAA are transported in this manner every 24 hr. Albumin is normally synthesized by the liver to the extent of 10 g/day, but this capacity can be increased 3- to 5-fold. The biological half-life of serum albumin in normal subjects is about 17 days. Each gram of albumin transports 0.3–1.0 mole of FAA, which are provided by adipose tissues circulating at a concentration of 0.3–0.7 mEq/liter with a biological half-life of 2–3 min. It is estimated that FFA supply 50–90% of the body's total energy requirement in the fasting state. The albumin molecule possesses three types of binding sites for FFA: 2 high binding sites, 5 intermediate binding sites, and 20 low affinity sites. Substances such as bilirubin, salicylates, and sulfonamides may compete for some of these sites and displace FFA. In patients with analbuminemia, a congenital disorder caused by an inability of the liver to synthesize this protein, FFA levels in the serum are markedly decreased. Concomitantly, these show increased levels of cholesterol and PL. Following albumin infusion, the cholesterol and PL levels return to normal.

Clinical Disorders of Lipid Transport in Serum

Disturbances of lipid transport in serum include: hyperlipoproteinemias, which may either be hereditary or acquired secondary to other disease processes, and hypolipoproteinemias, such as congenital abetalipoproteinemia and Tangier disease caused by a decrease in α-lipoproteins.

Hyperlipoproteinemias are clinical disorders which are characterized by increased circulating levels of cholesterol, triglycerides, or both. Diagnosis, therefore, requires the finding of increased levels of serum lipid. It is essential that serum samples are obtained after a 12- to 14-hr fast since TG levels are affected by food, even though cholesterol levels are not markedly affected by time of ingestion of foodstuffs. It is also important that basal studies are not made within 4–8 weeks after a myocardial infarction or other physical trauma, and that the patient should have been on his usual diet for about 2 weeks. Drugs which may affect serum lipoproteins, such as estrogens, steroids, oral contraceptive agents, and others, should be stopped 3–4 weeks before studies are made. Normal values of serum lipids are difficult to assign as these may depend on previous diets, race, geography, and age. Frederickson (8,9) recommends that a serum cholesterol concentration greater than 200 mg/100 ml plus the age in years be considered excessive. A serum triglyceride level greater than 150 mg/100 ml is also considered abnormal. Increased levels of cholesterol and TG should prompt the definitive work-up for identification of the hyperlipoproteinemia. Definitive work-up includes lipoprotein electrophoresis, acrylamide gel electrophoresis, ultracentrifugation, or quantitation of protein in the lipoprotein precipitated from serum. Of these tests, the most readily available to the clinician are paper or cellulose acetate electrophoresis and acrylamide gel electrophoresis. Patterns obtained by these procedures must be interpreted in the context of the cholesterol and TG levels. Six reasonably distinct entities have been described by the National Institutes of Health group (8,9): I, IIa, IIb, III, IV, and V. The features of these types are described in some detail later in this chapter and are also presented in Table 3.6.

It is necessary that all causes of secondary abnormalities in serum lipoproteins be excluded before hereditary or familial etiologies are implicated. By definition "primary hyperlipidemia is hyperlipidemia not clearly attributable to another recognized disease." Secondary causes of hyperlipidemia include hypothyroidism, nephrotic syndrome, obstructive jaundice, dysproteinemias, including multiple myeloma, macroglobulinemia, systemic lupus erythematosus and uncontrolled insulin-dependent diabetes mellitus. These entities are considered in Table 3.7.

Translation of Appearance of
Serum and Lipid Levels into Types of Hyperbetalipoproteinemia

Two relatively simple methods may be employed to determine the types of hyperbetalipoproteinemias. The appearance of the serum after storage at 4°C for 12–24 hr presents the following patterns:

1. A creamy layer on top of the serum with a clear infranatant indicates hyperchylomicronemia without an elevated VLDL (as in type I).

Table 3.6. Primary (Inherited) Hyperlipoproteinemias

	NIH type				
	I	II	III	IV	V
Chylomicrons	xxx				xxx
Beta (LDL S$_f$ 8–20)		xxx	xxx		
Pre-beta (VLDL 20–400)			xxx	xxx	xxx
Synonyms	Fat-induced hyperlipemia with hyperchylomicronemia and lipoprotein lipase deficiency; Burger-Grutz disease	Familial hyperbeta-lipoproteinemia with normal TG (IIa) or with TG (IIb)	Familial hyperbeta-lipoproteinemia with hyperprebetalipoproteinemia; broad β disease	Hyperprebetalipoproteinemia	Familial hyperprebetalipoproteinemia with hyperchylomicronemia
Inheritance	Autosomal recessive; mutant in some	Autosomal dominant	Autosomal recessive (?)	Autosomal dominant	?
Clinical features: Age of onset	Rare <10 years; increased CM in early weeks of life; bouts of severe abdominal pain, hepatosplenomegaly pancreatitis; eruptive xanthomas; lipemia retinalis	Common <30 years; tendinous and tuberous xanthomas; premature coronary, cerebral and peripheral atherosclerosis; IIb may be associated with obesity	Fairly common adulthood; tuberoeruptive and palmar xanthomas; premature atherosclerosis especially of peripheral vessels; worsened by alcohol	Very common adulthood; occasional eruptive xanthomas; no tuberous or tendinous hyperuricemia	Uncommon adulthood; bouts of abdominal pain, pancreatitis, eruptive xanthomas, hepatosplenomegaly, hyperuricemia; nonketotic diabetes mellitus common

Laboratory features:					
Cholesterol	Normal, ↑	↑↑↑	↑↑↑	↑	↑
Triglycerides	↑↑↑	Normal to ↑	↑	↑↑	↑↑↑
Phospholipids	Normal to ↑	↑	↑	Normal	↑
Uric acid	Normal	↑	↑	↑	↑
Glucose tolerance	Normal	Normal	↘	↘	↘
Fat tolerance	Abnormal	Normal	Very abnormal	Normal	Very abnormal
Bone marrow foam cells	+	−	+	+	+
Carbohydrate induction	−	−	+	+	+
Serum appearance	Creamy on top; clear below	Clear	Turbid	Turbid	Creamy on top; turbid below
Major diagnostic criteria	Type I LP pattern; decreased plasma PHLA	Type II LP; type II in a 1° relative or tendon xanthoma; homozygote: type II in both parents	Type III LP pattern in patient and in a 1° relative	Type IV LP pattern and 1 or more 1° relatives with type IV; no close relative with I, III, or V	Type V pattern; type IV or V in one or more parents or adult siblings

Continued

Table 3.6. *Continued*

	NIH type				
	I	II	III	IV	V
Minor criteria	Type 1 pattern in a close relative; bouts of abdominal crises as described before age of 20 years; exclusive of phenocopies	Plasma cholesterol 300–600 in adults with heterozygous form who also have TG 50–500 mg/100 ml; homozygotes have C >500 mg/100 ml and TG 50–500 ml xanthomas before 10 years of age; vascular disease before age 20 years	Planar or tubereruptive xanthomas; labile C and TG levels; type IV in adult 1° relative	At least 1 parent and one-half of siblings should have type IV	Usually each parent or two-thirds of siblings have IV or V; serum C and TG elevated; bouts of abdominal pain, pancreatitis, or family history of diabetes
Differential diagnosis	Dysproteinemias; pancreatitis; diabetes mellitus; hypothyroidism; oral contraceptives	Dietary excess of cholesterol; myxedema; porphyria; multiple myeloma; obstructive jaundice nephrosis	Myxedema; dysproteinemias; Diabetes mellitus	Diabetes mellitus; von Gierke's; Nephrotic syndrome; Werner syndrome; pregnancy	Multiple myeloma; macroglobulinemia; alcoholism; insulin dependent; diabetes mellitus; nephrosis; pancreatitis
Dietary therapy	Low fat 15–30 g; calories not restricted; alcohol not recommended; MCT	Low cholesterol; increased polyunsaturated fat caloric restriction in IIb	Low cholesterol; A.D.A. diet otherwise; calories to maintain ideal weight; limited alcohol	Controlled CHO (40–45% of total calories); moderately restricted cholesterol; calories to maintain ideal weight	Restricted fat (30%) controlled CHO (50%); moderate low cholesterol; calories to maintain ideal weight

Drug therapy				
None required	(1) Cholestyramine: initial dose, 4 g four times daily; maintenance, 4–8 g orally four times daily; excessive dosage may cause streatorrhea; other side effects include constipation, bloating; drug binds warfarin T4, digitalis. (2) D-thyroxine: 1 mg orally daily followed by 4–8 mg orally daily; may cause angina; may be contraindicated in ASHD. (3) Nicotinic acid: decreases LDL synthesis; initial dose, 100 mg orally 3 times daily; maintenance, 1–2 g orally 3 times daily with meals; side effects: flushing pruritis, hyperuricemia, hepatotoxicity	(1) Clofibrate: initial dose, 0.5–1.0 g twice daily orally; maintenance, 1 g orally twice daily; may cause blood dyscrasia, nausea, weight gain, abnormal liver function. (2) Nicotonic acid: decreases LDL synthesis; initial dose, 100 mg orally 3 times daily. (3) D-thyroxine, 1 mg orally daily followed by 4–8 mg orally daily; may cause angina; may be contraindicated in ASHD	(1) Nicotinic acid: decreases LDL synthesis; initial dose, 100 mg orally 3 times daily. (2) Clofibrate: initial dose, 0.5–1.0 g twice daily orally; maintenance, 1 g orally twice daily; may cause blood dyscrasia, nausea, weight gain, abnormal liver function	(1) Nicotinic acid: decreases LDL synthesis; initial dose, 100 mg orally 3 times daily

Table 3.7. Secondary Hyperlipidemias

Condition	Lipid changes			Lipoprotein changes	Mechanism; other features
	Cholesterol	Triglycerides			
Dietary excess of carbohydrate	±	Increased		Increased VLDL (pre-β)	Liver converts carbohydrate into TG; dietary sucrose and fructose especially. Patients with increased TG have abnormal GTT; the normal drop of FFA after glucose is less in these patients
Pregnancy	Increased; as well as increased PL in second trimester	Increased in third trimester		Increased α-lipo-proteins in second trimester. Increased VLDL in third trimester.	Due to estrogen Due to progesterone
Diabetes mellitus	Occasionally increased	In some, increased CM CHO induced TG synthesis Mixed types CM and TG Postacidosis increase in TG		CM increased VLDL increased VLDL and CM measured VLDL increased LDL (β) and VLDL (pre-β)	Due to decreased postheparin lipo-protein lipase activity; fat induced, treated with insulin Carbohydrate induced GTT abnormal; ketosis is rare; severe atherosclerosis; oral hypogly-cemic drugs

Ethanol excess	Increased	Increased VLDL	Ethanol decreases LPL activity
Pancreatitis	Increased	Increased LDL AND VLDL	Compare with Zieve's syndrome
Hypothyroidism	Increased CM in myxedema	Increased CM and LDL	Decreased plasma LPL activity
Nephrosis	Increased	Increased LDL and VLDL; albumin decreased	Increased lipid synthesis and decreased disappearance, increased hepatic synthesis of lipoproteins and decreased albumin synthesis. Note lipoproteins are not excreted through glomerulus
Multiple myeloma and macroglobulinemia	Increased; also increased PL	LDL and VLDL increased	β- or γ-myeloma peaks
Liver disease	Increased C and PL	LDL increased	Cholesterol increase is secondary to PL increase in biliary tract obstruction; tuberous and planar xanthomata

Table 3.8. Translation of Lipid Levels into Hyperlipoproteinemias

Lipid levels	Analysis of findings	Diagnosis	Differential diagnosis
High cholesterol	Consistent with ↗ LDL (hyperbetalipoproteins) II; Hyperbetalipoproteinemia (II); suggests IIa more specifically	IIa	Hypercholesterolemia associated with α-lipoproteins, e.g., after oral contraceptive pills
High cholesterol (TG 150–400 mg/100 ml)	Suggests increased LDL; suggests moderate increase in VLDL	IIb	Type IV (LDL and VLDL)
High cholesterol (TG 400–1,000 mg/100 ml)	Increased LDL; increased VLDL or CM; if CM test is positive, then type V; if negative, possible also to consider III	IV, V if CM+	Alcohol excess and glucose intolerances
High cholesterol (TG >1,000 mg/100 ml)	Increased LDL; increased VLDL or CM; if CM test is positive, with infranate turbid, then diagnosis is V	V	I; may require LP lipase activity to differentiate
Normal cholesterol (high TG)	Increased VLDL	IV	III occasionally

2. A clear serum without a creamy supernatant is consistent with the presence of LDL (as in type II).

3. A turbid infranatant layer suggests the presence of increased triglycerides associated with the VLDL (consistent with types III, IV, and V).

4. A turbid infranatant in the presence of a creamy layer floating on top is consistent with increased VLDL associated TG and CM, respectively (as in type V; see below). It is also possible to employ the levels of cholesterol and triglycerides to translate hyperlipidemia into hyperlipoproteinemias as shown in Table 3.8.

Inherited Hypolipoproteinemias

Congenital β-lipoprotein deficiency is an autosomal recessive disorder associated with a defective formation of triglyceride-β-globulin complexes in the intestinal mucosal cell as a result of which TG accumulation occurs in these cells. There is a defect of the β-apoprotein (apo-LDL) which serves a specific function in lipid, especially TG, transport. Fatty acids are readily absorbed and esterified to TG in the mucosal cell, but, because of a lack in the specific apoprotein, there is no chylomicron formation, and postprandial hyperlipemia does not occur. In patients with this disorder, the tissue fat composition is consistent with only endogenous sources of fat. Linolenic acid (not synthesized in man) is decreased in erythrocytes, intestinal mucosa, liver, and adipose tissue. Adipose tissues are high in palmitoleic acid, suggesting considerable endogenous lipid synthesis from carbohydrate sources. This disorder is characterized by steatorrhea, diarrhea, diffuse nervous system involvement, red cell acanthocytosis, low serum lipids, and absence of β-lipoproteins. The disorder becomes clinically manifest by age 2 years as failure to thrive, steatorrhea, diarrhea, abdominal distension—these symptoms being aggravated by lipid ingestion. About age 5 years, the patient develops an ataxia, intention tremors, athetoid movements, muscle weakness, nystagmus, and, often, absent deep tendon reflexes. Because of muscle weakness, these patients may develop lordosis, kyphosis, and pes cavus. They have normal intelligence but may exhibit emotional lability. Retinitis pigmentosa becomes a prominent finding later. Fatal cardiac arrhythmias have been reported as a cause of death in some of these patients.

Laboratory findings in this disorder include: evidence of autohemolysis and H_2O_2-induced hemolysis, but no marked anemia and a marked malabsorption of fat. Jejunal biopsy reveals a pathognomonic mucosal abnormality with presence of lipid droplets throughout the cytoplasm of the mucosal cells. The most characteristic abnormalities include decreased serum lipid levels, with cholesterol <90 mg/100 ml, and the triglyceride levels are the lowest reported for any disease, i.e., <20 mg/100 ml. Serum levels of vitamin A are low and those of vitamin E are the lowest reported in any disease. This deficit may be a factor in the lability of erythrocytes to peroxide hemolysis. It has also been suggested that the vitamin E deficiency may be causally related to the central nervous system disorder in abetalipoproteinemia.

The goal of therapy in early life is to maintain life and growth in these patients who tolerate fats poorly. The fat tolerance improves with age, but the patient is unable to tolerate more than 10% of the diet as fats at least until adolescence. Medium-chained triglycerides which do not require chylomicron formation are well tolerated. A recent report has suggested that some of the eye changes (retinitis pigmentosa and macular degeneration) may be reversed with vitamin A therapy.

Hypobetalipoproteinemia (familial low density lipoprotein deficiency) is presumably an autosomal dominant disorder characterized by a paucity of overt clinical findings, but with marked decreased levels of cholesterol, 55–146 mg/100 ml in the kindreds described, and TG ranging from 20–140 ng/100 ml. Levels of HDL are normal, but there are significantly low levels of LDL. In one patient, a demyelinating disorder was found after her fourth pregnancy. There are also suggestions of a lipid malabsorption in a few patients. A decreased synthesis of LDL is the probable basis of this disorder. It is well to note that low, but not absent, levels of cholesterol, TG, and lipoprotein may be found in patients with severe malabsorption syndromes and severe debilitating disorders.

Familial high density lipoprotein deficiency (Tangier disease) is a rare disorder that was first discovered in patients on Tangier Island in the Chesapeake Bay. This disorder is now considered to be inherited as an autosomal recessive trait. Two features that are considered pathognomonic of this disorder are a low plasma cholesterol in combination with normal or high TG and enlargement with orange coloration of the tonsils. Most of the patients studied have also exhibited features of a peripheral neuropathy. The HLD (α-lipoprotein) levels are decreased and the antigenic properties of Tangier-HDL differ from normal HDL; Tangier-HDL is also chemically different from HDL in other respects. The clinical manifestations are marked tonsillar enlargement with a distinctive orange coloration, lymphadenopathy and hepatosplenomegaly, and occasional lipid infiltration of the cornea. A peripheral neuropathy is seen in most of the patients. This is presumably caused by a loss of the myelin sheath. A dissociated loss of pain and temperature sensation, coupled with muscle wasting, is also found. The reticuloendothelial system, including the tonsils, have increased levels of lipids, especially esterified cholesterol; cholesterol oleate is found in tissues, and cholesterol linoleate in the plasma. Lipid infiltration in foam cells is seen on rectal mucosa, lymph nodes, and bone marrow. In this disorder, there is no defect in lipid absorption, and

Table 3.9. Clinical and Laboratory Features of Hypolipoproteinemias

Inheritance	Abetalipoproteinemia: autosomal recessive	Hypobetalipoproteinemia: autosomal dominant	Tangier disease: autosomal recessive
Clinical features			
Malabsorption	+	0	0
Retinitis	+	0	0
Neuropathy	+	Rare	+ in most patients
Acanthocytes	+	0	0
Abnormal tonsils and lymphadenopathy	0	0	+
Chemical features			
Plasma			
Cholesterol	Low	Low	Low
Triglyceride	Low	Low or normal	High (few N)
LDL	Absent	Low	Decreased
VLDL	Absent	Normal	Increased
CM	Absent	Normal	N
HDL	N	N	Low and abnormal

chylomicron formation is quite normal. Treatment is usually unnecessary except for the occasional need for tonsillectomy, although hypersplenism may necessitate splenectomy. The significant clinical and laboratory differential features of the hypolipoproteinic disorders are presented in Table 3.9.

CHOLESTEROL METABOLISM

Cholesterol is required for the formation of cell membranes and as substrate for the synthesis of steroid hormones and bile acids (10–12). The eventual sources of cholesterol include the diet, cholesterol from bile and intestinal mucosa, and cholesterol synthesized in the liver, intestinal mucosal cell, and other tissues including the adrenal cortex and arterial wall. In the intestinal lumen (Figure 1.13), dietary cholesterol mixes with cholesterol from the intestinal mucosa and bile and is absorbed from micelles by the intestinal mucosal cell. The process of absorption of dietary cholesterol requires intraluminal hydrolysis by pancreatic cholesterol esterases. It is estimated that less than 0.5 g of dietary cholesterol is absorbed from the diet daily, as this fraction must compete for absorption processes with 1–3 g of cholesterol excreted in bile daily. The absorbed cholesterol as well as locally synthesized cholesterol is re-esterified in the mucosal cell and is released slowly into lymph as chylomicrons. Peak levels of cholesterol in lymph do not occur until 9 hr after a meal, and the serum cholesterol peak takes up to 3 days to occur. Chylomicron cholesterol is taken up mainly by the liver, but may also be taken up by the adrenals, adipose tissue, and intestinal mucosa. In all tissues except the erythrocytes and the nervous system, cholesterol exists approximately 90% in the esterified form. In the adrenal cortex, the bulk of cholesterol is in the form of cholesterol esters. Cholesterol esters are hydrolyzed in the liver by a cytosol cholesterol esterase, with the esters containing unsaturated fatty acids being more rapidly hydroylzed than those with saturated FA.

The circulating cholesterol pool in man is estimated to be 10–12 g, with between 0.7 and 1.2 g being synthesized daily. Circulating cholesterol is transported mainly with the low density lipoproteins (LDL; β-lipoproteins) and there is relatively free exchange of cholesterol between the various lipoprotein fractions. The formation of cholesterol esters is dependent on the presence and activity of the enzyme plasma lecithin cholesterol acyltransferase. This enzyme is produced in the liver for action in the circulating plasma. The reaction requires the presence of lecithin which provides an unsaturated fatty acid to replace the hydroxyl group of cholesterol.

Endogenous Cholesterologenesis

Although several tissues are capable of synthesizing cholesterol, only the liver and intestinal mucosa contribute significantly to the total circulating pool of cholesterol. The steps involved in cholesterol synthesis have been established in considerable detail. The eventual source of endogenous synthesis is the acetyl-CoA pool. It is estimated that two-thirds of the carbons from carbohydrate and glycerol, one-half of carbons from amino acids, and all of the carbons from FA end up in the acetyl-CoA pool. The steps in the synthesis of cholesterol are presented in Chapter 1, Figure 1.12. It is shown that the initial reductive steps by which HMG-CoA is formed from three acetyl-CoAs require microsomal enzymes. This intermediate has an alternative fate, the formation of ketone bodies, in the presence of mitochondrial enzymes. The formation of mevalonic acid is the first step unique to cholesterologenesis. This reduction reaction (HMG-CoA reductase) is essentially irreversible and is the rate-controlling step in cholesterologenesis. Cholesterol is either degraded for bile formation or may be used for both certain biosynthetic reactions, e.g., steroid hormone synthesis. Both the synthetic and the degradative pathways are subject to feedback regulatory mechanisms.

Regulation of Cholesterologenesis in Liver and Intestinal Mucosa

Several studies have shown that there is an inverse relationship between dietary cholesterol and its synthesis in the liver. Excess dietary cholesterol suppresses HMG-CoA reductase. Bile acids have a major role as a secondary suppressor of cholesterol synthesis in the liver as well as in the intestinal cell, but it is not known whether this is a primary action or if it is dependent on the role of bile acids in cholesterol micellarization and absorption. Factors which produce an expanded bile acid pool cause an inhibition of cholesterol synthesis. In most species except the rabbit, absorbed cholesterol in excess of the amount synthesized by the liver is disposed of by the pathway of increased bile acid formation. In the rabbit, the excess cholesterol may enter the miscible pool of cholesterol. It is also known that decreased bile acids in the intestinal lumen result in an acceleration of both cholesterol and bile acid formation.

Diseases Associated with Altered Cholesterol Metabolism

Atherosclerosis is characterized by a focal thickening of the arterial endothelium with a variable amount of internal and subintimal deposit of lipids, mainly cholesterol and phospholipids. There is a fragmentation of the internal elastic membrane, connective tissue proliferation, followed by fibrosis of the media and intima. Occasionally, inflammation or necrosis may occur, leading to narrowing or occlusion of the arterial lumen. Local physical factors are undoubtedly involved in this process, as atheromas do not usually occur in areas of turbulent flow.

The pathogenesis of this process is not clear, but common denominators which may be of pathogenetic significance are: increased serum cholesterol levels, alteration in the ratio of cholesterol levels being carried in the α- and β-lipoproteins, with an increased amount being carried as β-lipoprotein, an increase in the glycine to taurine ratio in conjugated bile salts, and a smaller content of arachidonic acid conjugated to cholesterol. The participation of abnormal arterial intimal synthesis of cholesterol is also to be considered. Complications of atherosclerosis (AS) include coronary AS (which may progress to angina pectoris), myocardial infarction and congestive heart failure, cerebral atherosclerosis (which may lead to cerebrovascular insufficiency), cerebrovascular insufficiency, cerebrovascular thrombosis and/or hemorrhage, peripheral atherosclerosis (which may lead to impotence, claudication, and gangrene of extremities), and renal atherosclerosis (which may predispose to hypertension and renal failure). Xanthomas may appear on the upper and lower eyelids and in the corners of the eyes; xanthelasmas are associated with hypercholesterolemia. Xanthomas without lipemia may occur in a disorder where primary proliferation of the reticuloendothelial cells in the skin occurs with secondary cholesterol deposition leading to papular lesions resembling xanthomas localized to flexural and intertriginous surfaces, and to mucous membranes, despite normal serum lipids. The term xanthoma disseminatum has been used to describe this disorder which has been compared to histiocytosis X of Hand-Schuller-Christian type.

A recessively inherited lipid storage disorder with multiple tuberous and tendinous xanthomata in the presence of normal serum lipids has been described. Patients with the disorder cerebrotendinous xanthomatosis exhibit xanthomas in the tendons and in white matter of the brain, despite the presence of normal serum cholesterol levels. The disorder is an autosomal recessive characteristic with features of spasticity, ataxia, mental retardation, and cataracts ascribed to accumulation of cholesterol and dihydrocholesterol. No definitive treatment is known, and patients may survive to 6th decade with progressive disability. Cholesterol ester storage disease is a rare familial disorder in which large amounts of cholesteryl esters accumulate in the lamina propria of the intestine and in the liver. The patients have marked hepatomegaly, but liver functions are overtly normal. The patients are essentially asymptomatic. The disorder is diagnosed by the detection of excess cholesteryl esters in the liver, and there is no known treatment for it.

FATTY ACID SYNTHESIS AND DEGRADATION

These processes have been considered in Figures 1.9 and 1.10 (Chapter 1). Synthesis of FA occurs in the cell sap, microsomes, and mitochondria. Most de novo synthesis occurs in cell sap, requiring NADPH yielding palmitic acid as the final product. Two major processes are involved in this synthesis. Acetyl-CoA is carboxylated to malonyl-CoA by acetyl-CoA carboxylase and the fatty acid synthetase complex catalyzes the incorporation of 7 moles of malonyl-CoA and 1 of acetyl-CoA into 1 palmitic acid; the free carboxyl group of malonyl-CoA goes off as CO_2. The acetyl-CoA carboxylase requires ATP and is rate limiting for FA synthesis in cell sap. This enzyme, which is decreased in starvation and diabetes mellitus, is a biotin-containing enzyme and is inactivated by avidin. The enzyme is activated by tricarboxylic and cycle intermediates, especially citric acid. Subsequent steps involve the repetitive addition of two carbon fragments from malonyl S-acyl carrier protein. NADPH (obtained from pentose phosphate pathway and from isocitric dehydrogenase reaction) is required in the above steps. Mitochondrial and microsomal elements of the cells lengthen FA by addition of two carbon fragments, but not from de novo synthesis (13–15).

Fatty acid oxidation involves the β oxidation cycle which consists of four repetitive reactions, viz., acyl-CoA dehydrogenase, enoyl-CoA hydrase, β-OH acyl-CoA dehydrase, and β-ketoacyl-CoA thiolase. Each turn of the cycle produces one acetyl-CoA and one FA acyl-CoA which is 2 carbons less than the original. A preliminary reaction is "activation" of acyl group, i.e., thiokinase reaction which results in the formation of fatty acid acyl-CoA. This reaction requires Mg^{++}. FA oxidation occurs in mitochondria and is dependent on tricarboxylic acid intermediates; the ATP required for the thiokinase reaction is generated by the tricarboxylic acid cycle. Coenzyme A needed for this reaction is provided by condensation of acetyl-CoA with oxalacetic acid to yield citric acid and coenzyme A, and from the thiolase reaction whereby 2 acetyl-CoA molecules react to form acetoacetyl-CoA with the release of coenzyme A. α-Ketoglutarate can stimulate fatty acid oxidation even in the absence of ATP because GTP is derived from oxidation of α-ketoglutarate. Fatty acids are ultimately oxidized to H_2O and CO_2. In the fasting state, fatty acids account for 60% of energy production through their linkage to the electron transfer chain via flavin adenine dinucleotide (FAD) whereby 2 ATPs are produced. NADH is generated either by oxidation of β-OH, acetyl-CoA esters, or by oxidation of tricarboxylic acid cycle intermediates when acetyl-CoA condenses with oxalacetate to enter the tricarboxylic acid cycle, resulting in the formation of 3 ATPs. Oxidation of long-chained fatty acids and acetate is markedly stimulated by carnitine, but the oxidation of medium-chained triglycerides is little affected. A total of 23 molecules of O_2 are utilized, and 131 molecules of high energy phosphate bonds are formed during the complete oxidation of 1 molecule of palmityl-CoA to CO_2 and water. Approximately 700,000–1,000,000 g cal of energy result from this oxidation. The reaction is estimated to be between 29 and 42% efficient, as the calculated ideal energy production from this step is 2,400,000 g cal.

Diseases Affecting Fatty Acid Metabolism

In diabetes mellitus a decreased insulin effect leads to decreased carbohydrate utilization, and the most serious consequences in this disorder are related to changes in fatty acid metabolism. Because of the decreased carbohydrate utilization, there is increased dependence on fatty acid oxidation. To accommodate this need, the fatty acids are mobilized from adipose tissues, and their rapid oxidation leads to ketoacidosis. FA synthesis is depressed and the CoA is channeled to synthesis of cholesterol, leading eventually to degenerative changes. Insulin promotes the esterification of FA in adipose tissues, this requiring L-α-glycerophosphate which comes from the oxidation of carbohydrate. Hence, in insulin lack, there is mobilization of FA as well as decreased re-esterification of FA; accumulating FA and ketone bodies further antagonize insulin action. Insulin lack also causes a defect in fatty acid desaturation, probably through a defect in the oxygenase system; hence, synthesis of unsaturated FA ceases. A marked decrease in the hexose monophosphate shunt leads to decreased NADPH release. This limits the de novo synthesis of FA. A lack of phosphorylated sugars may contribute to the lack of FA synthesis via the malonyl-CoA pathway, as these phosphorylated sugars (especially G-6-P, G-1-P, F-1,6-P_2, and α-glycerophosphate) increase this pathway. Another disorder of fatty acid metabolism is diphtheria in which diphtheria toxin causes a decrease in myocardial carnitine levels. This leads to decrease in palmityl carnitine and palmitic acid synthesis and an accumulation of TG in the heart.

TRIGLYCERIDE METABOLISM

Triglyceride synthesis requires the successive addition of acyl moieties from 2 moles of acyl-CoA to L-α-glycerophosphate to form phosphatidic acid which is dephosphorylated to form 1,2-diglyceride. The addition of one additional acyl-CoA results in formation of TG. Sources of acyl-CoA may be dietary, the mobilization of FFA from adipose tissue, or de novo synthesis, most of which occurs in adipose tissue and liver. The steps in the oxidation include hydrolysis with FA release. The released FA enter the β

oxidation spiral leading to the formation of acetyl-CoA and acetoacetyl-CoA. The released glycerol can be phosphorylated by glycerol kinase and ATP in liver to form L-α-glycerophosphate which is reutilized. As glycerol kinase is missing from white adipose tissue, the glycerol released in this organ is transported to other tissues to be oxidized or to be phosphorylated.

Disorders of Triglyceride Metabolism: Fatty Infiltration of Liver

Normal liver contains 4% lipid of which one-fifth is TG. In man, fatty infiltration of liver (Figure 3.5) is seen in systemic disease, following ingestion of drugs and toxins, and in primary liver disease, and the moiety that increases in the TG fraction. The most common cause of fatty

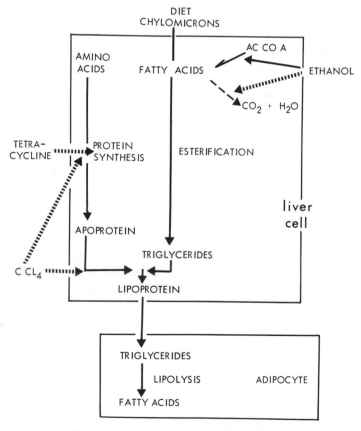

Figure 3.5. Fatty infiltration of the liver. The factors involved in the process include the amount of FA presented to the liver from the adipocyte or from depot stores, the rate of re-esterification, the rate of synthesis of fatty acids and TG, rate of oxidation of FA and TG, the synthesis of apoprotein in the liver, and the coupling of TG to apoprotein in the liver. Effects of drugs and chemicals are also presented.

infiltration of the liver is ethanolism, and the disorders most commonly misdiagnosed as fatty metamorphosis are Laennec's cirrhosis, neoplasm, granulomatous involvement, biliary tract disease, and viral hepatitis (15–16). Liver function tests are not extremely useful in the differential diagnosis. In one series, 65% had abnormal BSP, 40% elevated serum glutamic oxalacetic transaminase (never above 300), 36% showed hyperbilirubinemia (up to 20 mg/100 ml), 30% showed increased alkaline phosphatase, 10% had abnormal cephalic flocculation, and 7% had positive thymol turbidity tests. Fatty infiltration may be insidious or rapid, and the systemic complaints are nonspecific. Hepatomegaly is found, and liver is tender especially when the onset is rapid. Splenomegaly, occasional ascites and edema, as well as portal hypertension and esophageal varices, may occur. Fat embolism occasionally occurs and accounts for sudden death in alcoholics with fatty metamorphosis. Anemia, hypoalbuminemia, and various hyperlipidemias may also be found. Other causes of fatty metamorphosis of the liver include conditions associated with increased mobilization of FA, such as that following the infusion of catecholamines. Hypoglycemia may lead to mobilization of FA from adipose tissue and may be a factor in the pathogenesis of fatty metamorphosis. A similar process has been reported following exposure to cold temperatures. Increased hepatic uptake of FA mobilized from other organs undoubtedly plays a role in the pathogenesis of this disorder. The fatty metamorphosis of the liver found in obese patients may also be a result of increased hepatic uptake of FA.

Kwashiorkor is a cause of hepatic fatty infiltration in which the presumed mechanism involves decreased apoprotein synthesis due to amino acid deficiency in these patients. Tetracycline, even in therapeutic doses, has been observed to be followed by fatty infiltration of the liver. This is especially true in pregnant patients who receive the antibiotic. The mechanism of this complication probably involves the inhibition of apoprotein synthesis in the liver. Carbon tetrachloride and other chlorinated hydrocarbons may induce fatty infiltration of the liver by suppression of apoprotein synthesis as well as by a decrease in the ability of endoplasmic reticulum to couple TG with apoprotein. It has been suggested that this defect is due to a peroxidation of the membrane lipids. The fatty infiltration of the liver seen in phosphorus poisoning is ascribed to defective apoprotein synthesis.

PHOSPHOLIPID METABOLISM

Phospholipids (or, more correctly, phosphatides) are derivatives of phosphatidic acids in which phosphate is in a diester linkage with a second alcohol. These compounds are present in all cells, usually as components

Table 3.10. Classification of Phosphatides and Glycolipids

Name	Main alcohol component	Other alcohol components	P:N Ratio
Glycerophosphates			
Phosphatidic acids	Diglyceride (glycerol diester)		1:0
Lecithins	Diglyceride (glycerol diester)	Choline	1:1
Cephalins	Diglyceride (glycerol diester)	Ethanolamine, serine	1:1
Inositides	Diglyceride (glycerol diester)	Inositol	1:0
Plasmalogens (acetal phosphatides)	Diglyceride (glycerol diester)	Ethanolamine, choline	1:1
Sphingolipids			
Sphingomyelins	N-acetyl sphingosine	Choline	1:2
Cerebrosides	N-acetyl sphingosine	Galactose[a], glucose	0:1
Sulfatides	N-acetyl sphingosine	Galactose[a]	(1 H_2SO_4)
Gangliosides	N-acetyl sphingosine	Hexoses[a]; hexosamine; neuraminic acid	No P

[a] Not present as phosphoric acid esters, but present in glycosidic linkages; these substances = glycolipids.

of cell membranes and nerve tissue in particularly high levels. Two general classes are recognized (see Table 3.10) (17): glycerophosphatides and sphingolipids.

Glycerophosphatides

The fundamental component to this group of compounds is L-α-glycerophosphate, which arises from enzymatic reduction of dihydroxyacetone phosphate (glycolytic pathway). The sequential addition of two acyl-CoA moieties to the L-α-glycerophosphate yields phosphatidic acid; the enzyme phosphatidic acid phosphatase removes the phosphate group with the resultant formation of 1,2-diglyceride.

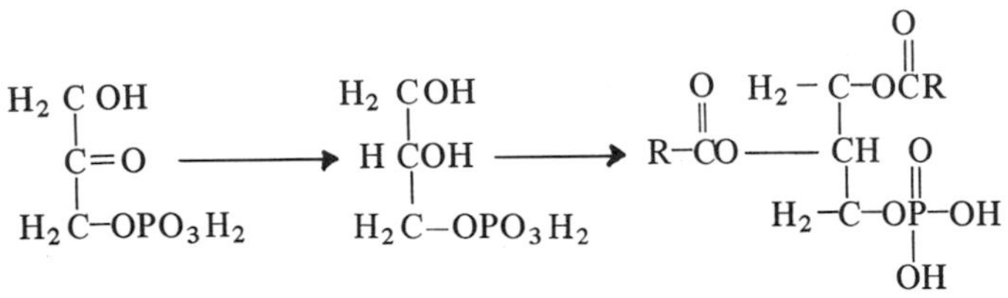

$$
\begin{array}{ccc}
\mathrm{H_2\,C\,OH} & \mathrm{H_2\,COH} & \mathrm{O \quad H_2-\overset{\displaystyle O}{\overset{\|}{C}}-OCR} \\
\mathrm{C=O} \longrightarrow & \mathrm{H\,COH} \longrightarrow & \mathrm{R-\overset{\|}{C}O -\!\!-\!\!- CH \quad O} \\
\mathrm{H_2C-OPO_3H_2} & \mathrm{H_2C-OPO_3H_2} & \mathrm{H_2-C-O\overset{\|}{P}-OH} \\
& & \mathrm{OH}
\end{array}
$$

The second acidic group of phosphoric acid may be esterified with amino alcohols, e.g., choline, to form lecithin (as presented in Table 3.1). Cytidine diphosphate derivatives are prominently involved in the pathways of these compounds, e.g., in the synthesis of:

(a) lecithins:

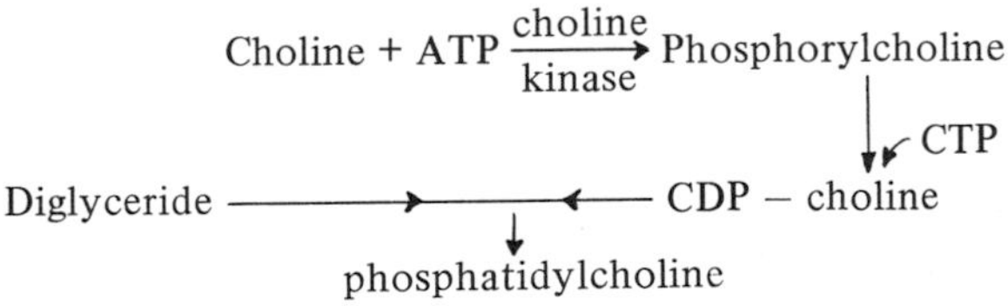

$$
\text{Choline + ATP} \xrightarrow[\text{kinase}]{\text{choline}} \text{Phosphorylcholine}
$$

$$
\text{Diglyceride} \longrightarrow \xleftarrow{} \text{CDP} - \text{choline} \;\big\downarrow\; \text{CTP}
$$

$$
\downarrow
$$

$$
\text{phosphatidylcholine}
$$

(b) cephalins, e.g.,

$$
\alpha,\beta\text{-Diglyceride + CDP-ethanolamine} \xrightarrow{\text{transferase}} \text{phosphatidylethanolamine}
$$

and (c) inositol phosphatides (inositides), which contain inositol, a cyclic hexahydroxy alcohol instead of a nitrogenous alcohol. A general scheme of phospholipid synthesis is given in Figure 3.6.

   Phospholipid (Phosphatide) Degradation These compounds are degraded by four major classes of phosphatidases as follows:

Phosphatidase B ~~~~~~~
$$H_2-C-O\!\!-\!\!C\ R \quad O$$

$$R-C \!\!-\!\! O-CH \!\!-\!\! O$$

Phosphatidase A ─ ─ ─ ─ ─ ─ $H_2\,C-O\!\!-\!\!P\!\!-\!\!O-$Choline

OH

Phosphatidase D ─ ─ ─ ─ ─ ─ ─ ─ ─ Phosphatidase C

A and *B* hydrolyze acyl groups at 1,2. *B* removes remaining fatty acyl groups. *D* attacks ester linkage between glycerol and phosphate, yielding 1,2-diglyceride. *C* liberates the base, and phosphatidic acid is thus formed. Phosphatidase A is found in venoms of snakes and bees and the end products released are lysolecithins which hemolyze erythrocytes. Phosphatidases A and B are present in the pancreas and other organs. Both phosphatidase C (from plants) and D (from *Clostridium tetani*) are phosphodiesterases.

Clinical Disorders of Glycerophosphatide Metabolism   Familial plasma lecithin cholesterol acyltransferase deficiency (plasma cholesteryl ester deficiency) is a clinical disorder described in seven members of three Scandinavian families (18). The disorder is transmitted presumably as an

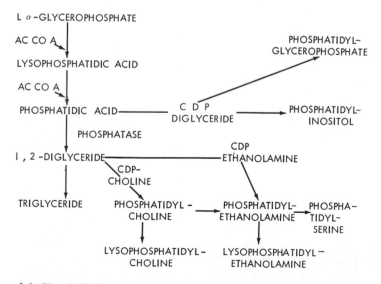

Figure 3.6. Phospholipid synthesis.

autosomal recessive defect characterized by renal, ocular, and hematological abnormalities. The clinical features include the presence of corneal
opacities which are discovered at puberty. The opacities are composed of
minute dots in the parenchyma, concentrated in the periphery giving the
appearance of arcus cornealis. An anemia which is evident at the end of
the 2nd decade is characterized by the presence of target cells in the
peripheral blood. High lecithin and free cholesterol levels are presumably
responsible for the presence of target cells. Hemolysis and decreased
erythropoiesis have also been found, and bone marrow aspirates show the
presence of foam cells. Proteinuria, microscopic hematuria, and the presence of hyaline casts have been described. One patient eventually died of
renal insufficiency, and, on autopsy, the glomerular tufts revealed the
presence of foam cells. The striking laboratory features are decreased
plasma cholesteryl esters and lysolecithin and increased levels of free
cholesterol and lecithin. Plasma pre-β-lipoproteins are absent and the
VLDL have been shown to migrate in the B-region. Hyperlipemia and
hyperglyceridemia are marked, and alterations in the migration properties
of other lipoproteins have been described. A high false positive ASO
(anti-streptolysin O) titer has been described when sheep red cells are used.
The metabolic defect in this disorder is ascribed to decreased hepatic
synthesis of the enzyme lecithin cholesterol acyltransferase. Treatment
with transfusions of plasma or concentrates of the enzyme promises to be
effective.

Biliary tract diseases may induce changes in glycerophosphatide metabolism. In biliary obstruction, there are increased levels of LDL with altered
immunological characteristics, increased levels of phospholipids (especially
lecithins), and increased levels of serum cholesterol. The detailed mechanisms for the above findings are not yet clear. Primary biliary cirrhosis is
a disease of unknown etiology which predominates in the adult female. It
is characterized by severe pruritus, darkening of the skin due to icterus and
increased melanin formation, hepatosplenomegaly and portal hypertension, and the presence of palmar, tuberous, and tendinous xanthomas. The
laboratory features include marked elevations of serum phospholipids
(400–1,700 mg/100 ml) and cholesterol (1,200–1,500 mg/100 ml), a large
proportion of which is unesterified, and the virtual absence of α-lipopro-
teins. Serum TG are often elevated, but the serum is never lipemic because
of the detergent action of PL. Late in the course of the disease the serum
lipids may decrease markedly, reflecting severe liver disease and its eventual inability to synthesize LP. Operative cholangiography is mandatory to
distinguish primary biliary cirrhosis from secondary biliary cirrhosis. There
is no specific treatment available for this disorder, but mercaptopurine
may retard progression, or, rarely, induce a remission. Severe pruritus may
be controlled by the use of cholestyramine therapy.

Sphingolipid Metabolism

This type of phospholipid differs from glycerophosphatides in the replacement of glycerol by the amino dialcohol sphingosine (17, 19, 20). The sphingolipids are found in membranous tissues throughout the body. A structure shared in common by these compounds is ceramide, which consists of sphingosine to which a long-chained fatty acid is linked through an amide bond on carbon 2 of sphingosine. The length of the fatty acid moiety varies with the type of sphingolipid.

$$H_3C-(CH_2)_{12}-CH=CH-\underset{\underset{OH}{|}}{CH}-\underset{\underset{NH_2}{|}}{CH}-CH_2OH$$

Sphingosine

$$H_2C-(CH_2)_{12}-CH=CH-\underset{\underset{OH}{|}}{CH}-\underset{\underset{\underset{\underset{\underset{CH_3}{|}}{(CH_2)\,16-22}}{|}}{\underset{\underset{C=O}{|}}{NH}}}{CH}-CH-CH_2OH$$

N-Acyl sphingosine (ceramide)

In subsequent discussions, the structure ceramide will be depicted by the symbol employed by others (20) (Figure 3.7). This structural unit ceramide is present in all mammalian sphingolipids, individual types being distinguished by the moiety esterified to the C-1 position of ceramide. For example: 1) in sphingomyelins, the moiety esterified to C-1 is phosphorylcholine; 2) in neutral glycosphingolipids, it is a mono- or oligosaccharide; 3) in galactocerebroside, the substituent is galactose; 4) in sulfatide, the substituent is galactose-3-sulfate; and 5) in gangliosides, the substituent is an oligosaccharide containing a sialic acid. An example of the synthetic pathway for a sphingolipid is depicted in Figure 3.7.

The metabolism of the various types of sphingolipids and clinical disorders associated with them are discussed under the general headings listed below. Sphingomyelin is the phosphorylcholine ester of N-acyl sphingosine (ceramide). The sphingosine base present in sphingomyelins from animal tissues and plasma is mainly the C-18 monounsaturated base (2-amino-4-octadecene-1,3-diol). Sphingomyelins in cytoplasm and plasma contain fatty acids of C-16 to C-18 length. In cell membranes there is a higher proportion of longer chain acids such as C-24. The fatty acid chain length of sphingomyelins of brain may vary with location and with aging; those in gray matter have a higher portion of C-16 to C-18 lengths compared with those in white matter with longer chain length. The

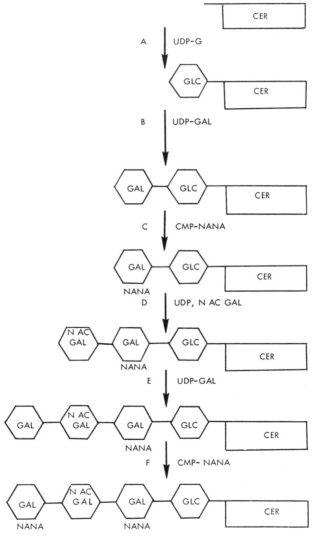

Figure 3.7. Sphingolipid synthesis. The synthesis of a prototype sphingolipid is depicted. *Enzymes A, B,* and *E* are transferases, e.g., *B* is glycolipid galactosyltransferase. *Enzymes C* and *F* are sialyltransferases, and *enzyme D* is glycolipid *N*-acetylgalactosamine transferase. End product inhibition of these enzymes involves binding of the metal ions required for enzyme activity.

neonatal brain contains little myelin, and, as myelination proceeds, the proportion of C-24:1 acids in sphingomyelin rises markedly while that of C-16 to C-18 falls. Sphingomyelins make up 5–25% of total lipid phosphatides, the content in specific tissues varying with species and age. In the liver, sphingomyelin accounts for less than 10% of lipid phosphorus, while, in plasma, sphingomyelin constitutes about 20% of total phospholipids. This group of compounds is especially useful in solubilization of TG.

Sphingomyelin Biosynthesis and Degradation Two pathways of sphingomyelin synthesis have been studied in liver and brain tissues; the relative importance of these two reactions has not been ascertained. In one synthesis, CDP-choline reacts with ceramide to form CMP and sphingomyelin. The alternative synthesis is essentially a two-step reaction, in the first of which sphingosine and CMP choline form sphingosylphosphorylcholine and CMP. In the second reaction, sphingosylphosphorylcholine and a fatty acyl-CoA form sphingosine. The initial step in the degradation of sphingomyelin is the hydrolytic cleavage by the enzyme sphingomyelinase (phosphatidylcholine choline phosphohydrolase) to phosphorylcholine and ceramide. The enzyme is located mainly in the lysosomes in liver and kidney, with some activity in mitochondria; intestinal mucosa and arterial wall also possess sphingomyelinase activity.

Clinical Disorders of Sphingomyelin Metabolism These disorders (21) are represented by the spectrum of disorders known as Niemann-Pick disease, which is characterized by the accumulation of sphingomyelin throughout the body. The patients are noted to have marked hepatomegaly with some splenomegaly, associated with severe central nervous system damage. A yellowish olive coloration of the skin is often noted, and, in 30% of the patients, a cherry-red spot is seen in the macular region of the eye. The disorder is inherited as an autosomal recessive characteristic which is found in various ethnic groups (with the largest number being found in patients of Jewish ancestry). In the type A (acute neuronopathic form, sphingomyelinase-deficient), the patients show a generalized loss of motor and intellectual functions by age 12 months. Behavior is unlearned, hepatosplenomegaly is noted by age 6 months, and death occurs by 4 years of age. In the type B (chronic form without central nervous system involvement, sphingomyelinase-deficient), the visceral signs seen in type A are present. Type C disorder (subacute form with questionably deficient enzyme) is characterized by a more prolonged course than type A, with the child normal up to age 1–2 years, at which time the neurological abnormalities start. The patients with this disease die in childhood or adolescence. Two forms, the Nova Scotia variant and an indeterminate adult form, have been described, but have not been clearly delineated.

Pathophysiology of Sphingomyelin Lipidosis (Niemann-Pick Disease) The reticuloendothelial cells in the liver, spleen, and bone marrow are enlarged with sphingomyelin which gives a waxy birefringence to the cells, which have a foamy appearance. The major source of sphingomyelin is the stroma of erythrocytes, the major components of erythrocyte stroma being sphingomyelin, lecithin, and phosphatidylethanolamine. However, since sphingomyelin is also known to be the major lipid in subcellular elements and in the plasma membrane of cells, it is likely that cellular destruction in other tissues may contribute to the total pool of undegraded sphingomyelin. There is a decreased degradation of this compound in Niemann-Pick disease secondary to diminished levels of sphingomyelinase; the synthesis of sphingomyelin is not increased. Laboratory studies in patients with this disorder reveal increased sphingomyelin content in several tissues, especially liver, and decreased sphingomyelinase activity in liver, spleen, kidney, leukocytes, and skin tissue culture plants. No specific treatment is yet available for this disorder, but Brady (19) suggests the feasibility of liver transplant to provide the missing enzyme.

Clinical Disorders of Neutral Glycosphingolipids Neutral glycosphingolipids include the glucocerebrosides and lactosylcerebrosides which are probably derived from the degradation of globoside, the major glycolipid from erythrocyte stroma. Globoside is degraded by a series of reactions resulting in the sequential release of 4 hexose molecules (Figure 3.8) by lysosomal catabolic enzymes. Defects in the various degradative steps caused by deficient or absent hydrolytic enzymes are characterized by reasonably distinct clinical and chemical patterns (19, 20, 22).

Gaucher's disease refers to a disorder in the degradation of glucocerebroside (or glucosylceramide) secondary to deficient activity of the enzyme β-glucosidase which catalyzes the cleavage of glucosyl from glucosylceramide. Excess Glc-Cer accumulates and is picked up by reticuloendothelial cells of the spleen, liver, and lymph nodes resulting in enlargement of these organs. The disease is a relatively common familial disorder which is characterized by accumulation of glucocerebroside (Glc-ceramide) in reticuloendothelial cells of various tissues, including the liver, spleen, and lymph nodes, as well as in bone. The disorder is manifested in three forms, viz., type I, chronic non-neuronopathic (adult Gaucher's disease); type II, acute neuronopathic Gaucher's disease; and type III, subacute neuronopathic (juvenile) Gaucher's disease which become manifest from birth to old age. Hematological abnormalities secondary to hypersplenism, including anemia, thrombocytopenia, and a brownish yellow discoloration of the skin which is darker on exposed surfaces, are major clinical findings. Erosion of the cortices of the long bones and pelvis may be the basis of the presenting complaint of bone pain or of a pathological fracture. The clinical evolution is quite variable, with some patients dying at an early age

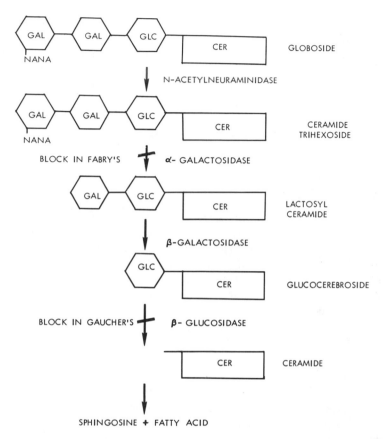

Figure 3.8. Degradation of neutral sphingolipids. Note the stepwise degradation by various enzymes. Sites of enzymatic defects in Fabry's disease and Gaucher's disease are identified.

because of bleeding secondary to thrombocytopenia while others may have a benign indolent course.

Acute neuronopathic Gaucher's disease is also called infantile malignant or cerebral Gaucher's disease and is characterized by a severe central nervous system disorder. The clinical features become apparent before 6 months of age, and the process is rapidly progressive. It is associated with cranial nerve and extrapyramidal involvement, including strabismus, muscular hypertonicity or spasticity, rigidity of the neck, trismus, dysphagia, and laryngeal stridor. Increased deep tendon reflexes, with positive Babinski, and seizures may occasionally occur, and a type of mental retardation may supervene preterminally. Splenomegaly, hepatomegaly, and bony lesions described under type 1 also occur, and the rapid progression of the disorder usually culminates in death within 1 month to 2 years. Subacute neuronopathic (juvenile) Gaucher's disease evolves in several respects similarly to type 2, but the course is more protracted with death occurring well after 2 years. Death in infancy or in the 3rd decade has been reported. In this disorder, the central nervous system manifestations appear later than in type 2. In the above forms of Gaucher's disease, pingeculae may be found, but the macular cherry-red spot found in some other sphingolipidoses is absent.

The underlying disorder in Gaucher's disease is a deficient β-glucosidase activity resulting in an accumulation of glucocerebroside (Glc-Cer) in various tissues rich in reticuloendothelial cells. Secondary lysosomes sequester the Glc-Cer, and the accumulation of Glc-Cer in lysosomes and similar cells gives the characteristic appearance of the Gaucher cell which may appear in "sheets" in the spleen and bone marrow. Kuppfer cells in the liver may also assume the characteristics of the Gaucher cell. The appearance of the cell is quite characteristic and, on supravital staining, the cytoplasm gives the appearance of "wrinkled tissue paper" or "crumpled silk." This material may be detected by the PAS stain and by histochemical methods for acid phosphatase. Accumulation of Glc-Cer in various tissue underlies the hepatosplenomegaly, lymph node enlargement, and bone destruction. The mechanism of the central nervous system disorder is not known, but it has been suggested by Svennerholm that there is a block in the normal catabolism of gangliosides in this disorder.

Laboratory studies reveal that vacuolated formed elements or foam cells are not found. An increased plasma acid phosphatase (not inhibited by tartrate) is a constant finding and is caused by spillage of acid hydrolases from lysosomes and Gaucher cells. The finding of elevated plasma acid phosphatase is not specific as it is also found in other lipidoses as well as in osteopetrosis and other disorders. Some patients with Gaucher's disease may have increased plasma cholesterol. No specific therapy for this disorder is available, but Brady has suggested the possible usefulness of spleen transplant to provide the missing β-glucosidase.

Ceramide lactoside lipodystrophy, presumably caused by a deficient or missing β-glucosidase, has been described in two patients by Brady, but the defect has not been authenticated by enzyme studies.

Fabry's disease is a systemic disorder of sphingolipid metabolism, transmitted by an X-linked gene. Original descriptions considered this disorder to be dermatological in nature and the term "angiokeratoma corporis diffusum" was employed to describe the numerous purplish papules occurring in the skin, especially around the scrotal area. There occurs a progressive accumulation of ceramide trihexoside (CTH) (galactosylgalactosyl glucosylceramide) in various tissues as a result of deficient galactoside required for CTH catabolism (Figure 3.8). Increased accumulation of dihexosylceramide (galactosylgalactosylceramide) has also been found in some tissues. Clinical manifestations which become evident in childhood or adolescence are characterized by periodic febrile crises, severe pain in the extremities, and vascular lesions in the skin conjunctiva and oral mucosa. Crystalline deposits may occur in the conjunctivae. Pain in the fingers, palms, and soles may be excruciating with a burning quality and is often precipitated by changes in environmental temperature, and may be followed by paresthesias in these areas. Skin lesions in this disorder include telangiectases which may occur quite early and progress with age. They develop small punctate, flat, or raised, dark red lesions which do not blanch with pressure. Clusters of these lesions occur between the umbilicus and the knees, with major locations on the scrotum, penis, buttocks, thighs, hips, and back. Similar lesions may occur in the conjunctiva and oral mucosa. Renal lesions are secondary to accumulation of CTH and CDH. There is early proteinuria with progressive signs of renal impairment. Azotemia may develop by middle age. A concentration defect occurs with specific gravity becoming fixed between 1.008 and 1.012. Casts, red cells, and birefringent lipid globules (intra- and extracellular) appear in the urine, and a pitressin resistant diabetes-insipidus has been described in some patients.

Accumulation of glycosphingolipids in the vascular system may lead to hypertension, cardiomegaly, myocardial ischemia or infarction, as well as to cerebrovascular thromboses and frank hemorrhage. Seizures, hemiplegia, and other neurological signs have been reported. Vessel involvement in the eyes affects mainly the cornea, retina, and conjunctiva. Sausage-like dilation of veins may be seen in the conjunctivae. Corneal opacities are often found. Occasionally, sphingolipid deposits in the respiratory tract may result in bronchitis, as well as in dyspnea caused by an alveolo capillary block. Death usually results from uremia or from cardiovascular problems and occurs usually between 40 and 50 years. This disorder may occur with milder clinical manifestations in heterozygous females in whom the ocular and dermatological manifestations predominate.

The clinical manifestations are secondary to the accumulation of excessive amounts of glycosphingolipids in tissues. Accumulation of CTH is ascribed to a deficiency of galactosidase in the plasma and various tissues. This enzyme, which is found in the kidneys, liver, brain, spleen, and gastrointestinal mucosa, is responsible for cleavage of a galactosyl from CTH. Increased tissue accumulation of ceramide dihexoside (galactosylgalactosylceramide) has also been reported to occur. The clinical diagnosis is usually suspected from the physical findings as well as from family history in many cases. The presence of pain in the extremities associated with an increased erythrocyte sedimentation rate may lead to the erroneous diagnosis of rheumatic fever.

Laboratory studies reveal the presence of doubly refractile lipid bodies

(Maltese crosses) in urinary sediment. Renal biopsy reveals accumulation of glycosphingolipid in the endothelial and epithelial cells of the glomerulus and of Bowman's space and in the epithelium of the distal tubule and Henle's loop. Lipid-laden cells may be found in the lining and in the tubular lumen. Increased levels of CTH in the plasma and urine and in cultural fibroblasts may antedate clinical manifestations of this disorder, and the level of galactosidase in the plasma, intestinal biopsy specimen, leukocytes, or cultured skin fibroblasts is low or absent. Infusion of normal plasma has improved the levels of galactosidase in the plasma for as long as 7 days. During this period, the levels of CTH in the plasma decreased progressively. Infusion of purified galactosidase has also been tried with some evidence of chemical improvement, and renal transplantation has resulted in chemical and clinical improvement.

   Clinical Disorders of Galactocerebroside Metabolism Galactocerebrosides are galactosyl esters of ceramide (*N*-acyl sphingosine). The acyl groups in this family of compounds are long-chained fatty acids C-14 to C-26, with a relative predominance of C-20 to C-26 chain length, lack of polyunsaturated FA, and presence of hydroxy acids. About two-thirds of FA in galactocerebrosides, and one-third in sulfatides are α-hydroxyl. It is of interest that α-hydroxy FA are not normally present in other lipids in the brain. The presence of long-chained FA is restricted to galactocerebrosides and sulfatides of brain and, to some extent, to sphingomyelins of white matter and myelin. Galactocerebroside is the characteristic sphingolipid of the nervous system; brain sulfatides are derived from galactocerebroside. In contrast, glucocerebrosides occur predominantly in systemic tissues other than the nervous system and are from this tissue after 1 year of age.

   Galactocerebroside is derived from ceramide and the galactosyl moiety from ceramide and galactosyl moiety from UDP-galactose according to the following scheme (Figure 3.9). The role of this structure in the synthesis of sulfatide is also shown. The sulfate group in sulfatide is derived from 3'-phosphoadenosine-5'-phosphosulfate (PAPS). Galactosylceramide is degraded to ceramide and galactose by a lysosomal hydrolase, galactocerebroside galactosidase. This enzyme has been purified from brain lysosome and is known to be inhibited by ceramide, sphingosine, lactosylceramide, and galactitol. The level of this enzyme in brain probably changes with the processes of cerebroside deposition and myelination. Galactosylceramide is the characteristic lipid of the brain, but the kidneys contain appreciable levels of this compound. In the brain, the white matter is especially rich in galactosylceramide and its sulfatide derivative. There are much smaller amounts of these substances in gray matter. There are good data to indicate that the bulk of these substances are localized in the myelin sheath and in oligodendroglial cells. The sum of galactocerebroside and

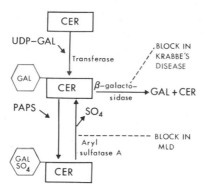

Figure 3.9. Synthesis and degradation of galactocerebrosides with identification of the biochemical lesions in metachromatic leukodystrophy and Krabbe's disease.

sulfatide is the most sensitive biochemical indicator of the amount of myelin in the brain, and there is a distinct positive correlation between the levels of these substances and the active myelination period. The myelin in adult brain contains galactocerebroside in a concentration range of 15–18%, the levels in myelin sheath of peripheral vessels being somewhat less. Most active myelination in the brain occurs between the perinatal period to age 18 months, and continues at a lower rate until about age 20 years, at which time it is essentially complete. After this time, there is a relatively slow turnover rate. The half-life of brain galactocerebroside and sulfatide is estimated to be 1 year or longer. The level of lysosomal galactosidase increases during the active myelination period, and the levels attained then are retained in the adult brain (19, 20).

Krabbe's disease (globoid cell leukodystrophy) is a rapidly progressive and fatal disorder of infancy. The disorder is inherited as an autosomal recessive characteristic lacking any sexual, racial, or geographical preponderance. The onset in most patients is between 3 and 6 months of age, prior to which time the patient develops normally. A rare patient may show symptoms from birth. The clinical manifestations are confined largely to the nervous system and have been described in three stages. Stage 1 is characterized by generalized hyperirritability, hyperesthesia, stiffness in the limbs, and an episodic fever of unknown origin. The child becomes hypersensitive to visual, auditory, tactile, and other external stimuli, with frequent crying without obvious cause; regression of psychomotor development is also noted at this time. Stage 2 is characterized by rapid and severe motor and mental deterioration. Marked hypertonicity is noted with extended and crossed legs, flexed arms, and backward-bent head. Deep tendon reflexes are hyperactive. Seizures may occur in this stage, and optic atrophy is observed. Stage 3 is achieved within a matter of several weeks; the child becomes blind, decerebrate, and deaf. This stage may last for months to 2 years, when death supervenes.

The extensive involvement of the nervous system is secondary to the severe involvement of the myelin sheath and oligodendroglia caused by the restricted localization of galactocerebroside in this tissue, and by the globoid reaction caused by galactocerebroside. There is severe myelin loss and astrocytic gliosis in the central nervous system and in peripheral nerves. The white matter is always more severely involved than the gray matter, the major abnormality being the presence of large numbers of globoid cells. The globoid cell reaction is produced by the accumulation of galactocerebroside. These cells are described as being mono- or multi-nucleated large cells of epithelioid origin. They occur in various areas of the brain and stain with the PAS and Sudan stains, but the cytoplasm does not exhibit metachromasia. The mechanism of the marked myelin abnormality is ascribed to the fact that, during the most active myelination, patients with this disorder lack the β-galactosidase to degrade galactocerebroside from catabolized myelin. The accumulating cerebroside elicits the globoid cell reaction and infiltration. There is eventual destruction of oligodendroglial cells with cessation of myelination. Eventually this leads to decreased cerebroside production secondary to the cessation of myelination. Globoid cell accumulation may also occur in the liver, spleen, kidneys, peripheral leukocytes, and fibroblasts. Definitive antemortem diagnosis is achieved by finding deceased levels of galactocerebrosidase in leukocytes or serum. No definitive therapy is available, but genetic counseling may be of aid on discovery of decreased β-galactosidase in amniotic fluid.

SULFATIDE METABOLISM

Sulfatides are sulfate esters of cerebrosides. The cerebrosides, for example, galactocerebrosides, contain almost exclusively C-18 sphingosine. Sulfotransferase catalyzes the transfer of a sulfate group from phosphoadenosyl phosphosulfate (PAPS) to C-3 of the galactosyl moiety of galactosylceramide. The fatty acid composition of the galactosylcerebrosides and the sulfates is distinctive in containing a high proportion of long-chain fatty acids and of α-hydroxy FA. Nearly all α-hydroxy FA in brain are present in galactocerebrosides and sulfatides. The FA patterns of sulfatides vary both with the type of tissue as well as with degree of maturity. For example, the FA in the sulfatides in brain contain a higher proportion of nervonic acid (24:1) than lignoceric (24:0), whereas, in the kidney, the reverse is true. Similarly, in the immature brain the medium-chain fatty acids (16:0, 18:0, and 18:1) predominate, whereas, in the mature brain, the longer chained FA are present. Sulfatides occur in highest concentrations in the white matter of the adult brain, representing approximately 4% dry weight. In adult gray matter, the sulfatide content approaches 0.8% dry weight. The next highest concentrations of sulfatides are found in the kidneys where they amount to 0.04% dry weight. Kidneys also contain a ceramide dihexoside sulfate, roughly one-half of the level of ceramide galactosyl sulfate. Lower levels are found in spleen and plasma.

The levels of sulfatides in brain tissue increase with maturation. The highest rate of increase occurs during the phase of most active myelination, in man during the first 2 years of life. Between age 2 and 10 years, there is a doubling of the amount of sulfatide in the brain, with a smaller increase up to age 40 years, when the highest level is achieved. Sulfatides, along with cholesterol, sphingomyelins, acetal phosphatides, and glycolipoproteins are components of the myelin sheath. The process of "ensheathment" of the nervous system is performed by the oligodendrocyte in the central nervous system, and by Schwann cell in the peripheral nerves. During myelination, there is a spiraling of a process of the myelinating cell so that the axon is ensheathed by multiple layers. There are data suggesting that sulfatides are involved with non-myelin structures also. Sulfatides exhibit the property of metachromasia, as they are anionic lipids which may react with certain dyes.

The first step in the degradation of sulfatide involves the desulfation to cerebroside (Figure 3.9) by cerebroside sulfatase. There are considerable data suggesting that this sulfatase activity is due to arylsulfatase A. Arylsulfatases are present in many tissues, with highest activity present in the liver. The brain contains approximately one-fifth of the levels in the liver; brain arylsulfatase is mainly of the "soluble" type. Arylsulfatase activity has been found in urine and on circulating leukocytes, mainly in the granulocytes. There is no activity in erythrocytes. Arylsulfatase A is active at a lower substrate concentration than is the B form. Platelets possess arylsulfatase A activity, as do cultured skin fibroblast cells and cells from amniotic fluid. This activity is located in the lysosomes (in brain and in liver), while arylsulfatase C (insoluble) is located in microsomes.

Clinical Disorders of Sulfatide Metabolism

Sulfatide lipidosis (metachromatic leukodystrophy) (MLD) describes an autosomal recessive inherited disorder in which there is myelin degeneration in the central nervous system and in peripheral nerves with an accumulation of cerebroside sulfate or galactosyl-3-sulfate ceramide. Three clinical forms of MLD are recognized: the late infantile form which is the most common type, the adult form in which the clinical features are evident after age 21 years, and the MLD variant which evolves differently from the other two forms and is ascribed to defects in several sulfatases.

Late infantile sulfatide lipidosis or late infantile MLD is a progressive neurological disorder which develops in children whose early development has been completely normal. The following features evolve in five stages starting at age 12-18 months. Stage 1 is characterized by weakness and hypotonia in the extremities, unsteadiness, and weak deep tendon reflexes, and genu recurvatum. These features may suggest a myopathy or peripheral neuropathy. This stage lasts for about 15 months. Stage 2 lasts 3−6 months and is a progression of the disorder in which there are advanced muscle weakness and the following pattern: mental regression, dysarthria, and aphasia, hypertonicity which replaces hypotonia, ataxia, and pain in the extremities. Stage 3 is characterized by the following features: the patient is quadriplegic and bedridden and muscle tone is variable; he may assume decorticate, decerebrate, or dystonic postures, and bulbar or pseudobulbar palsies may hinder feeding and maintenance of a patent airway. Optic atrophy may develop and, on funduscopy, the macula appears gray, with a red spot in the center. This stage may last 3−40 months, during which the child is barely able to respond to parental affection. In the final stage, the patient is oblivious of his surroundings, is blind and without speech. He may live in this vegetative state for months or years. There is a "juvenile" form which may evolve from 4−21 years of age. The major early manifestations in this form include emotional lability and visual disturbances.

The adult type of sulfatide lipidosis (adult MLD) is a rare disorder, with only 19 in the world literature, rarely diagnosed during life. The age of onset is 20−45 years, with a protracted course lasting up to 40 years in some cases. Early manifestations include dementia and delusions of grandeur, suggesting schizophrenia. Other features include generalized seizures, tremors and clonic movements, motor incoordination, and incontinence. MLD variant associated with various sulfatase deficiencies is a rare disorder in which the age of onset is 1−3 years, with the children showing delayed early development. The patients soon develop quadriplegia, nystagmus, seizures, and deafness. Certain skeletal abnormalities are also noted, including a convex sternum and flared lower ribs. Hepatomegaly is also present. The basic biochemical abnormality in the sulfatide lipidoses is the impaired degradation of sulfatides resulting from deficiency in cerebroside sulfatase activity. It is now known that the degradation of the galactosyl-3-sulfate ceramide structure is dependent on arylsulfatase A activity. Cerebroside sulfatase activity is normally low, with highest activity in the renal cortex. Small accumulations of cerebrosides apparently do not cause any significant damage, but toxic levels which accumulate after considerable time affect the Schwann cells and presumably oligodendrocytes. Because of the sulfatase defect in the kidneys, there is an accumulation of cerebrosides in the kidneys. Hepatic and gallbladder accumulations are also found. Clinical disorders of hepatic and renal functions are not described, however. There is good evidence to support the concept that these accumulations disrupt the myelin sheath in the central nervous system as well as in the peripheral nerves.

Several procedures are now available for the detection of these disorders, including methods to determine the enzyme activity as well as to quantitate excreted sulfatide. These are listed as follows:

1. Arylsulfatase A levels in urine: An assay method utilizing nitrocatechol potassium sulfate has been used quite successfully to determine sulfatase deficiency in urine.

2. Arylsulfatase A activity in leukocytes is quantitated by the above method. The results of this test should be confirmed by at least one procedure for quantitating excess sulfatides.

3. Metachromatic bodies in the urine sediment: Toluidine blue added to urinary sediment containing excessive amounts of sulfatides will reveal the presence of characteristic golden brown bodies. A similar procedure employing cresyl violet in an acid medium is regarded as more accurate.

4. Excess sulfatide in the urine: The lipids in urine sediment are extracted with organic solvent, and are then separated after equilibration of the solvent extract with water. The "white fluff" is applied to filter paper for a metachromasia test, or for chromatographic separation.

5. Peripheral nerve biopsy: Frozen sections of biopsy specimens of the sural nerve are treated with cresyl violet in an acid medium. The appearance of brown metachromatic granules within phagocytes surrounding the vasa nervorum, or just under the perineurium, indicates the presence of sulfatide.

There is no definitive therapy for this disorder. Ingestion of a low vitamin A diet resulted in lowered glycolipid excretion, but significant clinical improvement was not observed. Infusion of purified arylsulfatase A was followed by detectable levels of the enzyme in the plasma and liver for several hours. Whether this procedure can be of real clinical benefit remains to be determined.

GANGLIOSIDE METABOLISM

Gangliosides are sphingolipids in which an oligosaccharide containing a sialic acid is esterified to ceramide. The highest concentration of ganglioside is found in the gray matter of the brain, and only small amounts are present in non-neural tissues. The gangliosides in human neural tissue contain both C-18 and C-20 sphingosine bases, the relative amounts varying with age. For example, fetal tissue contains more C-18 sphingosine, the complement of C-20 increasing with age. The fatty acid composition of neural tissue differs from that of other sphingolipids, the neural tissue containing stearic (C-18) mainly, with some C-16, C-20, and C-26 fatty acids. In fetal brain, the gangliosides contain over 90% stearic acid, but the adult concentration of around 80% is achieved by 3 years of age. Hydroxy fatty acids are essentially absent from brain sphingolipids. The sialic acid of brain gangliosides is mainly N-acetylneuraminic acid (NANA). Gangliosides make up 2% dry weight of the gray matter of the brain and 0.4% of white matter. Smaller concentrations are found in the liver, spleen, kidney, retina, erythrocytes, plasma, gastrointestinal mucosa, mammary tissue, skin fibroblasts, and cardiac muscle. In neural tissues, significant amounts of the gangliosides are found in neuronal cell bodies, axons, synaptosomes, nerve endings, and peripheral nerves. Smaller amounts are found in glial cells. These substances function as structural elements in membranes and may be important in the process of impulse transmission. Gangliosides have been shown to have a rapid turnover before and during myelination and it is estimated that their half-life is about 20–24 days (19, 20, 23).

Biosynthesis and Degradation of Gangliosides

The structure of ceramide has been discussed previously. The glycosyl moieties and the NANA are added to ceramide essentially according to the scheme in Figure 3.10. Glycosyl groups are added by transferases to the ceramide structure one at a time. Sialic acid is added through cytidine monophosphate-N-acetylneuraminic acid (CMP-NANA). The degradative pathway involves sequential hydrolysis of oligosaccharide residues from G_{M1} by lysosomal glycosidases. These enzymes are present in the brain. The first step is the cleavage of the β-linked terminal galactose by a lysosomal β-galactosidase. The degradation scheme is presented in Figure 3.10 in which defects resulting in clinical disorders are also identified.

Clinical Disorders of Ganglioside Metabolism

Generalized gangliosidosis (G_{M1} gangliosidosis) type 1 is an autosomal recessive inherited disorder which is characterized by severe progressive cerebral degeneration leading to death within the first 2 years of life. There is an accumulation of a specific ganglioside in the brain and viscera and mucopolysaccharide in the viscera. From birth, a marked retardation of psychomotor development is seen in patients with this disorder. The infant exhibits poor sucking, poor appetite, and a failure to thrive. Hypotonia and hypoactivity are clearly evident. The following morphological features may be present at birth: frontal bossing with some degree of macrocephaly, depressed nasal bridge, large low-set ears, increased distance between nose and upper lip, downy hirsutism over forehead and neck, gingival hypertrophy, and macroglossia. Internal strabismus and nystagmus are evident and a cherry-red spot in the macula is present in 50% of

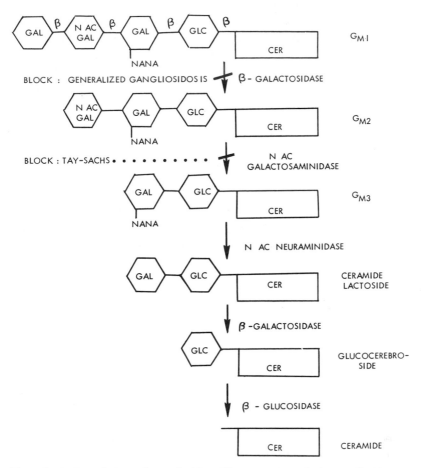

Figure 3.10. Degradation of gangliosides. The structures of the gangliosides are presented and the biochemical lesions in generalized gangliosidosis and Tay-Sachs disease are identified.

patients. Motor development is retarded; the infant is unable to crawl. Grasping is absent because of weakness and incoordination. The infant is inmobile and is considered a "good baby." At birth, the heart and lungs are normal, but soon these infants develop pneumonia. The liver and, occasionally, the spleen are enlarged by age 6 months. A dorsolumbar kyphosis may be noted, as are short and stubby fingers; a claw hand deformity is often present. Hard, nontender enlargement of the wrist and ankle joints may be noted, and the joints may be stiff with evident flexion deformities. Bone changes in this disorder are similar in some respects to those found in mucopolysaccharidosis I. Some of the changes may even be reminiscent of congenital syphilis. After age 6 months, the most significant radiological signs are in the spine and upper extremities, including rarefaction of the cortex and beaked vertebral bodies usually in the area of lumbar kyphosis. The humerus and other long bones are wider in the midshaft region, tapering in proximal and distal areas.

There is rapid deterioration after the first year of life with death by age 2 years. Tonic-clonic convulsions occur quite frequently. Respirations become labored; tube feeding becomes necessary because of difficulty with swallowing. Recurrent bronchopneumonia is a major problem. One patient was noted to have paroxysmal atrial tachycardia. Sudden death occurs commonly, bronchopneumonia being a frequent cause.

Ganglioside accumulation occurs in several tissues—there is a 10-fold excess in the gray matter and a 20- to 50-fold excess in the liver. An asialoganglioside ceramide tetrahexoside (G_1 ganglioside without NANA) also accumulates in the brain. Brain degeneration in this disorder is due to neuronal accumulation of these compounds. A fairly characteristic ballooning of the epithelial cells of the glomerulus is found in this disorder, resembling that of Fabry's disease. The brain defect in this disorder is a deficiency of lysosomal β-galactosidase (Figure 3.10). There is an associated disorder of mucopolysaccharide metabolism in generalized gangliosidosis. The mucopolysaccharide which accumulates is rich in galactose and glucosamine. Defective degradation of the mucopolysaccharide is ascribed to galactosidase deficiency. Laboratory studies reveal presence of vacuolated lymphocytes in the peripheral blood, with 10–80% of the cells showing 3–4 vacuoles/cell. Foamy mononuclear cells are found in the urine sediment. Urinary levels of acid mucopolysaccharides may be normal or slightly elevated. Urine β-galactosidase activity is decreased to as low as 10% of normal, and β-galactosidase deficiency is found in skin fibroblast cultures. Because of the similarities in clinical manifestations of generalized gangliosidosis, Tay-Sachs disease, infantile Niemann-Pick disease, mucopolysaccharidosis I and II, and acute neuronopathic Gaucher's disease, it is essential that the constellations of clinical and laboratory features be carefully evaluated before definitive diagnosis is made. No specific therapy is available for gangliosidosis (G_{M1}). Supportive therapy includes use of anticonvulsants for seizures, antibiotics for infections, and tube feeding to prevent starvation.

Juvenile G_{M1} gangliosidosis (type II) is a rare autosomal recessive inherited disorder which has no special ethnic or geographic preponderance. The clinical onset of this disorder appears later than in generalized gangliosidosis and progresses more slowly; bony deformities and visceromegaly are absent. In patients with this disorder, early development is overtly normal in all aspects. Locomotor ataxia is the first symptom and it appears at about age 1 year. Coordinated manipulative movements become more difficult. Speech becomes difficult and is soon lost. Physical examination at this time is completely normal except for the ataxia and gait disturbance. Some muscle weakness in upper and lower extremities develops. Deep tendon reflexes become hyperactive, and the Babinski is plantar until later when it becomes extensor. There is relatively rapid progression for the ensuing few months during which time mental and motor deterioration are quite evident. The child is lethargic and loses interest in his surroundings. Spasticity appears and progresses to spastic quadriplegia. Hyperacusis develops. By age 16 months, seizures may develop and, by 24 months, decorticate rigidity develops. Recurrent infections, especially bronchopneumonia, may eventually lead to death, which occurs between age 3–5 years or occasionally later.

The neurological problems are ascribable to defects similar to, but not identical with, the chemical changes in generalized gangliosidosis. Enzyme studies suggest that the β-galactosidase defect is not as extensive in this juvenile type. Hepatosplenomegaly and bony deformities are not characteristic of this form. No definitive therapy is available and supportive therapy is applied as in generalized gangliosidosis. The enzymatic defects may be detected in heterozygotes and homozygotes prenatally by enzyme assay of amniocentesis fluid. Family planning may then reduce the incidence of these gangliosidoses.

G_{M2} gangliosidosis (Tay-Sachs disease) is an abnormality of the nervous system due to a presumably autosomal recessive inherited characteristic. The clinical disorder becomes evident by age 5–6 months and is characterized by progressive retardation in development, dementia, and paralysis. The disorder is usually fatal by age 3–4 years. Ganglion cells and proliferating glial cells are noted to contain excessive amounts of gangliosides. There is associated extensive myelin degeneration in the nervous system. (It should be noted that gangliosidosis has been considered the basis of the amaurotic familial idiocies (AFI), but only two types of AFI, G_{M1} and G_{M2}, are true gangliosidoses.)

G_{M2} gangliosidosis has been found in Jewish and non-Jewish populations. The initial clinical manifestations may start at about 6–10 months of age, at which time the parents may note an inability of the infant to sit up. The children are overtly normal up to that time, but perhaps may have been somewhat apathetic. Weakness, retardation in development, and feeding difficulties occur early. Hypotonia, as well as spasticity, may occur by the 4th month. An exaggerated acoustimotor response in which sharp sounds elicit a rapid extension of both arms, as well as a startle reaction, may also be noted quite early. The infants may appear inattentive or listless, and may exhibit a fixed gaze; this may well be due to early visual difficulties. The macular area shows degeneration and the appearance of a cherry-red spot. Central blindness may occur before 18 months of age, with optic atrophy seen on physical examination. Epileptiform seizures may occur, but these are rarely seen before age 1 year. These seizures may be associated with inappropriate laughter (gelastic seizures) and episodes of autonomic dysfunction. Rarely, a few infants may show precocious sexual development which is ascribed to hypothalamic dysfunction secondary to gangliosidosis. The patients may reach a stage of marked hypotonia, and even the startle reaction may diminish. Macrocephaly may occur, but there is no visceromegaly.

Major morphological and chemical changes occur in the nervous system. These include atrophy of several parts of the brain and "ballooning" of these cells with displacement of their nuclei to the periphery. The number of cortical axons decreases, and astrocytes and microglia proliferate. Similar lipid infiltration is noted in the cerebellum. There is marked loss of Purkinje cells, and the few that remain may be distended with lipid and show degenerative changes. The myelin sheath is destroyed. Similar changes occur in the basal ganglia, brain stem, and spinal cord. Peripheral and autonomic nerves show myelin degeneration. Lesions in the retina, similar to those in the cortex, produce the cherry-red spot which consists of a grayish yellow zone in the macular region in which the fovea is seen as the red spot. The macular changes are caused by edema or degeneration of ganglion cells. Optic nerve demyelination is also seen. In a few patients, lipid-laden cells may be found in the spleen and lungs, and PAS-positive cells in the liver.

The changes described above are due to the accumulation of ganglioside G_{M2} (Tay-Sachs) ganglioside, and its NANA-free derivative, galactosylglucosylceramide. These compounds accumulate because of a deficiency of the enzyme N-acetylgalactosaminidase (hexosaminidase A). Absence of this enzyme has been found in the following tissues of patients with TSD: brain, liver, kidney, skin, fibroblast cultures, plasma, and leukocytes. The G_{M2} gangliosides accumulate in the ganglion cells and axis cylinders of nerves, glial cells, and in macrophages. The cells become filled with secondary lysosomes called membranous cytoplasmic bodies (MCB). Definitive diagnosis of this disorder requires demonstration of a marked decrease of N-acetylgalactosaminidase (hexosaminidase A) in plasma, leukocytes, or cultured fibroblasts takes from the skin. Similar decreases may be demonstrated in brain, skeletal muscle, liver, kidney, and spleen. The use of this enzyme assay makes it unnecessary to determine the ganglioside levels in brain biopsy specimen. No definitive therapy is available for this disorder, but supportive measures may prolong life somewhat. Several studies have shown that although Tay-Sachs disease occurs in non-Jewish as well as Jewish families, the disorder is 100 times more frequent in the Jewish population. It has been estimated that the carrier rate in the Jewish population in New York City is 1:30 compared with 1:300 in non-Jews. The highest carrier rates are in Jews whose antecedents

Table 3.11. Summary of Sphingolipodystrophies

Disease	Biochemical defect and key clinical features
Niemann-Pick	Deficient in sphingomyelinase; autosomal recessive disorder with hepatosplenomegaly, severe central nervous system involvement, and macular cherry-red spot. It is fatal in early childhood. Tissues show accumulation of sphingomyelin
Metachromatic leukodystrophy	Arylsulfatase A deficiency with myelin degeneration in central and peripheral nervous systems. Weakness, hypotonia, mental regression, quadriplegia are found, with the patient eventually becoming decorticate, decerebrate, and dystonic. A macular cherry-red spot is present
Krabbe's disease	Gal-cer β-galactosidase deficiency is an autosomal recessive disorder with disruption of myelin sheath, severe motor and mental retardation, with the patients becoming blind, deaf, and decerebrate. Fatal in infancy
Fabry's disease	Gal-Gal-Glc-cer α-galactosidase deficiency is an X-linked disorder characterized by periodic fever, purplish papules, paresthesias, telangiectases, renal lesions, uremia, and cardiovascular problems. Accumulation of ceramide trihexoside occurs
Gaucher's disease	Glc-cer β-glucosidase deficiency results in glucosyl ceramide accumulation in liver, spleen, lymph nodes, and bone. Hypersplenism, anemia, and thrombocytopenia are common. Some have severe central nervous system disorder. Serum acid phosphatase is increased
Generalized gangliosidosis	NAc-Gal-Gal-NANA-Glc-cer β-galactosidase deficiency is an autosomal recessive trait. Cerebral degeneration within 2 years with retarded psychomotor development occurs. Macrocephaly, macroglossia, and joint deformities are found. M1 deposits occur in brain, central nervous system, and liver. A macular cherry-red spot is characteristic. A milder form is type II
Tay-Sachs disease	Gal-NANA-Glc-cer N-acetylgalactosaminidase deficiency is an autosomal recessive disorder characterized by atrophy of several parts of brain with weakness, retardation, acoustimotor overreaction, and seizures. A macular cherry-red spot is present

lived in the Lithuanian and Polish provincies of Korno and Grodno during the late 19th century. It has been suggested that the hexosaminidase A assay of serum should be used for heterozygote detection. Such information may aid in pregnancy prevention measures when appropriate. Determination of enzyme activity in aminiotic fluid or cultured cells will also be useful for prenatal diagnosis.

Clinical variants of G_{M2} gangliosidosis have been described. In type 2, in addition to the storage of G_{M2}, there is also a more pronounced accumulation of its asialoganglioside than noted in Tay-Sachs disease. In type 3, the neurological problems appear 2–3 years later than in Tay-Sachs disease, and time of death may occur between ages 5 and 15 years. In this variant, macrocephaly and the retinal cherry-red spot are not seen. Retinitis pigmentosa may be present. This disorder is caused by a partial deficiency of the N-acetylgalactosaminidase. The various sphingolipodystrophies are presented in summary form in Table 3.11.

OTHER LIPID STORAGE DISORDERS

Wolman's disease is an autosomal recessive inherited disorder which is characterized by the accumulation of large amounts of cholesteryl esters and triglycerides in various tissues. The clinical features include vomiting and abdominal distension associated with diarrhea, steatorrhea, and malabsorption occurring within the first few weeks of life. Physical findings include hepatosplenomegaly. X-ray reveals adrenal calcification and enlargement. Adrenocortical response to stimulation is abnormal. A deficiency in acid lipase which catalyzes hydrolysis of esterified lipids has been described in this disorder, but the relationship to the pathogenesis is not clear. No definitive therapy is available, and the patients die by the age of 6 months.

Phytanic acid storage disease (Refsum's disease) is an autosomal recessive inherited lipid storage disorder which was first described by Refsum in five members of two inbred Norwegian families (24). The disorder is characterized by neurological, cutaneous, ocular, and osseous changes. Retinitis pigmentosa is the basis of decreased night vision, lenticular opacities, and altered visual fields. Peripheral neuropathy with motor and sensory deficits usually symmetrical occurs, and absent or decreased deep tendon reflexes are noted. Other neurological signs include cerebellar ataxia, intention tremor, nystagmus, nerve deafness, and anosmia. Ichthyosis-like cutaneous changes and epiphyseal dysplasia with short fourth metatarsal, hammer toes, pes cavus, and osteochondritis dessicans are also found.

Phytanic acid, a 20-carbon branched chain acid, accumulates in various tissues, especially in the liver and kidney. This acid may amount to 30% of total fatty acids in the plasma, compared with only trace amounts in the plasma of normal subjects. The phytanic acid is derived from dietary sources and from phytol which is a component of chorophyll. The metabolism of phytanic acid involves a unique first step hydroxylation reaction which converts phytanic acid to hydroxy phytanic acid. This is the initial step in the conversion to pristanic acid. The enzyme phytanic acid hydroxylase is missing in this disorder. The defect is demonstrable in skin fibroblast cultures. The best working hypothesis regarding the pathogenesis is that phytanic acid interferes with myelin formation. Treatment requires the exclusion of ruminant and dairy fats from the diet for 2–4 years.

LITERATURE CITED

1. Hoffman-Ostenhoff, O., W. E. Cohn, A. E. Braustein, J. S. Fruton, B. Keil, W. Klyne, C. Liebecq, B. G. Malmstrom, R. Schwyzer, E. C. Slater, and N. Tamiya. 1967. The nomenclature of lipids. J. Lipid Res. 8:523–528.
2. Johnson, J. M. 1963. Recent developments in the mechanism of fat absorption. Adv. Lipid. Res. 1:105–131.
3. Senior, J. R. 1964. Intestinal absorption of fats. J. Lipid Res. 5:495–521.
4. Wilson, F. A., and J. M. Dietschy. 1971. Differential diagnostic approach to clinical problems of malabsorption. Gastroenterology 61:911–931.
5. Boyd, G. S., and I. W. Percy-Robb. 1971. Enzymatic regulation of bile acid synthesis. Am. J. Med. 51:580–587.
6. Tyor, M. P., J. T. Garbutt, and L. Lack. 1971. Metabolism and transport of bile salts in the intestine. Am. J. Med. 51:614–626.
7. Garbutt, J. T., L. Lack, and M. P. Tyor. 1971. The enterohepatic circulation of bile salts in gastrointestinal disorders. Am. J. Med. 51:627–636.
8. Fredrickson, D. S., R. I. Levy, and R. S. Lees. 1967. Fat transport in lipoproteins—an integrated approach to mechanisms and disorders. N. Engl. J. Med. 276:34–44, 94–103, 148–156, 215–204, and 273–281.
9. Fredrickson, D. S., and R. I. Levy. 1972. Familial hyperlipoproteinemia. In J. B. Stanbury, J. B. Wyngaarden, and D. L. Fredrickson (eds.), The Metabolic Basis of Inherited Diseases. 3rd Ed., pp. 545–614. McGraw-Hill Book Co., New York.
10. Dietschy, J. M., and J. D. Wilson. 1970. Regulation of cholesterol metabolism. N. Engl. J. Med. 282:1128–1138, 1179–1183, and 1241–1249.
11. Tchen, T. T. 1960. Metabolism of sterols. In D. M. Greenberg (ed.), Metabolic Pathways. Vol. 1, pp. 389–429. Academic Press, Inc., New York.
12. Siperstein, M. D., and V. M. Fagan. 1966. Feedback control of mevalonate synthesis by dietary cholesterol. J. Biol. Chem. 241:602–609.

13. Green, D. E., and D. M. Gibson. 1960. Fatty acid oxidation and synthesis. *In* D. M. Greenberg (ed.), Metabolic Pathways. Vol. 1, pp. 301–340. Academic Press, Inc., New York.

14. Siperstein, M. D. 1960. Lipid derangements in diabetes. *In* R. H. Williams (ed.), Diabetes. pp. 102–120. Paul B. Hoeber, Inc., New York.

15. Leevy, C. M. 1961. Fatty liver: A study of 270 patients with biopsy proven fatty liver and a review of the literature. Medicine 41:249–276.

16. Feigelson, E. B., W. W. Pfatt, A. Karmen, and D. Steinberg. 1961. The role of plasma free fatty acids in development of fatty liver. J. Clin. Invest. 40:2171–2179.

17. Rossiter, R. J. 1960. Metabolism of phosphatides. *In* D. M. Greenberg (ed.), Metabolic Pathways. Vol. 1, pp. 357–388. Academic Press, Inc., New York.

18. Norum, K. R., J. A. Glomset, and E. Gjone. 1972. Familial lecithin: Cholesterol acyl transferase deficiency. *In* J. B. Stanbury, J. B. Wyngaarden, and D. L. Fredrickson (eds.), The Metabolic Basis of Inherited Diseases. 3rd ed., pp. 531–544. McGraw-Hill Book Co., New York.

19. Brady, R. O. 1969. The sphingolipodystrophies. *In* P. K. Bondy (ed.), Diseases of Metabolism, pp. 357–365. W. B. Saunders Co., Philadelphia.

20. Brady, R. O. 1965. The sphingolipidoses. N. Engl. J. Med. 225:312–318.

21. Fredrickson, D. S., and H. R. Sloan. 1972. Sphingomyelin lipidoses: Niemann-Pick disease. *In* J. B. Stanbury, J. B. Wyngaarden, and D. S. Fredrickson (eds.), The Metabolic Basis of Inherited Diseases. 3rd Ed., pp. 783–807. McGraw-Hill Book Co., New York.

22. Fredrickson, D. S., and H. R. Sloan. 1972. Glucosyl ceramide lipidoses. *In* J. B. Stanbury, J. B. Wyngaarden, and D. S. Fredrickson (eds.), The Metabolic Basis of Inherited Diseases, pp. 730–759. McGraw-Hill Book Co., New York.

23. Sloan, H. R., and D. S. Fredrickson. 1972. GM_2 gangliosidoses: Tay-Sachs disease. *In* J. B. Stanbury, J. B. Wyngaarden, and D. S. Fredrickson (eds.), The Metabolic Basis of Inherited Diseases, pp. 615–638. McGraw-Hill Book Co., New York.

24. Steinberg, D. 1972. Phytanic acid storage disease. *In* J. B. Stanbury, J. B. Wyngaarden, and D. S. Fredrickson (eds.). The Metabolic Basis of Inherited Diseases, pp. 833–853. McGraw-Hill Book Co., New York.

4
Clinical Disorders of Protein and Amino Acid Metabolism

PROTEIN METABOLISM

The processes involved in protein metabolism in man were summarized (1). Dietary protein undergoes transformation in the intestinal tract before absorption of its constituent oligopeptides and amino acids (AA). This intestinal phase of protein metabolism consists of the processes of digestion, absorption, and transport into the mucosal cell.

1. Digestion is the process by which proteolytic enzymes release the constituent amino acids and oligopeptides (Figures 4.1 and 4.2). Intact protein provides no nourishment as it cannot be absorbed as such except in newborns. The presence of proteolytic enzymes in the intestinal lumen is, therefore, essential for release of amino acids and oligopeptides. The process of digestion involves the following steps:

   (a) denaturation of protein in stomach by HCl;
   (b) acid-induced (HCl) conversion of gastric juice pepsinogen, parapepsinogen I, and parapepsinogen II to pepsin, parapepsin I, and parapepsin II, respectively;
   (c) trypsin conversion of procarboxypeptidase in pancreatic juice to carboxypeptidase A which attacks terminal aromatic or branched chained amino acids, and carboxypeptidase B which attacks terminal arginine or lysine;
   (d) conversion of proelastase in pancreatic juice to elastase which attacks neutral aliphatic amino acids;

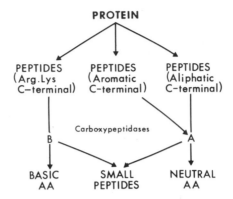

Figure 4.1. Sequential hydrolysis of protein in the duodenum by peptidases before absorption by the mucosal cell.

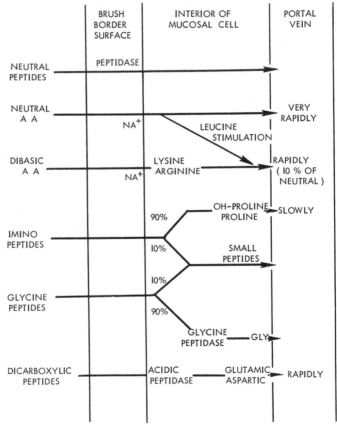

Figure 4.2. The mechanisms and rates of entrance of oligopeptides and amino acids into intestinal mucosal cell.

(e) conversion of chymotrypsinogen in pancreatic juice to chymotrypsin which attacks aromatic amino acids on the peptide chain;

(f) conversion of pancreatic juice trypsin by enterokinase from succus entericus (trypsin attacks the lysine and arginine in the peptide chain);

(g) aminopeptidases in the succus entericus attack the NH_2-terminal of the peptide; and

(h) dipeptidases in the succus entericus release free amino acids from oligopeptides.

2. Absorption is the process whereby free L-α-amino acids released by enzyme hydrolysis in the lumen reach the intestinal absorptive cells. After transcellular transport through these mucosal cells, they are delivered into the portal circulation. Amino acid absorption takes place mainly (80–90%) in the distal and proximal jejunum.

3. The transport of amino acids into the mucosal cell against concentration and electrochemical gradients is sodium dependent. The absorptive capacity of the mucosa is genetically controlled, and the transport mechanism matures with age. Amino acids are transported transcellularly from the intestinal lumen to the portal circulation, but the opposite process may also occur. In certain hyperaminoacidemic states, some of the amino acids are released into the intestinal lumen, resulting in decreased absorption of another amino acid. A clinical example of the phenomenon is seen in phenylketonuria (PKU), in which there is decreased tryptophan absorption in the presence of hyperphenylalaninemia.

Distribution of Amino Acids

The total free amino acids in the circulating plasma amount to 2 mM, plasma protein-bound amino acids amount to 20 mM, the free amino acid level in tissues is about 20 mM, and the protein-bound component is 30–60 times greater. Despite the fact that man is an episodic eater, there is little fluctuation in plasma amino acid levels because of the rapid tissue transport mechanisms. After intracellular accumulation, the liver metabolizes amino acids for protein synthesis and energy production. These plasma amino acid levels are lower in growing children than in adults. Plasma amino acid levels exhibit a circadian variation, with lowest levels at pre-dawn hours and highest levels in the mid-afternoon. The enzymes involved in protein metabolism show a similar circadian variation, presumably caused by enzyme induction either by hormones or by substrates. Free amino acids are readily filtered through the glomerulus, and all but 3–5% are reabsorbed by the renal tubules. In consideration of aminoaciduria, it is advisable to consider the renal excretion of amino acids in terms of clearance concepts. Amino acids occur in the cerebrospinal fluid

(CSF), both as a result of filtration through the choroid plexus and also from brain metabolism. The normal plasma:CSF ratio of amino acids is 8–10:1 and this ratio may be altered in certain aminoacidopathies. Amino acids are also found in sweat, tears, and saliva.

Amino Acid Metabolism

The carbons of amino acids are introduced into the Krebs tricarboxylic acid cycle, reversibly in many cases, so that the tricarboxylic acid cycle is involved in both amino acid anabolic and catabolic pathways (see Chapter 1). The initial reaction involves removal of the amino group by transamination or by oxidative deamination. The deaminated compounds enter the tricarboxylic acid cycle as previously described. Decarboxylation of amino acids results in the formation of amines, some of which are physiologically and pharmacologically active. Metabolites of amino acids produced by the above processes may occur in abnormal amounts, despite normal levels of the amino acids themselves, a situation found in many aminoacidopathies.

The nitrogen component of amino acids is metabolized as ammonia which may be taken up as the amide group in glutamine and asparagine. The glutamine is acted upon by glutaminase in the kidney with the release of NH_3^+ and in the presence of $H^+NH_4^+$ is formed and excreted. Ammonia may also enter the Krebs-Henseleit urea cycle. The majority of the catabolic reactions of amino acids require pyridoxal phosphate which is produced from pyridoxal and pyridoxine (vitamin B_6) by specific kinases. These kinases are subject to inhibition by vitamin B_6 analogues such as O-substituted hydroxylamines, hydrazines, and substituted hydrazines. The antituberculous drug isonicotinic acid hydrazine (INH) may impair amino acid metabolism through this mechanism. The dietary requirement of vitamin B_6 is dependent on the intake of protein. The requirement has been established to be 20 mg of pyridoxine/g of dietary protein. Figure 4.3 depicts the distribution of amino acids in the biological compartments.

The carbon compounds derived from the catabolism of amino acids have been listed in Chapter 1.

The minimum daily requirement of essential amino acids in man is as follows: L-isoleucine, 0.70 g/day; L-leucine, 1.10 g/day; L-lysine, 0.80 g/day; L-methionine, 1.10 g/day; L-phenylalanine, 1.10 g/day; L-threonine, 0.50 g/day; L-tryptophan, 0.50 g/day; and L-valine, 0.80 g/day.

Definitions in Protein Nutrition

Certain phenomena observed in protein and amino acid nutrition have been observed both clinically and experimentally and require definition (2).

Amino acid deficiency refers to inadequate availability of amino acids for metabolic or biosynthetic processes. This type of deficiency usually

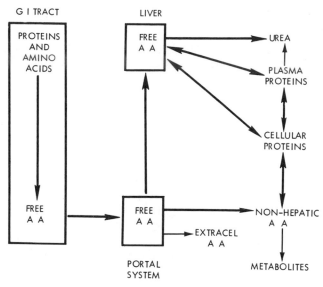

Figure 4.3. Distribution of amino acids in the biological compartments.

results from protein malnutrition, but may occasionally be seen with the use of synthetic diets which lack the full complement of essential amino acids. An unbalanced diet is present when the relative proportion of amino acids deviates from that of the reference whole protein. Thus, the intake of protein must be adjusted in accordance with the proportion of the limiting amino acid to restore balance. Protein imbalance occurs when the need for the limiting amino acid is actually increased because the diet contains an excess of another amino acid. For example, by administration of one amino acid in a marginal nutritional state, it is possible to induce a relative deficiency of a second limiting amino acid, thus leading to decreased growth and function. Amino acid antagonism refers to a competition with an analogous dietary essential for the site of metabolic activity, thus preventing the normal reaction from going to completion. An example of this is arginine-lysine interaction. This type of antagonism is alleviated by supplementation with a structurally related amino acid, but is not prevented by supplementation with the most limiting amino acid in the diet as it would be in amino acid imbalance. Amino acid toxicity occurs when there is an excess of amino acids which have diverse metabolic interrelationships. The amino acids with diverse metabolic interrelationships (e.g., methionine, tyrosine, tryptophan, and histidine) have greater toxicity than those with restricted catabolic pathways, e.g., branched-chain amino acids.

PROTEIN SYNTHESIS

The genetic control of protein synthesis has been summarized by Korner (3). Watson and Crick (4), on the basis of x-ray crystallography, showed that DNA is composed of two complementary helically coiled polynucleotide chains running in opposite directions and joined together by hydrogen bond linkages between bases: guanine base to cytosine base and adenine base to thymine base (G-C; A-T). At mitosis, each strand goes to one of the daughter cells and builds the complementary strand, thus reproducing genetic material of the mother cell. Mutation of one of the strands followed by pairing with appropriate nucleotide results in a new DNA form. Information stored by genetic material is transmitted to cell via formation of protein-synthesizing template. The whole purpose of the genetic apparatus is to supervise the synthesis of specific proteins, therefore, the cell is determined by the protein it contains. Each protein has a particular amino acid sequence with every molecule of that protein having the identical sequence, but errors may occur during biosynthesis, resulting in a certain amount of microheterogeneity. Each mammalian cell contains approximately 10,000 different types of protein.

By differential centrifugation of cell homogenates, it is possible to separate several components in the cell. Of importance to protein synthesis are the cell sap, microsomes, ribosomes, and endoplasmic reticulum. Microsomes are broken pieces of endoplasmic reticulum of cell which may have with them electron dense particles. These electron dense particles are the ribosomes which measure 15 nm in diameter and contain 50% RNA and 50% protein. Both microsomes and cell sap are necessary for amino acids to be incorporated into protein. Amino acids are assembled into the polypeptide chain in the ribosomes; the finished polypeptide chain is transferred from the ribosome via the lipoprotein membrane of the endoplasmic reticulum to the cell sap.

The steps in protein synthesis require activation of amino acids, transfer via soluble RNA (sRNA), and transfer to template RNA. Twenty amino acids are involved in protein synthesis, and there are 20 species of sRNA molecules which also are probably amino acid specific. The activation enzyme is also responsible for transfer of sRNA (Figure 4.4).

Pathological Changes in Protein Nutrition

Pathological changes in protein nutrition are conveniently considered under the following processes: abnormalities in the gastrointestinal tract, changes in intermediary metabolism associated with disease, conditions directly affecting the mechanism of protein synthesis, and changes in protein metabolism in individual organs and tissues. These categories will be considered briefly in the following discussion.

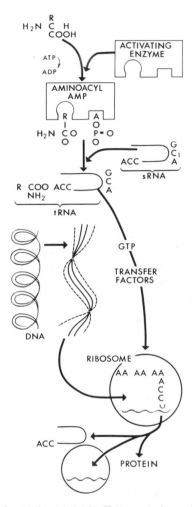

Figure 4.4. Process of protein synthesis. Twenty amino acids are involved in the synthesis of most proteins. They are glycine, alanine, valine, leucine, isoleucine, proline, phenylalanine, tyrosine, serine, threonine, aspartic acid, asparagine, glutamic acid, glutamine, arginine, lysine, histidine, methionine, cysteine, and tryptophan. Each amino acid has its specific activating enzyme, the amino acid becoming activated in the presence of ATP with the formation of aminoacyl-AMP on the surface of the enzyme. The complex is transferred to its specific sRNA in the cytosol (cytosol RNA is 10% of total cellular RNA). sRNA has a molecular weight of 20,000–35,000 and contains 75–100 nucleotides/chain. The amino acid is joined to sRNA at adenine if there are two adjacent cytosines. Template for protein synthesis is derived from DNA, and the mRNA in ribosomes is the site of synthesis. The sRNA identifies the template for its amino acid and, in the presence of GTP, GS-SG, and certain metal ions, the amino acid is attached to its site in the peptide chain. The finished protein is released via the rough endoplasmic reticulum. The cytosol sRNA re-enters that compartment unchanged.

Abnormalities in Gastrointestinal Tract   Disorders under this grouping cause impaired utilization of dietary protein or loss of protein from the gastrointestinal tract. The stomach functions as a holding organ regulating the transfer of foods. The process of digestion of proteins involves the release of oligopeptides and free amino acids by enzymatic action and their absorption by the intestinal mucosal cells by an active enzymatic process (Figure 4.2). Fecal excretion of nitrogen amounts of 0.5–2.0 g/day while the patient is on a diet of 60–100 g of protein. Malabsorption of amino acids may occur after gastrectomy, in pancreatic insufficiency of various etiologies, in pancreatic carcinoma, in congenital pancreatic fibrosis, in the presence of anatomic gastrointestinal lesions, and in idiopathic steatorrhea, sprue, celiac disease, and intestinal infections. Disorders which are associated with increased fecal nitrogen excretion usually cause increased fat excretion, but there are exceptions to this pattern. For example, in obstructive jaundice and hepatitis, there is an increased steatorrhea without azotorrhea, whereas, in ulcerative colitis, the excretion of nitrogen is increased while there is only slight steatorrhea.

In cystic fibrosis of the pancreas, there is a digestive defect wherein plasma amino acids increase after ingestion of a protein hydrolysate but fail to do so following a protein meal. In Hartnup disease, a gastrointestinal mucosal defect, as well as an associated defect in the renal tubules, is found. Unabsorbed tryptophan in the intestinal lumen is degraded to indole derivatives which are readily absorbed and excreted with resulting indoluria. In gluten sensitivity steatorrhea, high gluten peptides in the upper part of the small intestine may precipitate symptoms, and gluten products instilled further down into the lower ileum produce lesions typical of gluten enteropathy. In cystinuria, there is a competition between lysine, cystine, arginine, and ornithine for common absorptive sites. The unabsorbed amino acids in the gastrointestinal mucosa are degraded, resulting in the formation of agmatine from arginine, cadaverine from lysine, and putrescine from ornithine.

Under normal conditions, the proteins in the gastrointestinal lumen are derived from dietary sources and from proteins secreted into the lumen. These include mucins, enzymes, and traces of plasma proteins, amounting to approximately 35 g. Most of this is reabsorbed by the mucosal cells so that 0.5 g of protein nitrogen in the intestinal lumen is excreted. General protein loss may occur in tuberculosis of the intestines, ulcerative colitis, and carcinoma, often considerably in excess of 0.5 g of protein of nitrogen in 24 hr. Loss of plasma proteins into the gastrointestinal lumen may also occur in gastric carcinoma, hypertrophic gastritis, regional enteritis, ulcerative colitis, idiopathic steatorrhea, cardiac failure, constrictive pericarditis, and intestinal lymphangiectasia. A useful test in these conditions involves the intravenous infusion of [131]I- or chromium-labeled albumin and measurement of its fecal excretion. Normal individuals excrete <0.01% of the label by this route, whereas patients with the above types of enteric protein loss excrete amounts in excess of 0.78%. The fecal excretion of ^{131}I-polyvinylpyrrolidine given intravenously also serves as a measure of intestinal protein loss. Normal individuals excrete less than 1% of the test dose in 4 days, whereas the excretion is greater than 8% in patients with protein-losing gastroenteropathies.

Changes in Protein Metabolism Associated with Disease and Various Physiological States Physiological and pathological states affect protein metabolism by various mechanisms. The anabolic hormones, including growth hormone, testosterone, and insulin, increase the deposition of amino acid in tissue protein so that plasma amino acids are decreased in the presence of these hormones. The catabolic hormones include cortisol, thyroid hormone, estrogens, and progesterone. Cortisol, thyroid hormone, and estrogens (but not progesterone) activate deposition of protein and RNA in the liver and activate loss of carcass protein. Thyroid hormone and cortisol increase the turnover of serum albumin. Stress situations such as infections, injury, undernutrition, climatic stress, severe exertion, and psychological overstimulation are associated with increased activity of the catabolic hormones and their effects on protein metabolism. Protein loss may occur from skin disorders with desquamation. Normal loss of nitrogen by this process is about 1 g/day in the adult, but may increase to 3 g/day or more in desquamative disorders. Menstrual flow accounts for 0.3–0.6 g of nitrogen/day, and sputum in chronic bronchitis may amount to 1 g of nitrogen/day. Cutaneous burns may also cause considerable protein loss. Caloric undernutrition leads to a negative nitrogen balance which is exacerbated if there is an associated marked decrease in nonprotein foods. Obese subjects can maintain nitrogen equilibrium on caloric intakes which cause severe nitrogen loss in subjects with normal body fat. In neoplastic diseases, there is a translocation of nitrogen from the carcass to tumors, and plasma albumin is often decreased. Severe forms of this phenomenon lead to "malignant tumor cachexia." Protein undernutrition is associated with decreased resistance to stress, infections, and trauma. Protein deficiency without concurrent insufficiency of non-protein calories is termed kwashiorkor, whereas lack of both protein intake and calories leads to the state of marasmus.

Conditions Directly Affecting Mechanism of Protein Synthesis Defects in protein synthesis may be manifested in the following ways (Figure 4.5): 1) as defective enzyme protein synthesis as in the inherited metabolic disorders; 2) as alterations in amount of protein production, as in analbuminemia, hypogammaglobulinemia, and hemoglobinopathies; 3) as formation of a new and abnormal protein, as may occur in presence of viral DNA and RNA which may divert the pathways of normal synthesis;

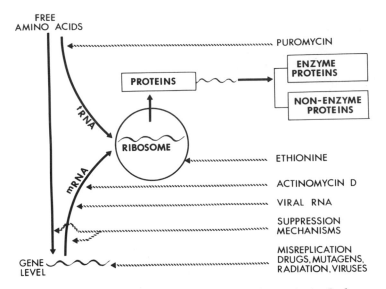

Figure 4.5. Abnormalities in the mechanism of protein synthesis. *Broken arrows* indicate inhibitory influences.

4) as the result of suppressor activity by which the cell has the capacity to suppress passage of a transcriptional message from the gene to ribosome through a mechanism which is itself genetically determined; and 5) as result of postgene control of protein synthesis. For example, the induction of the enzyme tryptophan pyrrolase by tryptophan is also activated by cortisol, but is blocked by actinomycin D and puromycin at two different sites. Another example of this phenomenon is a change in protein formation which follows substitution of a spurious message from an RNA virus.

Changes in Protein Metabolism in Individual Organs and Tissues There are several disorders of protein metabolism manifested by alterations in certain specific fractions of the body protein pool. These include the following: 1) diseases affecting plasma proteins such as analbuminemia and multiple myeloma; 2) diseases of the liver (such as hepatic cirrhosis where the postprandial elevation of plasma amino acids after protein ingestion is greater and more prolonged than normal—this elevation is a reflection of decreased protein synthesis and decreased entrance of ammonia into the urea cycle); 3) renal diseases such as uremia which is related to decreased glomerular filtration rate, aminoacidurias caused by reabsorption defects in the tubules, and proteinuria in which reabsorption of increased filtered protein is not sufficient to compensate for the increased loss through the glomerulus; 4) disorders of the reticuloendothelial (RE) system affecting antibody protein production. Antibodies are produced by the RE system, e.g., lymphocytes, and circulate as γ-globulins. The levels of these globulins may increase in infections, autoimmune disorders, and in other pathological states. A pathological overproduction of plasma cells in multiple myeloma is accompanied by increased levels of certain globulin fractions; 5) diseases of collagen metabolism are associated with alterations in the levels of certain amino acids (for example, the amino acid hydroxyproline, which is a component of collagen and elastin, is decreased in pituitary dwarfism and increased in acromegaly, in certain bone disorders, and, occasionally, in the Marfan syndrome); and 6) diseases of muscle, such as muscular dystrophy, are associated with increased protein turnover.

DISORDERS OF AMINO ACID METABOLISM

More than 40 conditions associated with increased excretion of amino acids have been described (Tables 4.1, 4.2, and 4.3). These are conveniently classified as prerenal or overflow aminoacidurias (which encompass the general metabolic disorders leading to increased amino acid levels in the plasma, with resultant aminoaciduria) and renal aminoacidurias (caused by defects in renal transport mechanisms). In these disorders, the plasma amino acids are normal.

Prerenal aminoacidurias are classified as congenital and acquired.

Congenital Prerenal Aminoacidurias

Clinical Disorders of Glycine Metabolism   Glycine has more metabolic fates than any other amino acid (5). It is a key substrate for creatine, porphyrins, and constitutes 25% of gelatin, collagen, and elastin. About 1 g of glycine/day is utilized in several conjugation reactions, e.g., with benzoate to form hippuric acid, with bile acids (glycocholate), and with salicylates, steroids, and bromsulfalein. Dietary intake in the U. S. is approximately 3–5 g. The glycine pool is 80 mg/kg, and the turnover rate is 1 mg/kg/24 hr, i.e., the glycine pool turns over 10–12 times in 24 hr. The plasma glycine level is 1 mg/100 ml at age 5–14 years, and 0.65 mg/100 ml in children <5 years. CSF glycine is approximately $1/10$ of plasma value.

Serine is the principal source of nondietary glycine, the conversion being mediated by the enzyme serine aldolase (serine hydroxymethylase) in the liver in the presence of pyridoxine and tetrahydrofolate. Glycine is also formed from the degradation of threonine and from glyoxylate. The metabolic fates of glycine are: 1) pyruvic acid via serine, 2) condensation with succinyl-CoA in presence of a cytosol enzyme to form α-amino-β-ketoadipic acid which is converted to δ-aminolevulinic acid (DALA), 3) condensation with acetyl-CoA by a mitochondrial enzyme to form

Table 4.1. Defects in Amino Acid Metabolism Associated with Neurological Symptoms

Disease	Clinical features	Biochemical defect and findings
Hyperglycinemia Ketotic	Vomiting, lethargy, retardation associated hypogammaglobulin and thrombocytopenia; leucine in diet induces ketosis. Treated by decreased dietary protein	Propionyl-CoA carboxylase; block in conversion of glycine→serine; elevated plasma glycine; ketosis
Non-ketotic	Defective growth; seizures; spastic paraplegia	Biochemical defect unknown; hyperglycinemia and hyperglycinuria, ? hyperoxaluria
Sarcosinemia	Mental retardation; death <1 year	Decreased sarcosine dehydrogenase; ↗ sarcosine in blood and urine
Hyperprolinemia	Deafness, seizures, cerebral dysfunction (renal disease)	↓ Proline dehydrogenase; elevated plasma and urine proline
Phenylketonuria	Mental deficiency in infancy; convulsions, muscle hypertonicity, tremors, hypertension, dermatitis	Phenylalanine hydroxylase deficiency; increased phenylalanine in plasma, increased urine phenylpyruvic acid; associated tryptophan defect
Familial dysautonomia (Riley-Day)	Decreased or absent tears; poor motor coordi-	Dopamine β-oxidase; decreased VMA:

Table 4.1. *continued*

Disease	Clinical features	Biochemical defect and findings
	nation; difficulty swallowing; breath-holding; hypertension; shock; hypersensitivity to epinephrine and norepinephrine	HVA:VMA ratio to urine 4 or greater
Familial goitrous cretinism	Physical and mental retardation; with deafness (Pendred's)	Biosynthetic defects in thyroid: dyshormonogenesis, concentration, organification or coupling defects
Congenital tryptophanuria	Physical and mental retardation; dwarfism; cerebellar ataxia; photosensitivity	Defect in conversion of tryptophan to kynurenine
Hartnup (hereditary pellagra)	Hereditary pellagra-like skin rash with temporary cerebellar ataxia, constant renal amino aciduria and other bizarre biochemical features	Defective transport of neutral amino acids; increased urinary neutral amino acids; indoles, decreased nicotinamide synthesis
Hyperhistidinemia	Moderate mental retardation; speech defect caused by short auditory memory span	Histidine deaminase; increased histidine in plasma; increased keto-acids in urine; positive ferric chloride and phenistix tests

continued

Table 4.1. *continued*

Disease	Clinical features	Biochemical defect and findings
Hyperammonia disorders Carbamyl synthetase deficiency	Lethargy caused by increased ammonia; Rx: low protein	Carbamylphosphate deficiency; increased ammonia
Ornithine transcarbamylase deficiency	Lethargy, failure to thrive, stupor, cerebral atrophy, retardation; Rx: low protein diet helps	Ornithine transcarbamylase deficiency: increased ammonia in blood and CSF; increased ammonia and glutamine in CSF
Argininosuccinic acid synthetase deficiency	Vomiting, seizures; mental deterioration; low protein diet helps	Argininosuccinic synthetase deficiency: increased ammonia and citrulline in plasma and CSF
Argininosuccinase deficiency	Severe retardation, seizures, ataxia, nodularity of hair	Decreased liver, brain, and RBC argininosuccinic acid in plasma and urine; PP rise in ammonia
Lysine intolerance	Stupor, lethargy secondary to increased ammonia	Lysine depresses arginase activity in these patients; increased serum ammonia after protein (lysine) diet
Hyperlysinemia	Hypotonia, seizures; may be normal	Increased plasma and urine lysine; biochemical defect unknown
Isovaleric acidemia (sweaty feet syndrome)	Recurrent acidosis, coma, un-	Defect in isovaleryl-CoA de-

Table 4.1. *continued*

Disease	Clinical features	Biochemical defect and findings
	usual urine and body odor	hydrogenase → increased plasma and urine isovaleric acid; short-chained fatty acids
Hypervalinemia	Vomiting, failure to thrive, nystagmus, mental retardation	Defect in valine transaminase, increased blood and urine valine, no increased keto acids
Methylmalonic acidemia	Autosomal recessive; metabolic acidosis, irritability, pallor, apnea, flaccidity-coma, hepatomegaly, and mental retardation, respiratory failure early in infancy	Defect in isomerase converting MMCoA to succinyl-CoA; vitamin B_{12}-dependent: keto-acidosis, increased MMA, increased glycine and ammonia
Homocystinuria	Autosomal recessive; mental retardation in 50%; light complexion, growth failure, ectopia lentis, optic atrophy, glaucoma may occur; seizures, schizophrenic reaction; abnormal EEG	Defect in cystathione synthetase; increased homocysteine and homocystine in plasma and urine; positive cyanide-nitroprusside test
Cystathionuria	Autorecessive; occasional mental	Defect in cystathionase; in-

continued

Table 4.1. *continued*

Disease	Clinical features	Biochemical defect and findings
	retardation and convulsions	creased cystathione (may be pyridoxine dependent)
Sulfite oxidase deficiency	Familial disorder; bilateral ectopia lentis; multiple neurological abnormalities; death at <3 years	Decreased sulfite oxidase → increased S-sulfocysteine, sulfite, and thiosulfate
Hyperlaninemia	Intermittent cerebellar ataxia and choreoathetosis	Decrease in pyruvate decarboxylase; increased serum alanine, lactate, and pyruvate
Hyperbetaalaninemia	Seizures starting at birth; somnolence	β-alanine α-ketoglutarate transaminase is decreased; increased plasma and urine β-alanine and β-aminoisobutyric acid; increased urine γ-aminobutyric acid
Carnosinemia	Grand mal and myoclonic seizures; mental retardation; dysrythmia on EEG; autosomal recessive; death at <2 years	Deficiency of carnosinase; increased serum and urine carnosine; increased CSF homocarnosine
β-Hydroxyisovaleric aciduria and β-methylcrotonylglycinuria	Similar to infantile spinal muscular atrophy; urine smells like that of a cat	? Defect in methylcrotonyl-CoA carboxylase: increased β-hydroxyisovaleric acid and β-methylcrotonylglycine

Table 4.2. Hereditary Aminoacidopathies

Catabolic defect	Amino acids involved
Best detected by plasma studies	
Phenylketonuria	Phenylalanine
Hyperphenylalaninemia	Phenylalaine
Hypertyrosinemia	
Neonatal	Tyrosine
Hereditary	Tyrosine, methionine
Tyrosinosis	Tyrosine
Tyrosinemia	Tyrosine
Hyperhistidinemia	Histidine
Branched-chain ketoaciduria (maple syrup urine)	Leucine, isoleucine, valine
Intermittent branched-chain ketoaciduria	Leucine, isoleucine, valine
Hypervalinemia	Valine
Homocystinuria	Homocystine and methionine
Hypermethioninemia	Methionine
Hyperglycinemia (nonketotic)	Glycine
Sarcosinemia	Sarcosine
Hyperprolinemias	Proline
Hydroxyprolinemia	Hydroxyproline
Diseases of urea cycle	Glycine, ammonia, glutamine, ornithine citrulline
Hyperlysinemia	Lysine; arginine; glutamine
Best detected by urine studies	
Cystathionuria	Cystathione
β-Aminoisobutyric aciduria	β-AIB
Hyperbetaalaninemia	β-Alanine
Carnosinemia	Carnosine
Detection possible in plasma and urine	
Hyperprolinemia	Proline
Hyperbetaalaninemia	β-Alanine
Hyperlysinemia	Lysine
Defect in reactive transport site with detection in urine only	
Cystinuria	Cystine and dibasic amino acids
Hypercystinuria	Cystine only
Renal iminoglycinuria	Proline, OHP, and glycine
Hartnup	Neutral monoamino acids, monocarboxylic acids (except amino acids and glycine)
Blue diaper syndrome	Tryptophan
Methionine malabsorption	Methionine
Inhibition of transport process with detection best in urine	
Fanconi syndrome	Generalized aminoacidurea plus other solutes
Oculocerebrorenal syndrome	Generalized
Busby syndrome	Generalized

Table 4.3. Other Renal Aminoacidurias

Generalized type	Associated tubular defect
Hepatolenticular degeneration	Glucose, phosphorus, uric acid
Galactosemia	Phosphorus
Vitamin D deficiency	Phosphorus
Vitamin D-resistant rickets	Phosphorus
Scurvy	Tyrosine
Congenital renal tubular Acidosis (Lightwood syndrome)	
Poisons: lead, cadmium; DNB, uranium fluoride	
Lactosuria and aminoaciduria of infancy	Lactose
Familial hypolipidemia	Indole
Severe potassium depletion	
Salicylate intoxication	
Congenital fructose intolerance	
Sickle cell anemia	
Pernicious anemia	
Thalassemia	
Progeria	
Specific aminoacidurias	
Cadmium poisoning	Threonine, serine
Pregnancy	Histidine
Hereditary pancreatitis and pancreatitis	Lysine, leucine

α-amino-β-ketobutyric acid which is converted to aminoacetone. Amino acetone is degraded to NH_3 and CO_2.

Clinical Disorders with Hyperglycinemia Non-ketotic hyperglycinemia is an inborn error of metabolism characterized by a large accumulation of glycine in the blood and cerebrospinal fluid. An increased excretion in the urine is also noted. Plasma levels provide the best diagnostic data. Clinical features include severe mental retardation, hypotonia, myotonic seizures, grand mal convulsions, and spastic cerebral palsy. This disorder is usually fatal in the early months of life. The metabolic defect is in the glycine decarboxylase reaction which converts glycine to CO_2, NH_3, and a tetra-hydrofolate derivative (Figure 4.6). No effective therapy is known for this disorder. Treatment with methionine to provide 1-carbon groups is followed by lowered glycine levels, but it is too early to assess the clinical response.

Hyperglycinemia is also found transiently in methylmalonic aciduria. This disorder is discussed with branched chain aminoacidurias. The hyperglycinemia found in carbamylphosphate deficiency is discussed under disorders of urea cycle enzymes. Hypersarcosinemia is a rare disorder

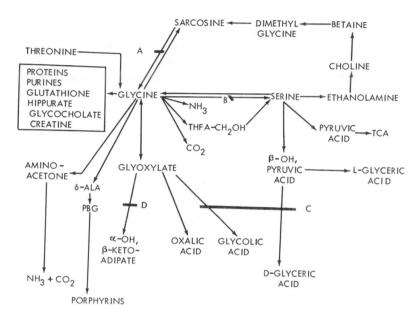

Figure 4.6. Glycine metabolism with locations of the biochemical lesions in clinical disorders of glycine metabolism. *A,* sarcosine dehydrogenase is deficient in sarcosinemia; *B,* glycine decarboxylase is deficient in non-ketotic hyperglycinemia; *C,* D-glycerate dehydrogenase, deficient in type II hyperoxaluria; *D,* glyoxylate: α-ketoglutarate carboligase, defective in type I hyperoxaluria.

transmitted by an autosomal recessive gene with variable expressivity. Clinical features include slight mental and motor retardation, but this is not invariably present. Plasma levels of sarcosine are elevated, as are levels of glycine and, occasionally, serine. The metabolic defect is probably due to deficiency of sarcosine dehydrogenase (Figure 4.6).

Primary Hyperoxaluria and Oxalosis Primary hyperoxaluria (6) describes autosomal recessive disorders characterized by a continuous excess synthesis of oxalic acid from glyoxylate. The three sources of glyoxylate are glycine (and serine), glycolic acid, and, to a lesser extent, ketohydroxyglutarate derived from hydroxyproline. The reaction from glycoxylic acid to glycine is enhanced by pyridoxal phosphate. Glyoxylic acid is reversibly derived from glycolic acid by the action of glyoxylic acid oxidase which is found in the liver, kidneys, and other tissues. This interconversion may also be catalyzed by lactic dehydrogenase. Glyoxylate may also be irreversibly decarboxylated to α-hydroxy-β-ketoadipate by the enzyme ketoglutarate: glyoxylate carboligase (3), and it is also oxidized to oxalic acid (Figure 4.6). Oxalic acid readily forms a salt with calcium, and the salt has low solubility at neutral or alkaline pH. Small amounts of oxalic acid may be derived from ingested ascorbic acid. Two forms of hyperoxaluria are recognized, type I or primary oxaluria which is also termed glycolic aciduria, and type II oxaluria with glyceric aciduria.

Type I primary oxaluria or glycolic aciduria is characterized by an increased excretion of oxalic acid and glycolic acids. Clinical manifestations include growth retardation, recurrent calcium oxalate nephrolithiasis, and nephrocalcinosis progressing to renal insufficiency and uremia. Symptoms of renal calculi may start at less than 5 years of age, and the disorder may progress to death by age 20 years. Crystal accumulation in joints may cause arthritis. Cardiac symptoms may be caused by oxalate crystal accumulation in the conduction system. Accumulation of oxalate crystals in several organs is termed oxalosis. The metabolic defect in primary oxaluria has been identified as deficiency of a ketoglutarate: glyoxylate carboligase, which is a soluble enzyme normally found in liver, kidney, spleen, and other tissues. The accumulation of oxalate crystals occurs in several organs, including bone marrow.

Type II primary oxaluria with glyceric aciduria (6) is characterized by nephrocalcinosis and nephrolithiasis similar to type I. There are excessive amounts of oxalic acid and L-glyceric acids in the urine. The metabolic defect (Figure 4.6) is secondary to a deficiency of the enzyme D-glyceric dehydrogenase, an enzyme normally present in liver, kidney, spleen, leukocytes, and other tissues. The disorder may be detected by a decrease in the leukocyte enzyme activity. This enzyme may be identical with glyoxylate reductase. An increased synthesis of oxalate from glyoxylate has been ascertained. The reduction of β-hydroxypyruvate to D-glycerate is coupled normally to the reduction of glyoxylate to glycolic acid, and hydroxypyruvate to L-glyceric acid, with resultant hyperoxaluria and L-glyceric aciduria.

Therapy includes measures to inhibit oxalate synthesis for which pyridoxine in large doses has been employed with some success. This vitamin decreases the glyoxylate pool by increasing its transamination back to glycine or by decreasing the deamination (oxidation) of glycine to glyoxylic acid. The solubility of calcium oxalate is increased by the use of magnesium and phosphate to permit excretion. Renal transplantation is helpful in patients with nephrocalcinosis and renal failure.

Disorders of Histidine Metabolism Histidine is not an essential amino acid in human nutrition and the daily requirement is about 35 mg/kg body weight. The amino acid has several metabolic fates (Figure 4.7). It is concentrated in keratohyaline granules in the skin and has been implicated in the keratinization process. Histidase (α-deaminase) is absent in the skin of squamous and basal cell carcinoma, but is increased in benign skin tumors. Urocanic acid derived from histidine serves as a sun screen. The derivative of histidine formiminoglutamic acid is important in 1-carbon transfer in nucleoprotein synthesis.

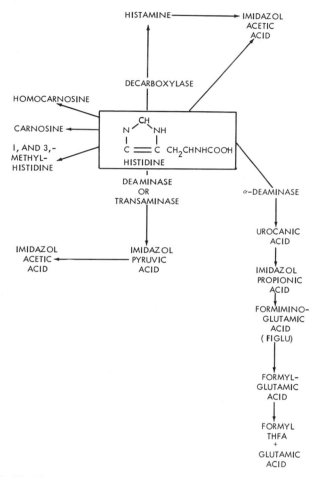

Figure 4.7. Histidine metabolism. Histidinemia is caused by a defect in the enzyme histidine α-deaminase.

Hyperhistidinemia is a rare recessive familial disorder which is due to a defect in histidine α-deaminase. Fifty percent of patients with this disorder are mentally retarded, and this manifestation is ascribed to a short memory span. Fifty-four cases have been described, and, in most, patients are under 8 years of age. Increased plasma and urine histidine is found in this disorder, but it is not diagnostic as such levels are also found in pregnancy, cerebromacular degeneration, and renal tubular acidosis. The phenistix and ferric chloride tests in the urine are positive in this disorder, but definitive diagnosis is made by finding decreased enzyme in skin and liver. No definitive therapy is available for hyperhistidinemia.

Clinical Disorders of Aromatic Amino Acid Metabolism The meta-

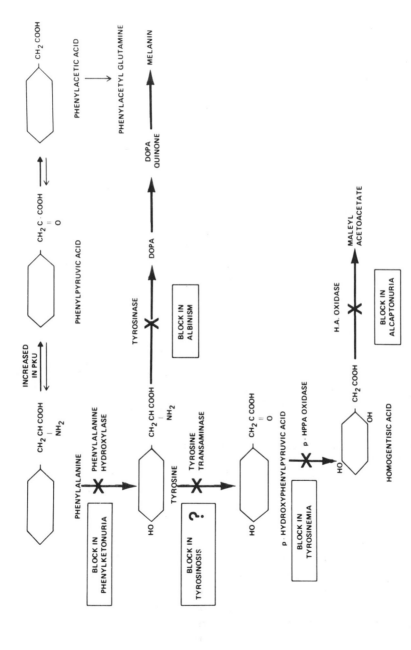

Figure 4.8. Aromatic amino acid metabolism with locations of biochemical defects in their metabolism.

bolic pathways of aromatic amino acids (7) are presented in Figure 4.8, in which the biochemical lesions in the amino acidopathies are indicated.

Tyrosinosis is a rare disorder caused by a deficiency of the enzyme p-hydroxyphenylpyruvic acid oxidase which converts p-hydroxyphenyl-pyruvic acid to homogentisic acid. The disorder is characterized by a persistent excretion of p-hydroxypyruvic acid. No treatment is needed in this disorder.

Tyrosinemia is a congenital disorder characterized by congenital cirrhosis, renal tubular defect, phosphatemia, hyperphosphaturia, and vitamin D-resistant rickets. The afflicted infants exhibit failure to thrive, vomiting, diarrhea, dyspnea, hemorrhage, edema, ascites, and hepatosplenomegaly. The acute form of this disorder is noted by the 1st month of life, with death occurring by 3–8 months. A chronic form of this disorder starts later, and the children live longer. Afflicted subjects exhibit glycosuria, proteinuria, and aminoaciduria. The metabolic block in this disorder is in the transaminase which converts tyrosine to p-hydroxy-phenylpyruvic acid. Treatment of this condition requires ingestion of proteins with decreased tyrosine and phenylalanine.

Phenylketonuria is an hereditary disorder which is found in approximately 1/25,000 Northern European births. Affected infants appear normal at birth. Soon there is mental retardation with delayed milestones and locomotor problems. Muscular hypertonicity, adventitious hyperkinesis, and seizures may occur. Microcephaly, eczema, enamel hypoplasia, hypertension, and hyperpigmentation are prominent features. Chemical features include the occurrence of excessive amounts of phenylalanine in the plasma, cerebrospinal fluid, and urine. There is also an accumulation of phenylacetic, phenyllactic, and phenylpyruvic acids. An associated secondary defect in tryptophan metabolism results in decreased nicotinic acid and decreased serotonin. Indican and indolepyruvic acid accumulate. Plasma tyrosine and catecholamine levels are decreased. The metabolic defect resides in the hepatic deficiency of phenylalanine hydroxylase. The ferric chloride test in the urine is positive. Therapy requires early institution of a diet low in phenylalanine.

Alcaptonuria is an autosomal recessive disorder which is often first detected by discoloration of the diapers. The disorder is caused by a deficiency of homogentisic acid oxidase which is normally present in the liver and kidneys. The defect is manifested by increased urinary homogentisic acid. Retained homogentisic acid leads to formation of homogentisic acid melanin. In adult life, there is discoloration of the connective tissues, ochronosis, and arthritis. Ochronotic arthritis is characterized by narrowing and calcification of the intervertebral discs. Ochronotic nephritis has also been reported in these patients. A low protein diet has been tried with limited therapeutic success.

Albinism is characterized by cutaneous and ocular manifestations. The ocular manifestations include poor vision, photophobia, horizontal nystagmus, astigmatism, and the iris may be blue, pink, or red. The cutaneous manifestations include albinism, keratosis, and melanoma, and the hair may show albinism. The clinical forms of the disorder are the generalized form inherited as an autosomal dominant characteristic and the ocular form transmitted as an X-linked trait. The disorder is caused by a deficiency of the enzyme tyrosine hydroxylase. In one form of albinism caused by decreased availability of tyrosine, the enzyme level may be normal. Albinism is found in 1 in 5,000–25,000 births. The diagnosis is made on clinical grounds, and therapy involves protection of iris of the eyes.

Familial dysautonomia (Riley-Day syndrome) is an autosomal recessive disorder found almost exclusively in Ashkenazic Jews, and it is estimated to be present in 1 in 10,000–20,000 births. Clinical features include feeding and swallowing difficulty with associated regurgitation and aspiration. By age 3–4 years, there is a lack of tearing, relative insensitivity to pain, emotional lability, breathholding, episodic vomiting, unexplained fever, skin blotching, excessive sweating, and motor incoordination. There may be erratic temperature control, orthostatic hypotension, and paroxysmal hypertension. Patients show a marked hypersensitivity to epinephrine and norepinephrine. By the age of 10 years, a marked kyphoscoliosis is noted, and growth is poor. A typical facies with transverse mouth and facial drooping is present, and the patient exhibits cerebellar ataxia, lacks the gag reflex, and has a nasal voice. Charcot neuropathic joints may also be present. A classic clinical sign in these patients is the absence of the triple response to scratching. The patient shows only a thin red line without a flare. Twenty-five percent of this group of patients die by age 10 years, and 50% by age 22 years.

The pathological process involves autonomic, sensory, hypothalamic, brain stem, autonomic ganglia, and the central nervous system. The metabolic basis of this disorder is a deficiency in dopamine β-oxidase which converts dopamine to norepinephrine. Increased catecholamine levels are found in the blood and urine because of the accumulation of dopamine. The urinary vanilmandelic acid (VMA) is decreased, whereas the homovanillic acid (HVA) level is increased. Zetterstrom's syndrome is a disorder in which decreased catecholamine effects are noted after hypoglycemic challenge. The mechanism of this disorder is not known, but adrenal medullary insufficiency is considered to occur in these patients. These patients do well on ephedrine therapy.

Clinical Disorders of Tryptophan Metabolism The alternative metabolic fates of tryptophan are presented in Figure 4.9. Under normal conditions, the 5-hydroxylation of tryptophan to 5-hydroxytryptophan,

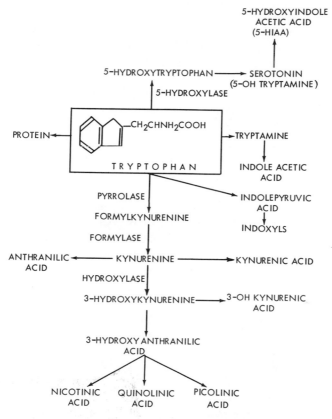

Figure 4.9. Pathways of tryptophan metabolism. Clinical disorders are described in the text.

the precursor to serotonin (5-hydroxytryptamine), utilizes 1% of dietary tryptophan. In the carcinoid syndrome, about 60% of tryptophan is utilized by this pathway, with resulting increased serotonin and decreased nicotinic acid levels. The decreased level of nicotinic acid produced from this substrate is the basis of pellagra in some patients with carcinoid syndrome. This hydroxylation step is also decreased on phenylketonuria, resulting in decreased serotonin and disturbed brain function. Congenital tryptophanuria is the basis of dwarfism, physical and mental retardation, photosensitivity, and cerebellar ataxia. It is ascribed to a defect in tryptophan pyrrolase activity.

Hartnup Disease (Hereditary Pellagra) Hartnup disease is a "hereditary pellagra-like skin rash with temporary cerebellar ataxia, constant renal amino aciduria and other bizarre biochemical features" (8) which is transmitted by a rare autosomal allele. Patients with this disorder have a skin rash, indistinguishable from pellagra, which may be red, scaly, dry, or weeping, and occurring intermittently. Inconstant and reversible episodes of cerebellar ataxia, chronic headaches, fainting, delirium, emotional instability, and increased or decreased intelligence are characteristic findings. These symptoms may be precipitated by fever, stress, sunlight, sulfa therapy, and poor nutrition. The chemical features include increased excretion of: monoamino monocarboxylic, amino acids with neutral or aromatic side chains; branched-chain amino acids (leucine, valine, and isoleucine); aromatic amino acids (tryptophan, phenylalanine, and tryosine); hydroxyamino acids (serine, theronine); and histidine, alanine, asparagine, and glutamic acid. These aminoacidurias are caused by increased renal clearance approximating the glomerular filtration rate. The mixed aminoaciduria is the only consistent feature of this disorder and is the only certain diagnostic test. Tryptophanuria is the basis of decreased nicotinamide and the symptom of pellagra but without nutritional deficiency, particularly if cutaneous and psychiatric symptoms are accompanied by cerebellar signs. Amelioration of the disorder comes with adulthood. For treatment, an increased protein diet may be helpful. The skin manifestations respond to nicotinic acid therapy.

Metabolic Disorders Involving Urea Cycle   Amino nitrogen in mammalian organisms is in dynamic equilibium. The various processes involved are transamination, deamination, and reamination. Deamination results in release of ammonia which is gotten rid of via reutilization in protein synthesis via reversal of the deamination reaction, incorporation into glutamine, aspartate, carbamylphosphate, and glycine, and, eventually, the synthesis of purines and pyrimidines, formation of glutamine from ammonia and glutamic acid in the presence of ATP. Glutamine is responsible for 60% of ammonia in the urine, but this is only a small part of ammonia kinetics. The conversion of ammonia to urea takes place largely in the liver and, to a lesser extent, in the central nervous system. The reaction in the kidneys requires citrulline supplied from plasma. The liver is the only organ with the complete urea cycle. The enzymes involved in the urea cycle are: carbamylphosphate synthetase, ornithine transcarbamylase, argininosuccinic acid synthetase, argininosuccinase, and arginase. Details of this cycle are presented in Chapter 1.

Argininosuccinic acid synthetase is the rate-limiting enzyme in this cycle, followed in order by argininosuccinase and carbamylphosphate synthetase. In defects in this cycle, the serum ammonia levels may increase considerably (compared with normal values of less than 70 μg/100 ml.). This is caused by decreased urea synthesis. In addition, in chronic hepatocellular disease, portosystemic shunting diverts ammonia from the cycle. A significant ammonia pool comes from bacterial action in the gastrointestinal tract.

Clinically recognizable syndromes (9) not explainable by liver disease are found in: carbamylphosphate synthetase deficiency, ornithine transcarbamylase deficiency, argininosuccinic acid synthetase deficiency, argininosuccinase deficiency, and congenital lysine intolerance where there is an interference with arginase action. Hyperammonemia may also occur in lysine dehydrogenase deficiency, hyperglycinemia, and defective intestinal and renal transport of dibasic amino acids and ornithine.

Carbamylphosphate synthetase deficiency is characterized by episodic vomiting, dehydration, and lethargy, precipitated by a high protein intake. The disorder is characterized by hyperammonemia. Fatty infiltration of the liver and hyperlipidemia are also found in this disorder. Liver biopsy in this disorder reveals decreased carbamylphosphate synthetase. One patient showed an associated defect in glycolysis cycle enzymes. Therapy with a low protein diet may lead to some improvement.

Ornithine transcarbamylase deficiency is characterized by failure to thrive, episodic vomiting, screaming, lethargy, slow development, stupor, seizures, cortical atrophy, and abnormal electroencephalographic changes. Hyperammonemia in plasma and cerebrospinal fluid is characteristic. Cerebrospinal fluid glutamine is also elevated. The disorder may be found in offsprings of consanguineous marriages. Therapy with a low protein diet has been somewhat helpful, but three out of eight patients have died thus far.

Argininosuccinic acid synthetase deficiency is characterized by postprandial hyperammonemia and citrullinemia. Neurological manifestations include vomiting, seizures, and mental deterioration. Cyclic neutropenia is often seen. The plasma and cerebrospinal fluid show increased levels of citrulline. It is likely that there is a defect in urea synthesis in the central nervous system in this disorder. The urine shows a positive Ehrlich's aldehyde test. A low protein diet may be helpful. It is likely that thyroid hormone therapy may also be helpful as the enzyme is inducible by thyroxine.

Argininosuccinic aciduria is a disorder that has been found in over 20 patients, often in siblings. Two clinical patterns are recognized. In the early onset type severe retardation, seizures, ataxia, abnormal electroencephalogram (EEG), nodularity of the hair (trichorrhexis nodosa), hepatomegaly in early months, and early deaths are characteristic. In the late onset type slow development, seizures, intermittent ataxia, and occasional survival to adulthood are known. Serum and urine argininosuccinic acid are elevated. Postprandial hyperammonemia is characteristic. Argininosuccinic acid, normally absent in the urine, is found in large amounts. Cerebrospinal fluid argininosuccinic acid exceeds plasma concentration by four times. Dietary management with low protein diet started early may be helpful.

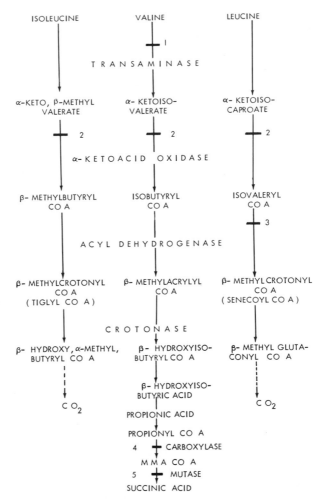

Figure 4.10. Metabolism of branched-chain amino acids with locations of the bio-chemical defects in clinical disorders. *1* is site of defect in hypervalinemia, *2* locates the defect in maple syrup urine disease, *3* is site of defect in isovaleric aciduria, *4* is site of defect in neonatal ketoacidotic disorder, and *5* is site of the defect in methylmalonic aciduria.

Arginase deficiency has been described in two sisters with spastic diplegia and seizures. In these patients, erythrocyte arginase levels were found to be low and hyperammonemia was a characteristic finding. Congenital lysine intolerance may be associated with decreased arginase activity. Hyperammonemia may also occur in lysine dehydrogenase deficiency, hyperglycinemia, and in defective intestinal and renal transport of dibasic amino acids and ornithine.

Clinical Disorders of Branched-Chain Amino Acid Metabolism The metabolic pathways of the amino acids isoleucine, leucine, and valine are presented in Figure 4.10.

Hypervalinemia is characterized by vomiting, lethargy, and mental and physical retardation. The disorder is secondary to a defect in the transamination of valine. A low valine diet has been tried in the management of this disorder.

Maple syrup urine disease exists in the classic and intermittent forms, both of which are inherited as autosomal recessive characteristics. The disorder is reported to occur 1 in 300,000 live births. The clinical manifestations include vomiting, hypertonicity, flaccidity, apnea, and convulsions. The neurological manifestations are ascribable to the accumulation of metabolities in the central nervous system rather than to the enzyme defect per se. The changes in the central nervous system include the presence of spongy white matter, gliosis, and defective myelination. A maple syrup odor of body and urine is noted. The disorder is caused by decreased levels of α-ketoacid oxidase, with resultant branched-chain ketoacidosis. The ketoacids may be detected by a positive dinitrophenylhydrazine reaction. Treatment consists of a decrease of dietary amino acids to basal level.

Isovaleric aciduria is inherited as a rare autosomal recessive trait. Accumulation of short-chain fatty acids leads to metabolic acidosis and neurological manifestations. The disorder is also called the "sweaty feet syndrome" and should be suspected in an acutely ill patient with unexplained acidosis and strange smell. The disorder is caused by a defect in acyldehydrogenase with resulting impaired degradation of isovaleric acid which comes from leucine. This disorder is the first type of aminoacidemia not identified by amino acid screening of urine by the ninhydrin reaction. The plasma isovaleric acid may be 1,500 times normal. Treatment includes a low protein diet and special measures to prevent debility and infections.

Deficiency of propionyl-CoA carboxylase results in a ketoacidotic state in neonates which is lethal unless treated with alkali and low protein diet.

Deficiency in the mutase system which converts methylmalonic acid (MMA) to succinic acid is responsible for a ketoacidosis. The disorder is inherited as an autosomal recessive trait. One form is vitamin B_{12}-dependent. The form nonresponsive to the vitamin is caused by a defect in the production of an apoenzyme for MMA-CoA mutase. Clinical features in both forms include irritability, pallor, apnea flaccidity, coma, and respiratory failure in infancy. The patient also exhibits hepatomegaly and mental retardation. A megaloblastosis is found in the B_{12} responsive form. Therapy includes a low protein diet, with the use of B_{12} injections in the responsive form.

Metabolic Disorders of Sulfur Amino Acids   In mammals, the need for sulfur is met by sulfur-containing amino acids L-cysteine, L-cystine, and methionine, and by the vitamins biotin and thiamin. The structures of these amino acids and their related metabolities are presented below.

```
                                                                Adenine
                                                                  |
CH3                                                             Ribose
 |                                                                |
SH            SH          S- - - -S                               S
 |             |          |       |                               |
CH2           CH2        CH2     CH2         SH                   CH2
 |             |          |       |           |                    |
CH2           CH2        CH2     CH2         CH2                   CH2
 |             |          |       |           |                    |
HC NH2        HC NH2     HC NH2 HC NH2       HC NH2               H C NH2
 |             |          |       |           |                    |
COOH          COOH       COOH   COOH         COOH                 COOH

Methionine   Homocysteine    Cystathione    Cysteine    S-Adenosylmethionine
```

In addition to being constituents of proteins, the sulfur amino acids participate in many vital biochemical systems. For example, because methionine is an important methyl donor, it is involved in the synthesis of choline, acetylcholine, creatine, and epinephrine. Cysteine is involved in synthesis of glutathione, coenzyme A, and taurine. Inorganic sulfate from sulfur amino acids is involved in the synthesis of sulfated mucopolysaccharides and other conjugated sulfur esters. The end products of sulfur amino acids are involved in diseases, e.g., fetor hepaticus is caused by accumulation of methyl mercaptan as a result of abnormal methionine metabolism. Accumulation of inorganic sulfate contributes to metabolic acidosis in renal failure.

The transsulfuration pathway describes the mechanism whereby methionine and homocysteine are precursors of cystine. The process involves activation of methionine to S-adenosylmethionine. The subsequent steps involve S-adenosylhomocysteine to homocysteine and adenosine. Homocysteine may be converted to methionine to homocystine or to H_2S and α-ketobutyrate, or it may, in the presence of cystathione synthetase, form cystathione which is later cleaved to cysteine and serine. There is a high content of cystathione in the brain. Cysteine may be converted to cystine or may be incorporated into glutathione. Other pathways include cysteine sulfinic acid (oxidation of sulfhydryl group) or taurine or hypotaurine. Taurine is involved in bile activity. Cysteine may also be transaminated to mercaptopyruvate or desulfhydrated to pyruvate and H_2S. Sulfite is oxidized to sulfate by enzyme sulfite oxidase. These transformations (9) are depicted in Figure 4.11 which also presents the inherited disorders of sulfur amino acid metabolism: homocystinuria, cystathionuria, cystinosis, and sulfite oxidase deficiency.

Homocystinuria is an autosomal recessive trait in which the clinical

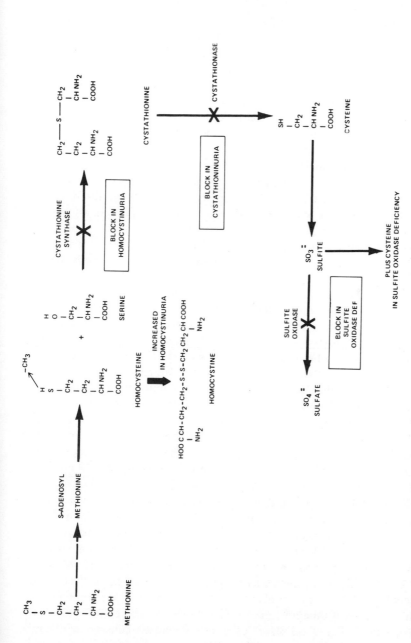

Figure 4.11. Sulfur amino acid metabolism with the sites of defects associated with clinical disorders identified. The clinical disorders are described in the text.

phenotype exhibits growth failure and light complexion. One-half of the patients may have mental retardation. Cutaneous manifestations include wide pores, telangiectasis with aging and malar flush with livedo reticularis. The patients exhibit a flat-footed gait, pectus excavatum, and arachnodactyly. Some patients have been kyphoscoliotic. Ectopia lentis is the most common abnormality, with secondary myopia, optic atrophy, glaucoma, and retinal detachment. Cardinal vascular signs are arterial and venous thromboses, and carotid and coronary occlusions; gangrene and hypertension are also prevalent. The patients may have occasional seizures, schizophrenic reaction, and may often have abnormal EEG findings. The pathological process includes thin media of coronary, carotid, iliac, and renal arteries in which the muscle fibers are separated by overgrowth of ground substance. The metabolic defect is a deficiency of the enzyme cystathione synthetase which catalyzes the conversion of homocysteine to cystathione. Diagnosis of this disorder is made on the basis of positive cyanide nitroprusside test on the urine. Treatment with a diet low in methionine, high in cystine, supplemented with pyridoxine may be helpful.

Cystathionuria is inherited as an autosomal recessive trait. Clinical manifestations include mental retardation in some patients, various endocrinopathies, e.g., diabetes insipidus. The patients may also exhibit convulsions, anemia, thrombocytopenia, and nephrogenic diabetes insipidus. Phenylketonuria may be an associated abnormality. The chemical defect in this disorder is a deficiency of cystathionase. This enzyme catalyzes the conversion of cystathione to cysteine, the only function of cystathione being the transfer of sulfur from methionine to cystine. Affected patients may have 0.2–0.6 mg of cystathione/100 ml of serum, whereas there are no detectable amounts in normal subjects. The amino acid may be detected in the urine in excessive quantities. Therapy with pyridoxine is followed by decreased cystathione levels without marked clinical improvement.

Cystinosis is an autosomal recessive inherited disorder in which the patients have an inability to maintain cysteine in the reduced form. Two clinical forms are recognized. The childhood form is characterized by vitamin D-resistant rickets, chronic acidosis, polyuria, dehydration, growth failure, cystine deposition in the kidneys, and death before 10 years of age. In the adult form, the patients complain of headaches and burning and itching of the eyes. Corneal cystine deposits may lead to photophobia. In this form, renal function is not affected, and the adult form does not limit longevity. The diagnosis of cystinosis should be considered in any child with vitamin D-resistant rickets, Fanconi syndrome, or glomerular insufficiency. No specific therapy is available for this disorder.

Sulfite oxidase deficiency is a familial disorder characterized by bilateral ectopia lentis, multiple neurological abnormalities, and death at less than 3 years of age. The serum and urine contain increased amounts of S-sulfocysteine, sulfite, and thiosulfate, but no sulfate.

Clinical Disorders of Imino Acid Metabolism (9)   Hydroxyprolinemia has been described in one patient with an accumulation of free hydroxyproline (OHP) in plasma and urine. OHP serves one known function. This disorder may be a basis for mental retardation and is caused by deficiency of "OHP oxidase" which oxidizes hydroxyproline D'-pyrroline-3-hydroxy-5-carboxylic acid (HPC) as follows:

$$\text{OPH} \xrightarrow{\text{``OHP oxidase''}} \text{HPC} \xrightarrow{\hspace{2cm}} \text{glyoxylic acid}$$

Bound OHP is elevated in the urine of patients with the Marfan syndrome, rapid growth, and in other conditions of rapid collagen turnover.

Hyperprolinemia is an autosomal recessive disorder characterized by increased plasma proline and increased excretion of proline, glycine, and OHP. The urine levels depend on the excess in the plasma. Two types of this disorder are described, viz., type I with deafness and, rarely, retardation, but several are asymptomatic. The biochemical defect is a deficiency of proline oxidase. Type II is characterized by central nervous system disturbances, seizures, abnormal EEG, and mental retardation. The basic defect is a deficiency in pyrroline-5-carboxylic acid (PC) dehydrogenase. The reaction is presented below:

$$\text{Proline} \xrightarrow{\text{``proline oxidase''}} \text{PC} \xrightarrow{\text{dehydrogenase}} \text{glutamic semialdehyde}$$

In both disorders, the diagnosis requires chromatographic analysis of the urine. There are increased levels of proline in type I, and of proline and pyrroline-5-carboxylic acid in type II. Low protein diets have been tried without success in therapy of these disorders.

Hyperlysinemias   The principal end product of lysine is acetyl-CoA. Lysine is converted to saccharopine via lysine ketoglutaric reductase present in the liver, kidney, heart, adrenal, thyroid, brain, and skin. This amino acid also enters the pathway to citrulline and homoarginine. Lysine and ornithine are the most potent inhibitors of arginine, and competitive inhibition in man interferes with ammonia elimination via the urea cycle. A description of the clinical entities (10) associated with hyperlysinemia follows.

Periodic lysinemia with hyperammonemia was described in one 3-month-old female infant. The disorder is characterized by vomiting in the neonatal period which may progress to dehydration, coma, and spasticity. The EEG was diffusely abnormal and a challenge with lysine led to hyperammonemia and coma. Hereditary hyperlysinemia was described in a 14-year-old characterized clinically by abdominal pain, vomiting, ptyalism, profound muscle weakness, and lethargy.

Persistent hyperlysinemia is a rare metabolic abnormality characterized by hyperlysinemia and hyperlysinuria without ammonemia. The clinical features include mental retardation and retarded physical development in 50% of the patients, lax ligaments in 3/7, convulsions in 2/7, and abnormal EEG in 3/7. There is no episodic pattern in this disorder. Plasma and cerebrospinal fluid lysine is increased as is the urine lysine. Serum ammonia remains within normal limits. Mental retardation of unknown origin is the reason for screening for this disorder. Low protein diets have not been of benefit in therapy.

Clinical Disorders of β-Amino Acids β-Alanine is an insignificant fraction of free amino acids in plasma. The presence of free β-amino group is associated with inefficient membrane transport; hence, the renal clearance is high. β-Alanine is present mainly in the form of β-alanylhistidine or carnosine. Muscle tissue contains free β-alanine to carnosine in the ratio 1:500. β-Alanine is incorporated into pantothenic acid to form coenzyme A. β-Alanine is also derived from dihyrouracil:

$$O=C-CHCH_2 - COOH \xrightarrow[\text{aminase}]{\text{trans}} H_2N\,CH_2\,COOH \xrightarrow{\text{carnosinase}} \text{carnosine}$$

Hyperbetaalaninemia is a disorder found in one male infant. Clinical features included somnolence and seizures not controlled by anticonvulsant therapy. There was an increased excretion of β-aminoisobutyric acid, taurine, alanine, and β-aminobutyric acid. These compounds were also elevated in plasma and cerebrospinal fluid. It is presumed that the neurological disorder is largely caused by accumulation of γ-aminobutyric acid. Pyridoxine may possibly be a helpful therapeutic measure in this disorder.

Carnosinemia is an autosomal recessive disorder characterized by severe mental retardation, muscle twitching, myoclonic epilepsy, and dysrhythmia on EEG. Death occurs within 2 years. No definitive therapy is at hand.

β-Aminoisobutyric acid (β-AIB) is derived from stepwise degradation of the pyrimidine thymine. The aminotransferase system serves the transamination of β-AIB and β-alanine. Excessive urinary excretion of β-AIB is a common form of human polymorphism, being formed in 5–10% of Caucasians and in 95% of mongoloids. The basis of the disorder is prerenal. The high excretor trait is an autosomal recessive characteristic. Acquired high excretion of β-AIB is caused by limited capacity for β-AIB transformation. This occurs in conditions of tissue destruction, neoplastic diseases, leukemia, tuberculosis, liver diseases, march hemoglobinuria, and radiation. Splenectomy in thalassemia major is followed by a sharp decrease in AIB excretion.

Cystinuria Cystinuria is an inheritable disorder of the transepithelial transport mechanism in the renal tubule and gastrointestinal mucosal cell affecting the amino acid cystine as well as the dibasic amino acids lysine, arginine, ornithine, and cysteine-homocysteine mixed disulfides. It is inherited as a recessive characteristic in both sexes, with greater clinical severity in males. It is estimated that 1 in 250 people has increased cysteine in urine, with 1 in 100,000 homozygous for the trait. The disorder may be manifested over a wide age range, from 1 year to the 9th decade.

The major clinical manifestations include renal colic with renal infection, renal insufficiency, and hypertension as sequelae. Cystine stones which have a yellow-brown color and a maple sugar crystal surface form readily in acid urine. These crystals are firmer than uric acid and are radioopaque (because of sulfur) but are smoother and less dense than calcium stones on x-ray. Cystine stones may occur in staghorn formation or as multiple recurrent stones. Microscopic examination of urine may show the characteristic appearance of cystine crystals. The cyanide nitroprusside test also detects homozygous stone formers who excrete >250 mg/g of creatine. Cystinuria is occasionally associated with hyperuricemia, hemophilia, retinitis pigmentosa, muscular dystrophy, muscular hypotonia, mongolism, hereditary pancreatitis, and hypocalcemic tetany. Patients with cystinuria tend to be shorter than average as cystine is essential to fetal development.

The basic defects in cystinuria reside in the renal tubule and in the gastrointestinal mucosal cell. Excessive losses of cystine and dibasic amino acids occur with normal or below normal plasma levels of the amino acids. These amino acids share a common transport mechanism so that increasing the filtered load of one amino acid in the group reduces the reabsorption of the others in normal individuals. Glycine, methionine, cystathione, homocysteine, and cysteine disulfide may also be lost. Cystine excretion in cystinuria usually exceeds 250 mg/g of creatinine in the urine. Cystinuria is, thus, the classic example of a disorder of renal tubular function. In the gastrointestinal tract, cystine and dibasic amino acids share a common transport system. Three clinical types of cystinuria have been described, based on the relative severity of the renal and gastrointestinal defects.

Treatment of cystinuria includes the following measures: procedures to increase solubility of cystine by increasing fluid intake to 4–5 liters/day and increasing water intake at bedtime, attempts to increase urine pH to 7.15, and institution of penicillamine therapy. This is recommended in patients in whom conservative measures have failed, and who may have lost one kidney from calculus disease.

Acquired Disturbances in Amino Acid Metabolism

Premature and newborn infants tend to have a generalized aminoaciduria which is more pronounced in premature infants. In adults, the α-amino nitrogen accounts for 2% of total urinary nitrogen, but in newborns this may amount to 10%. Part of the aminoaciduria is caused by immature renal function, but may also be caused by metabolic defect since increased plasma AA are also found. Hydroxyproline and homocitrulline occur in the plasma of this group, but not in adults. Plasma tyrosine levels are higher in this period.

Aminoacidemia and aminoaciduria may occur in conditions of excessive tissue destruction, e.g., burns, postoperative state, diabetic ketoacidosis, severe infections, leukemia, and progressive muscle dystrophy.

Liver disease is frequently associated with a metabolic aciduria. In milder cases, this is a reflection of impaired deamination of amino acids by liver; in massive liver necrosis, it is also secondary to breakdown of liver tissue. Most frequently there is a rise in several amino acids, but in some cases specific amino acids may be elevated, e.g., cystine alone or with β-aminoisobutyric acid, methylhistidine, or phosphoethanolamine. This pattern is more characteristic of cirrhosis and fatty metamorphosis. In acute liver failure, there is a massive generalized aminoaciduria. Aminoaciduria of hepatolenticular degeneration (Wilson's disease) is both metabolic and renal. Renal involvement occurs early because of copper deposition in the renal tubules. The metabolic derangement occurs later when liver damage supervenes.

Kwashiorkor refers to a severe protein deficiency which leads to an abnormal pattern of plasma amino acids. In incipient deficiency, several unessential amino acids (alanine, proline, histidine, serine, taurine, and aspartic acid) are increased whereas levels of essential amino acids (tyrosine, arginine, citrulline, and α-amino-n-butyric acid) tend to be depressed. In more severe depletion states, all of the plasma amino acids are depressed. Branched-chained amino acids are particularly depressed.

LITERATURE CITED

1. Munro, H. N. 1964. A general survey of pathological changes in protein metabolism. *In* H. N. Munro and J. B. Allison (eds.), Mammalian Protein Metabolism. Vol. 2, pp. 267–319. Academic Press, New York.

2. Harper, A. E. 1964. Amino acid toxicities and imbalances. *In* H. N. Munro and J. B. Allison (eds.), Mammalian Protein Metabolism. Vol. 2, pp. 87—134. Academic Press, New York.

3. Korner, A. 1964. Protein biosynthesis in mammalian tissues. *In* H. N. Munro and J. B. Allison (eds.), Mammalian Protein Metabolism. Vol. 1, pp. 177—242. Academic Press, New York.

4. Watson, J. D., and F. H. C. Crick. 1953. Molecular structure of nucleic acids. Nature 171:737—738.

5. Nyhan, W. L. 1972. Nonketotic hyperglycinemia. *In* J. B. Stanbury, J. B. Wyngaarden, and D. S. Frederickson (eds.), The Metabolic Basis of Inherited Disease. 3rd Ed., pp. 464—471. McGraw-Hill Book Co., New York.

6. Williams, H. E., and L. H. Smith. 1968. L-glycericaciduria, a new genetic variant of primary oxaluria. N. Engl. J. Med. 278:233—239.

7. Holt, L. E., Jr., and S. E. Snyderman. 1964. Anomalies of amino acid metabolism. *In* H. N. Munro and J. B. Allison (eds.), Mammalian Protein Metabolism. Vol. 2, pp. 321—372. Academic Press, New York.

8. Baron, D. N., C. E. Dent, H. Harris, E. W. Hart, and J. B. Jepson. 1956. Hereditary pellagra-like skin rash with temporary cerebellar ataxia, constant renal amino aciduria, and other bizarre biochemical features. Lancet 2:421.

9. Rosenberg, L. E., and C. R. Scriver. 1969. Disorders of amino acid metabolism *In* P. K. Bondy (ed.), Diseases of Metabolism, pp. 366—516. W. B. Saunders Co., Philadelphia.

10. Ghadimi, H. 1972. The hyperlysinemias. *In* J. B. Stanbury, J. B. Wyngaarden, and D. S. Frederickson (eds.), Biochemical Basis of Inherited Disease. 3rd Ed., pp. 393—403. McGraw-Hill Book Co., New York.

5

Clinical Disorders of Purine and Pyrimidine Metabolism

Purines and pyrimidines are organic bases which serve as substrates in the synthesis of nucleic acids and as end products from degradation of cellular nuclear material. Nucleic acids are polymers of nucleotides made up of ribose, phosphoric acid, and purine or pyrimidine bases. Two types of nucleic acids exist: 1) deoxyribonucleic acids (DNA) containing 2-deoxyribose (these transmit genetic information); and 2) ribonucleic acids (RNA) containing ribose (these are involved in all phases of protein synthesis). The organic bases in nucleic acids are either pyrimidines (cytosine, uracil, and thymine) or purines (adenine, guanine, and hypoxanthine). Nucleosides are made up of a base and a sugar linked through the N-glycoside bond (C–N) as depicted in Figure 5.1. Nucleotides are made up of a sugar, a base, and phosphoric acid in ester linkage. When the pyrimidine bases cytosine, uracil, and thymine are in nucleoside structures, they are, respectively, cytidine, uridine, and thymidine. Similarly, when the purine bases adenine, guanine, and hypoxanthine are present in nucleoside structures, they are called adenosine, guanosine, and inosine, respectively.

PURINE METABOLISM

The body pool of purines is derived from dietary purines and from cellular synthesis from smaller molecules. Dietary purines are released from their nucleotides by intestinal and pancreatic hydrolytic enzymes. The absorbed purines have several alternative biosynthetic fates whereby purine nucleo-

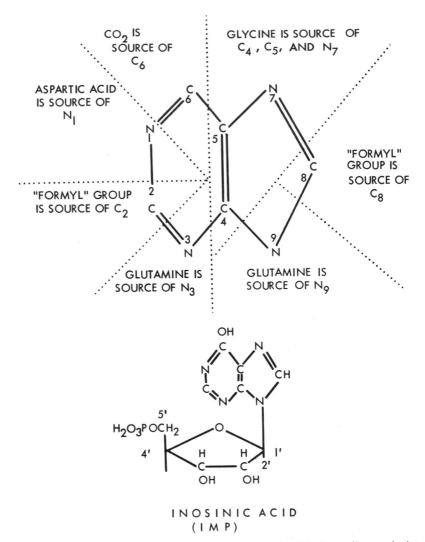

Figure 5.1. Sources of the components of the purine ring. The lower diagram depicts structure of a typical nucleotide. Note that the positions in the ribose component are numbered as *1′, 2′*, etc.

tides can be made in certain tissues. However, exogenous hypoxanthine, guanine, and xanthine are less readily incorporated into nucleic acids since they are subject to degradative reactions in the intestinal epithelium by enzymes such as guanase and xanthine oxidase to form uric acid. Serum uric acid levels are influenced to a small extent by dietary purine intake. Patients with hyperuricemia may exhibit a decrease of serum uric acid of greater than 1 mg/100 ml when given a diet free of purines. In the synthesis of purine nucleotides, glycine contributes the skeletal carbons and nitrogens of the purine structure (Figure 5.1). The metabolic origins of the carbon and nitrogen atoms have been established by tracer studies (Figure 5.1). Ribose phosphate derived from the hexose monophosphate shunt (pentose phosphate pathway) is converted to phosphoribosyl pyrophosphate (PRPP) by transfer of the terminal pyrophosphate from ATP (1). PRPP is then utilized for the formation of phosphoribosylamine. PRPP has two possible alternative fates, viz., formation of imidazol acetic ribonucleotide or the formation of pyrimidine NAD and NADP. The first reaction unique to purine biosynthesis is the formation of phosphoribosylamine from PRPP, glutamine, and inorganic pyrophosphate. This reaction is committed to purine synthesis and it is subject to feedback control by adenine and guanine, the end products of the purine synthetic pathway. The formation of phosphoribosylamine is the determining reaction for de novo purine synthesis. Subsequent reactions (1) in the purine synthetic pathway are presented in Figure 5.2.

The purine biosynthetic, reutilization, and feedback pathways (2), as well as the formation of uric acid, are depicted in Figure 5.3. In the de novo synthetic pathway, ribose phosphate, amino acids, folic acid, and CO_2 contribute to the synthesis of inosinic acid. The indispensable step in this synthesis is the formation of PRPP. Beyond this biosynthetic intermediate the conversion to phosphoribosylamine (PRA) commits the pathway to the synthesis of inosine monophosphate (IMP) by an irreversible transferase reaction. This series of reactions completes the de novo purine synthetic pathway. Increased activity of this synthetic pathway is a cause of increased uric acid formation and the basis of hyperuricemia in some forms of gout.

In the reutilization pathway, purine bases released from the de novo pathway as well as from ingested nuclear material are converted to their nucleotides. This pathway requires the presence of PRPP and the appropriate phosphoribosyltransferase (PR-transferase), such as adenine-phosphoribosyltransferase (A-PR-transferase) and hypoxanthine-guanine-phosphoribosyltransferase (HG-PR-transferase). This reutilization pathway is of considerable quantitative importance in incorporating purines into further synthesis and diverting them from excess uric acid formation. For example, in the entity xanthinuria, where there is decreased degradation of xanthines to uric acid, hypoxanthine is utilized for nucleic acid synthesis to the extent of about 1 g daily. Purine reutilization may be achieved by reversal of the nucleoside phosphorylase reaction, and a purine base and ribose 1-phosphate form a nucleoside which is subsequently converted to ribonucleotide by a kinase reaction. An alternative and quantitatively quite significant mechanism of reutilization involves the direct reaction of

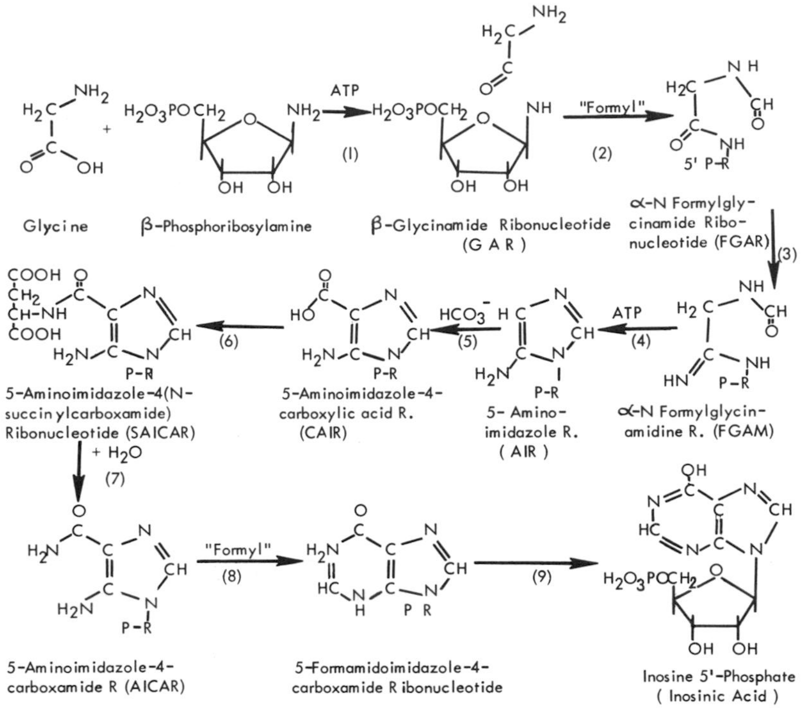

Figure 5.2. Synthesis of the purine ring showing detailed steps, cofactors, and substrates involved.

the purine base with PRPP in the presence of the appropriate phosphoryl-transferase, e.g., A-PR-transferase and HG-PR-transferase. A-PR-transferase converts adenine to adenylic acid (adenosine monophosphate, AMP) and HG-PR-transferase catalyzes the transfer of ribose 5-phosphate moiety of PRPP to hypoxanthine and guanine to form, respectively, inosinic acid (IMP) and guanylic acid (guanosine monophosphate, GMP). There are significant clinical disorders which may result from defects in the reutilization pathways, e.g., the Lesch-Nyhan syndrome which is second-ary to complete HG-PR-transferase deficiency.

In the purine degradation pathway, the free purines of endogenous origin or from the diet are degraded to xanthine, e.g., guanine converts to xanthine. Hypoxanthine and xanthine are oxidized to uric acid by the enzyme xanthine oxidase which is present in greatest abundance in the liver and intestinal mucosa. Degradation of endogenous purines accounts for 600–700 mg of uric acid in the normal adult man, whereas the degradation of dietary purines to uric acid accounts for less than one-half of this amount.

The de novo purine synthetic pathway is controlled by feedback

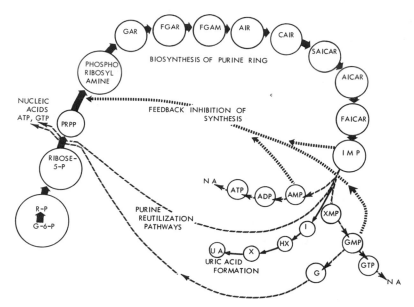

Figure 5.3. Purine biosynthetic, feedback, and reutilization pathways. The negative feedback pathway is depicted as *broken lines*. For abbreviations, see Figure 5.2.

inhibition (Figure 5.3), by which the end products of the pathway inhibit the activity of PRPP-amidotransferase, the initial enzyme unique to, and rate limiting in, this pathway. AMP and GMP, end products of the synthetic pathway, may inhibit the amidotransferase activity at different allosteric sites whereby their effects may be additive. Additional, but minor, sites of feedback inhibition of the pathway exist. Purine and pyrimidine ribonucleotides may inhibit PRPP formation from ribose-5-P and ATP. Products of PR-transferase reactions may inhibit the reactions by competing for the side of attachment of PRPP to the enzyme surface.

Purine nucleotides may be inconverted by complex regulatory mechanisms, including both negative and positive feedback controls. For example, the conversion of IMP to AMP or GMP is subject to regulation by the availability of nucleotide triphosphate cofactors. IMP interconversion to AMP is inhibited by high concentrations of the latter, and the interconversion of IMP to GMP is inhibited by GMP.

URIC ACID: METABOLIC AND CLINICAL ASPECTS

Uric acid is the most highly oxidized purine compound. It is weakly acid, and, at plasma pH of 7.4, exists largely as monosodium urate (MSU). Uric acid is less water-soluble than MSU, and it may appear in acid urine. Uric acid remains soluble in plasma at the level of approximately 7 mg/100 ml, and above this level the solution is supersaturated. The uric acid pool in normal subjects is estimated to be 1,000 mg, and the metabolic turnover rate is 600 mg/day. Normal serum uric acid ranges from 6.9–7.5 mg/100 ml in males and 5.7–6.6 mg/100 ml in females. Two groups of gouty patients are recognized on the basis of uric acid pool size and turnover rates, viz., patients with pool size of 1,300 mg and a normal turnover rate and patients with a pool size of 2,400 mg with a turnover double the normal rate. Serum uric acid is excreted mainly through the renal route, to the extent of 66–75%. The bulk of remainder is discharged into the gastrointestinal tract where it is degraded by enzyme of the bacterial flora. Small amounts of serum uric acid may be degraded by verdoperoxidase in leukocytes.

Renal Clearance of Uric Acid

The processes involved in uric acid clearance are glomerular filtration, tubular reabsorption, and tubular secretion. Uric acid and other organic acids are freely filtered at the glomerulus. Reabsorption in the proximal convoluted tubule, as well as over the rest of the nephron, and secretion by the tubular epithelium follow. The relative rates of reabsorption and secretion are largely dependent on the pK_a of uric acid, pH of the tubular fluid, and the rate of urinary flow. (pK_a is the pH at which the compound is equally distributed between the ionized and unionized states.) Ionized organic acids are less freely diffusible. Despite ready filtration of uric acid, the clearance is less than 10% that of inulin. It is estimated that at least 90% of filtered uric acid is reabsorbed. The normal estimated rate of uric acid reabsorption is 15 mg/1.73 m^3/min.

There are data to suggest that reabsorption is more important than secretion in uric acid excretion. Uricosuric drugs at low doses inhibit both secretory and reabsorption mechanisms. The drug pyrazinamide has been shown to selectively inhibit the secretion mechanism. Some studies indicate that 98% of filtered urate is reabsorbed, and most of the uric acid appearing in urine is secreted. The 2% that escapes reabsorption represents 20% of total excretion; hence, secretion accounts for the remainder of uric acid excreted. The fraction of the filtered load is relatively constant, but the secretory process responds to variations in uric acid. The concentration of uric acid in the renal tubular lumen is, therefore, the result of dominance of one mechanism over the other.

Plasma uric acid levels increase relatively slowly as glomerular filtration rate (GFR) decreases. Patients with mild to moderate renal impairment (creatinine clearance less than normal but greater than 15 ml/min) retain a relatively normal uric acid secretory mechanism, responding appropriately to the serum uric acid. When the GFR drops below 10 ml/min, the filtered load of urate drops markedly, and the secretory mechanism becomes defective. Hyperuricemia results, despite a decrease in reabsorptive capacity. In some patients with gouty arthritis, urate clearance is decreased because of an inability of the secretory site to respond normally to a given uric acid load.

Drug Effects on Purine Synthetic, Reutilization, and Degradation Pathways

Several patterns of drug effects (4–6) on the purine metabolic pathways have been described, and some of these have been applied in clinical situations. Xanthine oxidase is inhibited by 6-pteraldehyde and by purine analogues such as allopurinol. Allopurinol decreases uric acid formation from purine precursors. These precursors inhibit PRPP-transferase by the feedback pathway, hence resulting in a decreased de novo purine synthesis. The amidotransferase which is responsible for the synthesis of phosphoribosylamine is affected by several pharmacological agents. The compounds 4-amino-5-imidazole carboxamide and adenine-8-C support the feedback inhibition of amidotransferase. These agents also possibly deplete intracellular PRPP. Azathioprine is partly converted to 6-mercaptopurine which may function as an inhibitor of purine synthesis. Similarly 6-thioguanine, 8-azaguanine, 6-mercaptopurine ribonucleotide acid, and 6-mercaptopurine ribonucleoside inhibit purine synthesis.

GOUT AND HYPERURICEMIC STATES

Gout is a form of arthritis characterized by recurrent, paroxysmal, acute attacks of severe inflammation usually involving a single peripheral joint, followed by complete remission. The inflammatory reaction is caused by a deposition of monosodium urate crystals in and about joints. The monosodium urate is derived from body fluids supersaturated with uric acid; hence, hyperuricemia is the principal biochemical requirement for gout. Hyperuricemia is either caused by increased synthesis of purine precursors of uric acid or by diminished renal excretion of normal or increased purine synthesis, or by a combination of both. Hyperuricemia is often asymptomatic throughout a lifetime, but between 15 and 25% of subjects with it may develop acute attacks of gouty arthritis. The causes of gout are presented in Table 5.1. Most patients with the classic manifestations are considered to have primary gout. Secondary gout develops as a complication of the other diseases. Primary gout constitutes 4–5% of arthritis patients, and it is estimated that 0.27–0.30% of the general population have gout. It is most likely that the disorder is of polygenic inheritance. The incidence is higher in certain racial groups, such as Filipinos and the Maoris of New Zealand. A much greater incidence is seen

Table 5.1. Causes of Hyperuricemia and Gout

I. Idiopathic gout: familial and non-familial
II. "Secondary" gout and/or hyperuricemia
  A. Hematological disorders
    1. Hemolytic diseases
    2. Myeloproliferative disease
  B. Endocrine defects
    1. Hypothyroidism
    2. Hypoparathyroidism
    3. Hyperparathyroidism
  C. Vascular diseases
    1. Hypertension
    2. Myocardial infarction
  D. Renal disease
    1. Glomerulonephritis and pyelonephritis
    2. Lead poisoning (late effect)
III. Hereditary diseases
  A. With excessive purine synthesis
    1. Glycogenosis I (glucose-6-phosphatase deficiency)
    2. X-Linked deficiency of hypoxanthine-guanine phosphoribosyltrans-
      ferase
      a) Complete (Lesch-Nyhan)
      b) Incomplete (with gout)
  B. Possible phosphoribosyl pyrophate amidotransferase deficiency
  C. Mental retardation with autistic behavior
  D. Encephalopathy
  E. With decreased renal uric acid clearance
    1. Hereditary nephropathy
    2. Glycogenosis I
  F. Down's syndrome
  G. Pitressin resistant nephrogenic diabetes insipidus
  H. Obesity, starvation, psoriasis, idiopathic hypercalciuria
IV. Drug-induced hyperuricemia and/or gout
  Pyrazinamide
  Diuretic drugs
  Salicylates at some dosages

in males, but postmenopausal females may also be subject to gout. While hyperuricemia is the essential biochemical component of gout, the duration and degree of the elevation are important factors. There is a general correlation of hyperuricemia with intelligence and achievement, suggesting that this is a reflection of response of such subjects to stresses of environment. Some studies suggest an autosomal dominant form of inheritance, but it is more likely caused by polygenic familial factors. A few cases of X-linked transmission have been reported. Several epidemio-logical studies have shown that hyperuricemia is a major factor in the precipitation of gout. It is also known, however, that several other factors may be involved in its development. These include variations of protein binding of urates which may explain differences in gout incidence in patients with comparable levels of serum uric acid.

No single cause for hyperuricemia has been identified in primary hyperuricemia. Excess synthesis of uric acid is responsible for the hyperuricemia in about 10% of gouty patients with myeloproliferative disorders. Excess purine synthesis is the basis of increased levels of uric acid in about 30% of hyperuricemic patients. In other patients, diminished renal excretion, in the presence of normal synthesis, is responsible for hyperuricemia. In most patients, a combination of the above pathogenetic factors is probable.

The natural history of primary gout evolves essentially in three forms. In mild cases, the manifestations are limited to a few acute attacks throughout a lifetime. Severe cases present a fulminating course, starting early, with essentially an unremitting course to eventual renal insufficiency. Most patients experience a milder course which is intermediate between the two extremes. Gout generally evolves through the following stages: hyperuricemia, followed by acute gouty arthritis, which may progress to chronic tophaceous gout, which may be associated with gouty or hyperuricemic nephropathy. Previous impressions that uric acid nephropathy was the most common cause of death in patients with gout are only partly true. Probably about 50–60% of patients, especially with mild to moderate gout, die of cardiovascular or cerebrovascular disease. Another disorder which is strongly correlated with gout is hypertension, but the mechanism of the association is not clear.

ACUTE GOUTY ARTHRITIS

An acute attack of gouty arthritis is the presenting symptom indicating transition from the stage of essential hyperuricemia to gout. The sudden attack is usually monarticular in a peripheral joint, usually the first metatarsophalangeal joint occurring in 50% of cases. (Eventually this joint is involved in 90% of patients with gout.) Within a few hours the patient experiences excruciating and incapacitating pain, swelling, erythema, red shiny skin, and heat over the joint. Associated systemic findings include fever and leukocytosis. The skin may later develop a violaceous hue and dilated veins. Ordinarily the first attack subsides within 2 weeks even if untreated. A symptomatic period of intercritical or interval gout is characterized by persistent hyperuricemia. Repeated recurrence of acute arthritis usually involving the same joint is the rule. More severe cases may have polyarticular involvement and, in extremely severe cases, the intercritical period is essentially nonexistent. With recurrent attacks, there are residual changes in the affected joints, consisting of stiffness, swelling, and chronic pain, with x-ray evidence of tophaceous deposits.

Mechanism of Acute Gouty Arthritis

While hyperuricemia and monosodium urate monohydrate formation are essential requirements for gouty arthritis, there are additional factors which are necessary for the deposition of monosodium urate crystals. Phagocytosis of urate crystals by leukocytes of synovial fluid is a most important pathogenetic component. The activation of Hageman factor, which subsequently activates kinins, is involved as an initial step (Figure 5.4). Accumulation of uric acid itself does not initiate this pattern of events. Neither does a solution of monosodium urate induce the inflammatory reaction of acute gouty arthritis. The presence of micro-crystals of monosodium urate is essential to this process. The predominant occurrence of the gouty arthritis in relatively avascular joints suggests a major metabolic component in this reaction. Local metabolic factors and lactate and pH changes are important in the initiation and progression of the inflammatory process (Figure 5.4).

Precipitating factors in gouty arthritis include changes in host reaction, lowering of threshold of the inflammatory reaction, and changes in the size and aggregration of crystals. Surgical operations and trauma lead to a nonspecific response and increased anaerobic glycolysis with generation of lactic acid which alters the local pH. Other factors include emotional upsets, violent exercise, ketonemia of starvation and ethanol excess leading to ketonemia, lactic acidemia, and decreased pH. Acute ACTH, pyrazin-amide, and antihypertensive therapy may also precipitate hyperuricemia. Mercurial diuretics, decholin, vitamin B_{12} , thiamin, and administration of liver extract may all precipitate increased uric acid levels, thus increasing the potential for precipitation of acute gouty arthritis.

Tophaceous Gout

The appearance of tophaceous gout, which may be quite slow, is indicated by progression to a phase of gross and excessive storage of urates caused by the inability of the patient to excrete the rapidly synthesized uric acid. In primary gout, this is probably caused by decreasing excretory mechanisms, but, in secondary forms, it is ascribable to increased formation of urates. About 40% of patients with gout develop tophi within 5 years after the initial attack, 60% within 10 years, with a slow increase in occurrence thereafter. The most common site of visible tophi is in the great toe. Other common areas of involvement are the ear lobes, the elbows, the heels, and the knees. Removal of a few drops from the deposit for microscopic examination reveals the presence of monosodium urate

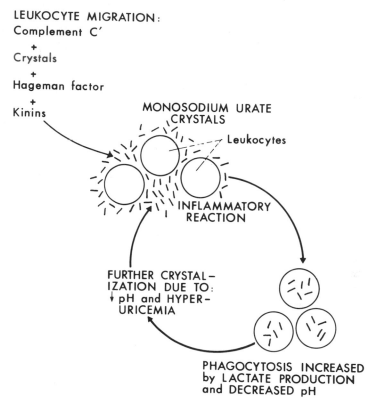

LEUKOCYTE MIGRATION:
Complement C′
+
Crystals
+
Hageman factor
+
Kinins

MONOSODIUM URATE
CRYSTALS

Leukocytes

INFLAMMATORY
REACTION

FURTHER CRYSTAL-
IZATION DUE TO:
↓ pH and HYPER-
URICEMIA

PHAGOCYTOSIS INCREASED
by LACTATE PRODUCTION
and DECREASED pH

Figure 5.4. Mechanism of the acute inflammation in gout. Details are given in the text.

crystals. Rarely, subcutaneous tophi may develop after several years of hyperuricemia. X-ray changes of tophaceous gout are the characteristic punched-out areas of affected joints caused by presence of radiolucent urates.

Approximately 20% of patients with gout develop uric acid nephrolethiasis which may be in the form of gravel, small calculi, or staghorn calculi. Gouty nephropathy is one of the common causes of severe morbidity and of mortality in gout. Renal damage results from small to large tophi in the kidneys.

HEREDITARY DISEASES WITH HYPERURICEMIA

Hyperuricemia is found in several relatively rare inborn diseases of metabolism. In glycogen storage disease I (classic von Gierke's disease), there is an absence or deficiency of the hepatic enzyme glucose-6-

phosphatase, which is normally responsible for conversion of hepatic glucose 6-phosphate to glucose. These patients are subject to hypoglycemia as a result of the deficiency. Increased lipolysis leads to increased fatty acids and ketone bodies. The patients also are subject to lactic acidemia. These factors all compete with the uric acid for renal excretion. In addition, the presence of high intracellular levels of glucose 6-phosphate eventually leads to overproduction of PRPP, which is substrate for increased purine synthesis.

The most severe excess of the de novo synthetic pathway for purine synthesis is found in the Lesch-Nyhan syndrome (3), which is an X-linked disorder with specific enzyme defect. The deficiency of the enzyme hypoxanthine-guanine phosphoribosyltransferase (HG-PR-transferase) occurs in all body tissues of the affected patients. The enzyme is essential for the reutilization of hypoxanthine and guanine through combination with PRPP. This enzyme, which is normally present in greatest amounts in the basal ganglia of the brain, is absent in these areas in the afflicted patients. The nonutilization of PRPP in this synthesis results in its intracellular accumulation and induction of increased amidotransferase activity, and hence, an increase in purine synthesis. The clinical manifestations of this disorder include choreathetosis, spasticity, mental retardation, and a compulsive aggressiveness and self-destructiveness. These patients may compulsively bite through their lips, tongue, and fingers while being fully aware of their actions. They often ask to be restrained to prevent the self-destructiveness.

Incomplete HG-PR-transferase deficiency is the basis of a hyperuricemia state found in a small number of patients. There is a direct correlation with the degree of enzyme deficiency and the severity of the clinical manifestations which include hyperuricemia, neurological dysfunction, and severe gouty arthritis. The degree of gouty arthritis and nephropathy is more severe than in patients with primary gout. A defect in the feedback regulation of PRPP-amidotransferase by purines is responsible for increased purine synthesis and hyperuricemia in a small group of patients. Other hereditary causes of hyperuricemia are listed in Table 5.1. In hereditary nephropathy, and in conditions in which there is an accumulation of ketoacids (e.g., branched-chain ketoaciduria), or ketone bodies (e.g., glycogenosis I), hyperuricemia is the result of the decreased renal clearance.

SECONDARY HYPERURICEMIA

Hyperuricemia and acute gout attacks are often early indicators of an occult disorder. Approximately 10% of hyperuricemic patients have myeloproliferative disorders which include leukemias, multiple myeloma, polycythemia vera, secondary polycythemia, myeloid metaplasia, Waldenstrom's macroglobulinemia, lymphoblastoma, lymphosarcoma, Hodgkin's disease, hemolytic anemia, pernicious anemia, sickle cell anemia, thalassemia, and nontropical sprue. Other disorders associated with increased cellular proliferation (e.g., psoriasis) may also show hyperuricemia. Hyperuricemia is also found in myxedema, hypoparathyroidism, and in hyperparathyroidism, situations wherein there is decreased renal clearance of uric acid. Other disorders associated with hyperuricemia include pitressin-resistant diabetes insipidus and idiopathic hypercalciuria. The association of hyperuricemia with hypertension and other cardiovascular disorders was noted previously. Drug effects as causes of hyperuricemia have been discussed previously. Diuretic agents (except spironolactone and triamterene) decrease renal clearance of uric acid. Pyrazinamide suppresses tubular secretion of uric acid.

TREATMENT OF HYPERURICEMIA

The measures for treatment of hyperuricemia states in general are discussed in this section. The management of acute gouty arthritis is discussed in a subsequent section. It is essential to recognize that in idiopathic hyperuricemia the emphasis in therapy is management of hyperuricemia and its sequelae. In the secondary hyperuricemia states, therapeutic emphasis is directed to the underlying disorders. Management of hyperuricemia requires measures to decrease uric acid production, to increase uric acid excretion, or a combination of both. The measures to decrease uric acid production include dietary restriction of excessive purines and the use of the drug allopurinol. This drug serves as a substrate for and competition inhibitor of xanthine oxidase which catalyzes the reactions:

$$Hypoxanthine \rightarrow xanthine \rightarrow uric\ acid$$

In addition, the drug allopurinol is excreted as oxipurinol which is also an inhibitor of xanthine oxidase. Blockage of xanthine oxidase results in the accumulation of xanthine and hypoxanthine. These compounds deplete PRPP via the reutilization pathway with the result of decreased de novo synthesis of purines. Allopurinol may also utilize hypoxanthine-guanine phosphoribosyltransferase (HG-PR-transferase) to form allopurinol ribonucleotide. This product blocks the enzyme amidotransferase which is essential in the de novo synthetic pathway (Figure 5.3). These drug effects are depicted in Figure 5.5.

Measures to increase uric acid excretion include the induction of osmotic diuresis to increase urine volume, thereby increasing uric acid excretion, and the use of drugs that interfere with the tubular transport of

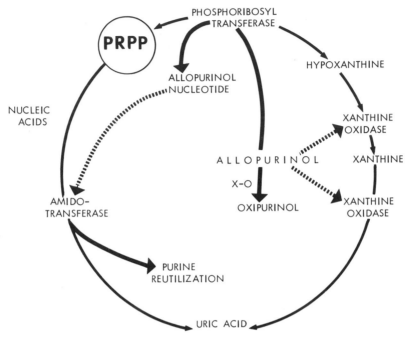

Figure 5.5. Mechanism of drug actions on hyperuricemia. Inhibitory pathways are depicted by *broken lines*. Allopurinol blocks the action of xanthine oxidase, thus decreasing uric acid formation from xanthine and hypoxanthine. The accumulated hypoxanthine may enter the reutilization pathway, but this step is also inhibited by the allopurinol nucleotide derived from the reaction of PRPP with allopurinol.

uric acid. Some drugs decrease tubular excretion of uric acid and, thereby, lower serum uric acid while others decrease tubular secretion and increase serum uric acid. Drugs that possess both activities usually affect secretion at low doses, and affect reabsorption at high doses, the latter being quantitatively more important. The drugs probenecid, sulfinpyrazone, phenylbutazone, and glucocorticoids act by the combined mechanism discussed above. In small doses, salicylate drugs inhibit secretion with resultant increased serum urate levels. Doses of salicylates >4 g daily induce uricosuria. The uricosuric agents do not decrease uric acid production. Alkalinization of the urine increases the excretion of uricosuric agents which are organic acids and fails to increase uricosuria. The uricosuric agents are contraindicated in the treatment of hyperuricemia associated with uric acid nephropathy.

Measures designed to reduce uric acid production and increase excretion of uric acid include the combined use of allopurinol and a uricosuric agent. It is important to note that the uricosuric agents also increase the excretion of oxipurinol which is derived from allopurinol.

Hence, this combination may occasionally result in reduction of the inhibition of uric acid production. The overproduction of uric acid associated with gout or uric acid nephropathy is best treated with allopurinol. Uricosuric agents should not be employed until the serum uric acid falls into the normal range. In addition, uricosuric agents are contraindicated as adjuncts to hypouricemic therapy in neoplastic diseases. The drug of choice in this situation is allopurinol.

TREATMENT OF ACUTE GOUTY ARTHRITIS

The drug of choice in treatment of the initial attack of acute gouty arthritis is colchicine. This drug is an alkaloid of complicated ring structure derived from the seeds and corms of *Colchicum autumnale.* The configuration of the side chains in the molecule confers its marked anti-inflammatory action. The drug given in appropriate dosages rapidly enters the polymorphonuclear leukocytes and inhibits their migration and random mobility. In an established attack of acute gouty arthritis, the patient is given 0.5–0.6 mg of colchicine hourly until therapeutic benefit is seen or gastrointestinal toxicity appears. The dose requirement is related to the severity of the symptoms and to body weight of the patient. With this regime the patient should have disappearance of symptoms within 12–24 hr or earlier. Thereafter, the patient should be essentially symptom free of gouty arthritis for several months. The dose effective in the initial attack may be employed in subsequent attacks. An alternative method of management, especially in patients who are unable to take the oral medication because of recent surgery or other procedures, is the intravenous infusion of colchicine. Because the intravenous administration of colchicine is not accompanied by gastrointestinal manifestations, the required dose may be given in a single intravenous injection over a 5-min period. In this manner, 3 mg is given with special care to avoid extravasation of the drug which is quite irritating to tissues.

Should colchicine fail to induce improvement, a rare event, the patient is treated with an anti-inflammatory agent such as phenylbutazone which is given at the dose of 600–800 mg the first day and 200–400 mg daily for the next 2 days. Because of the side effects from these drugs, they should be stopped on cessation of the acute attack. Occasionally intramuscular injections of ACTH are necessary to abort an attack of acute gouty arthritis. The required dose is usually 80–120 units daily for 2 or 3 days.

PROPHYLACTIC MANAGEMENT OF ACUTE GOUTY ARTHRITIS

It is prudent to institute a prophylactic program for patients with hyperuricemia and recurrent attacks of acute gouty arthritis. A program of prophylactic therapy with 0.5–1 mg of colchicine daily is recommended in patients with previous severe attacks. In some patients with asymptomatic hyperuricemia, colchicine chemoprophylaxis may prevent attacks permanently. The use of allopurinol and uricosuric agents is also an excellent prophylactic measure. It is important to recognize that the use of allopurinol may precipitate acute attacks of gouty arthritis in patients with hyperuricemia or tophaceous gout by mobilizing the stores of urates. It is prudent, therefore, to maintain the patient on small doses of colchicine for several months after institution of therapy, even until disappearance of tophi.

HEREDITARY XANTHINURIA

Hereditary xanthinuria is an autosomal recessive relatively benign disorder which is associated with hypouricemia and hypouricaciduria. Clinical manifestations include occurrence of xanthine crystals in the ureter, occasional muscle cramps, and synovitis caused by accumulation of xanthine and hypoxanthine in tissues. Xanthine crystals usually give a positive murexide test, and are of reddish brown color. Diagnosis is usually confirmed by duodenal or liver biopsy and assay for xanthine oxidase. Because of xanthine oxidase deficiency, there is decreased uric acid formation, but the accumulated hypoxanthine and xanthine fail to regulate purine synthesis via feedback suppression. There is, however, a substantial amount of hypoxanthine reutilization, with relatively little reutilization of xanthine or guanine. Treatment of this disorder requires a high fluid intake alkali therapy, restriction of dietary proteins, and the use of allopurinol which perhaps substitutes the more soluble hypoxanthine for the sparingly soluble xanthine.

CLINICAL DISORDERS OF PYRIMIDINE METABOLISM

Orotic acid is a dietary constituent present in milk and milk products. It is a highly insoluble pyrimidine compound and it is not readily absorbed. Active transport of this substance takes place in the small intestine. Dectectable levels have not been demonstrated in human plasma, and there is no tubular reabsorption of orotic acid, but drug-induced orotic aciduria is associated with decreased uric acid excretion, suggesting a competition for renal transport.

In vivo synthesis of this pyrimidine has been demonstrated in man and in bacteria. Carbamylphosphate is synthesized from the substrates CO_2 and NH_3 in the presence of $Mg^{++}ATP$ and a mitochondrial enzyme carbamylphosphate synthetase. The enzyme aspartate carbamylase is the first enzyme unique to pyrimidine biosynthesis and catalyzes the irreversible carbamylation of L-aspartate to carbamylaspartate. This enzyme is of highest concentrations in liver, testis, spleen, bone marrow, and intestine. Carbamylaspartate is converted to dihydroorotic acid in the presence of the enzyme dihydroorotase. Dihydroorotic acid (DHO) contains the closed ring structure and is precursor to the pyrimidine ring. DHO is reversibly oxidized to orotic acid (OA) by the enzyme DHO dehydrogenase which is present in leukocytes, intestinal mucosa fibroblasts, and reticulocytes. The enzyme is probably lost during maturation as it is absent from mature erythrocytes.

Although orotic acid is not detectable in plasma, the urinary excretion amounts to 1.2–1.8 mg/24 hr. The turnover rate in man is estimated to 0.6 g/24 hr. This compound has two alternative fates, either reversal to DHO or conversion to orotidylic acid with the intermediate formation of orotidine 5′-phosphate. This transformation is catalyzed by the enzyme orotate phosphoribosyltransferase. This reaction requires the presence of PRPP (see purine metabolism). Orotidine 5′-phosphate decarboxylase catalyzes the conversion to uridine 5-phosphate (UMP). UMP may also be produced from other pyrimidines through a "salvage pathway." The fates of UMP include formation of RNA, DNA, and coenzymes.

Hereditary orotic aciduria is an autosomal recessive disorder which is characterized by a hypochromic megaloblastic anemia resistant to iron, folic acid, and vitamin B_{12}. The disorder develops in the first year of life and is associated with growth and developmental retardation. Marked oroticaciduria leads to obstructive uropathy. The urine becomes cloudy in cooling, and crystals attach to the container. The urine orotic acid may exceed 1,000 times normal. The disorder is caused by deficiency of the enzymes orotate phosphoribosyltransferase and orotidine 5′-phosphate decarboxylase in leukocytes, erythrocytes, fibroblasts, liver, and perhaps other tissues. It is likely that the enzyme deficiencies are caused by a single mutation with the probability that most homozygotes do not survive intrauterine or neonatal development. Definitive diagnosis is established by decreased levels of the enzymes orotate phosphoribosyltransferase and orotidine 5′-phosphate decarboxylase in erythrocytes, leukocytes, or skin biopsy fibroblasts. Treatment of orotic aciduria requires use of uridine at dosages to be calculated according to age and weight. Acquired orotic aciduria has been found in patients receiving 6-azauridine for the treatment of malignant neoplasms. There are pathogenetic similarities between the congenital orotic aciduria and the species enzyme deficiency leading to scurvy in man and also to the adenine responsive anemia in some patients with the Lesch-Nyhan syndrome. Excessive orotic acid may cause faulty infiltration of the liver because of failure to release β-lipoproteins needed for transport of triglyceride and other lipids.

LITERATURE CITED

1. Karlson, P. 1963. Introduction to Modern Biochemistry, pp. 116–143. Academic Press, New York.
2. Seegmiller, J. E. 1969. Diseases of purine and pyrimidine metabolism. *In* P. K. Bondy (ed.), Diseases of Metabolism, pp. 516–599. W. B. Saunders Co., Philadelphia.
3. Lesch, M., and W. P. Nyhan. 1964. A familial disorder of uric acid metabolism and central nervous system function. Am. J. Med. 36:561–570.
4. Kelley, W. N., F. M. Rosenbloom, and J. E. Seegmiller. 1967. The effect of azathioprine (Imuran) on purine synthesis in clinical disorders of purine metabolism. J. Clin. Invest. 46:1518–1529.
5. Levenberg, B., I. Melnick, and J. M. Buchanan. 1957. Biosynthesis of the purines. XV. The effect of aza-L-serine and 6-diazo-5-oxo-L-norleucine on inosinic acid biosynthesis *de novo*. J. Biol. Chem. 225:163–176.
6. Grayzel, A. I., J. E. Seegmiller, and E. Love. 1967. Suppression of uric acid synthesis in gouty human by use of 6-diazo-5-L-norleucine. J. Clin. Invest. 39:447–454.

6

Clinical Disorders of the Connective Tissue Complex

The connective tissue complex (Figure 6.1) is made up of the macro-molecules 1) collagen, 2) elastin, 3) glycoproteins and glycolipids, and 4) protein-mucopolysaccharides arranged in a structurally and functionally interdependent unit (1–3). Each macromolecular component is a product of biosynthetic reactions (Table 6.1, Figure 6.2) and these steps determine both the nature of the macromolecules and their distribution in the complex, and, hence, the characteristics of the particular connective tissue. It is possible to have disorders which affect different connective tissue components manifested by similar clinical effects; hence, similarities in phenotypic expression do not necessarily indicate similar etiologies. The basic structure specified by the protein synthetic mechanism is considerably altered by a number of intra- and extrafibroblastic synthetic steps. On this basis, collagen structure may be altered by disease processes. There is a relatively low metabolic activity in connective tissue macromolecules, but catabolic processes for repair, regeneration, and remodeling do occur, and changes in degradation may result in altered structure and function.

COLLAGEN

Collagen is found in all multicellular forms studied thus far and represents an evolutionary adaptation to the structural requirements of multicellularity; e.g., bacteria contain no collagen, while 25% of mouse protein is collagen. Collagen fibrils (microfibrils) (diameter 500 Å or less) are associated in bundles to form fibers which are visible in the light

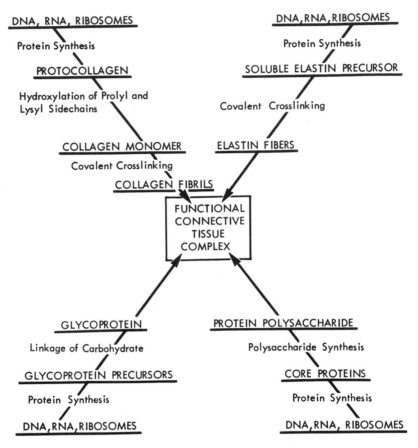

Figure 6.1. The connective tissue complex depicting the synthetic steps for the major components.

Table 6.1. Mucopolysaccharide Production by Cell Types

Cells	Mucopolysaccharide produced
Fibroblasts	Collagen, hyaluronate, chondroitin sulfate
Synovial cell	Hyaluronate
Mast cell	Heparin
Chondroblast	Collagen
Osteoblast	Collagen, chondroitin sulfate

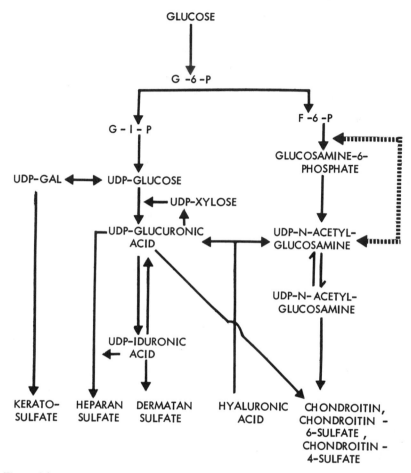

Figure 6.2. Uridine nucleotides required for mucopolysaccharide biosynthesis. Negative feedback pathways are depicted by *broken arrows*.

microscope, showing a characteristic banding pattern. Arrangement of collagen fibers varies according to functional requirements, as follows: 1) in parallel in tendons to provide greater tensile strength; 2) in laminated layers in fishes and aquatic animals, but in random bundles in terrestrial animals; 3) in alternating helical orientation in glandular ducts, blood vessels, and sarcolemma; 4) in a fibrillar network in cartilage to supply rigidity and resiliency; 5) in a matrix in bone for deposition of hydroxyapatite crystals; 6) in network pattern in the basement membrane of blood vessels and in the glomerulus; 7) in a network (vitrosin) dispersed in a hyaluronate gel in the vitreous humor; 8) in regularly spaced fibers to permit transparency of the cornea; and 9) in irregular fibrous arrangement to permit opacity of the sclera to light.

Collagen in denatured form is gelatin and in artificially cross-linked form is leather. The collagen molecule consists of three polypeptide chains which are parallel in direction. Each chain is oriented in a left-handed minor helix and the three helices are twisted about a central axis to form a right-handed major helix. Every third amino acid in each of the three chains is glycine. The native fibril contains collagen molecules arranged so that there is a characteristic banding pattern caused by a staggered array of the molecules. This arrangement is ultimately caused by the amino acid sequence of the molecule. When soluble collagen is denatured, the hydrogen bonds which stabilize the triple helical structure are broken, yielding chains in random coils. The proportion of single (α), double (β), and triple (γ) chain species depends on the tissue of origin and the covalent interchain cross-linking characteristic of the tissue.

The temperature at which transition from collagen to gelatin (denaturation) occurs in solution differs with species, but is usually close to body temperature. In the febrile state, and in the presence of a local increase in temperature because of inflammation, there is denaturation of collagen, with the consequent enzymatic degradation or appearance of antibodies to the denatured protein. Whether this actually occurs in vivo is questioned especially since virtually all collagen is in fibrillar form.

Glycine constitutes one-third of all amino acids in collagen, and is necessary for the formation of the triple helix. Proline and 4-hydroxyproline constitute one-fourth of the amino acids in collagen, and 3-hydroxyproline and 5-hydroxylysine are also present. Mammalian collagen contains little tyrosine and tryptophan and no cysteine and cystine; hence, there is no sulfhydryl cross-linkage. The paucity of the aromatic amino acids may account for the poor antigenicity of collagen.

Collagen Biosynthesis

Collagen biosynthesis takes place in fibroblast cells in essentially two phases (Figure 6.3): 1) intracellular steps involving modification in the covalent structure of the protein after peptide bond synthesis and 2) extracellular transformation of soluble collagen to an insoluble polymer.

The intracellular biosynthetic steps take place in the fibroblasts. For this process, the amino acids are activated and proline and lysine are hydroxylated to hydroxyproline and hydroxylysine, respectively. Exogenous hydroxyproline is not incorporated into collagen, but proline serves as precursor of collagen hydroxyproline; similar considerations probably apply to lysine and hydroxylysine (4). Hydroxylation of these two amino acids takes place on relatively large polypeptide chains (Figure 6.3). Peptide subunits of about 250 amino acids and molecular weight

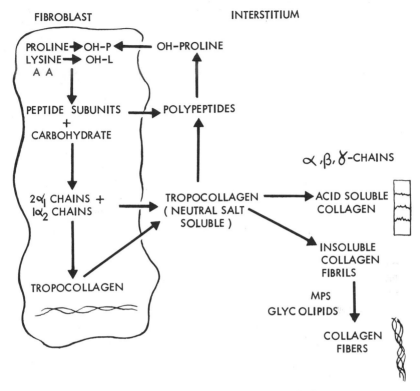

Figure 6.3. Intra- and extrafibroblastic steps in collagen synthesis.

30,000 are assembled on the ribosome. Carbohydrate of unknown composition is added to aspartic acid residues at one end of the peptide and serves to link it with another peptide; thus, α chains (2 α_1 and 1 α_2) each containing four of these peptides (molecular weight 120,000) are formed. The three chains spontaneously associate to form coiled coil of tropocollagen of molecular weight 360,000. Tropocollagen is secreted via vesicles or via communications with the rough endoplasmic reticulum (Figure 6.4). The amino acid sequence in protocollagen chain determines which prolines are hydroxylated; when proline is on the amino side of glycine, i.e., position 3, the prolyl is hydroxylated, whereas prolyl residues on the carboxyl side of glycine are not hydroxylated. The function of hydroxyproline in the collagen molecule is not known. Perhaps it plays a role in formation of intermolecular interchain hydrogen bonds which contribute to the stability of the fiber. The hydroxyl groups of hydroxylysine serve as point of attachment of disaccharides in collagen. These carbohydrates may signal completion of the molecule and trigger

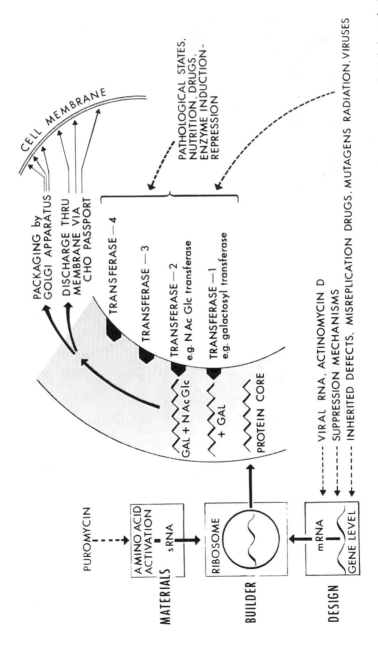

Figure 6.4. Synthetic steps in the formation of a representative acid mucopolysaccharide. As the protein core traverses the tubular endoplasmic reticulum, various membrane-bound glycosyltransferases determine the type and location of the carbohydrate substituents. The carbohydration step may confer certain biological properties to the molecule, as well as serve as a "passport" for trans-membrane transfer.

secretion of the protein from fibroblast; hence, they are a very important control mechanism (5).

The extracellular tropocollagen is soluble in cold neutral salt solutions. With development of stronger bonds between the α units, they form β and γ components, progressively more insoluble with eventual formation of insoluble collagen fibrils. The fibrils form collagen fibers in the presence of mucopolysaccharides, lipids, and the cofactors which, either by occlusion or chemical interaction, become part of the fiber. The relative metabolic inertia of collagen is well known, but during bone remodeling and in the involuting postpartum uterus there is rapid breakdown. The process involves catabolism of insoluble collagen to tropocollagen and eventually to peptides and amino acids. In the biosynthetic pathway, free hydroxy-proline or peptides containing it appear as by-products at various stages up to tropocollagen. Some may appear in the urine; hence, urinary hydroxy-proline may be used as a measure of collagen synthesis. However, hydroxyproline may also come from breakdown of collagen. Ascorbic acid is required for the activity of collagen hydroxylase (peptidyl hydroxylase). Ascorbic acid deficiency and scurvy are accompanied by several defects which are apparently caused by an inability to form soluble collagen; the defect is caused by inability to hydroxylate proline and lysine. Ascorbic acid functions to aid the "hydroxylase" to function as a mixed function oxidase. Neurolathyrism is characterized by a spastic paraplegia of the lower extremities and was described by Hippocrates. Degeneration of the lateral pyramidal tracts of the cord is caused by neurotoxins (β-cyano-L-alanine, and L-α,γ-diaminobutyric acid) in species of Lathyrus plants (lathyrus factor) and Vicia Sativa. Ingestion of seeds of these plants in cereals and bread results in the disorder. Treatment consists of removal of these factors from the diet, but the neurological changes are essentially irreversible. Osteolathyrism occurs in animals and is characterized by extensive changes in connective and vascular tissues, with skeletal and large vessel disease being most prominent. Skeletal changes include malformations and exostoses of long bones, kyphoscoliosis of spine, and rib deformities. Vascular changes are aortic aneurysm and rupture. The disorder is induced by sweet pea meal (*Lathyrus odoratus*) in which the active toxin is β-aminopropionitrile (β-APN). The locus of involvement of this toxin in collagen synthesis is the step after normal tropocollagen formation. Stabilization of collagen does not occur because of inadequate cross-linking. Lathyrogenic activity is found in nitriles such as β-APN and aminoacetonitrile, ureides such as thiosemicarbazide, and hydrazides such as isonicotinic acid hydrazide and hydrazine. These agents are carbonyl-blocking agents and disrupt the aldehyde linkages necessary for cross-linking of the protein because of inhibition lysyl aldehyde formation. It is possible that compounds such as penicillamine may act similarly. Because of this action in inhibiting cross-linking of collagen, β-APN has been tried in scleroderma and in rheumatoid arthritis, resulting in chemical evidence of increased soluble collagen, but toxic side effects probably preclude its extensive clinical usefulness. β-APN has also been tried fairly successfully to inhibit joint stiffness following immobilization and other orthopedic procedures and it has been suggested to be of possible usefulness in toxic hepatic cirrhosis (fibrosis).

Collagen Degradation

Vertebrate collagenases participate in repair and remodeling of connective tissues in growth and development. It is suggested that trophic skin ulcers, in the absence of bacterial infection, may be caused by pressure in local areas releasing active collagenases. Collagenases have been found in several tissues including granulocytes, and in the postpartum myometrium. Perhaps the granulocytic collagenases participate in the inflammatory reaction. Collagenases presumably play a role in the invasive properties of certain malignant tumors. These enzymes are also found in synovial fluid in rheumatoid arthritis but not in osteoarthritis. Increased levels of collagenase are found in the recessive form of epidermolysis bullosa.

Urinary hydroxyproline is useful in following changes of collagen metabolism. When gelatin-containing foods, such as meat and fish, are excluded from the diet, hydroxyproline in biological fluids reflects collagen metabolism. Factors which affect urinary hydroxyproline include rate of conversion between soluble and insoluble collagen and changes in the rate of degradation in these foods either to hydroxyproline-containing compounds or urea and CO_2. Normal values vary with age, with peak values probably at puberty. Increased urinary hydroxyproline is found in patients with severe burns, Paget's disease of bone, acromegaly, hyper-parathyroidism, hyperthyroidism, Klinefelter's syndrome, malabsorption syndromes (perhaps secondary to the bone changes), congenital hydroxy-prolinemia, and occasionally in rheumatoid arthritis, scleroderma, derma-tomyositis, and Marfan syndrome. Decreased hydroxyproline is found in hypothyroidism, dwarfism (pituitary and non-pituitary), after pharmaco-logical doses of estrogens, and occasionally in malnutrition.

ELASTIN

Elastin is less widely distributed phylogenetically than collagen and is perhaps an evolutionary product of divergent collagen gene. The sub-stance, which is difficult to isolate, plays a prominent role in ligaments, media of large vessels, and in dermis, as well as in elastic cartilage of eustachian tubes, epiglottis, pinnae, and pulmonary tract. Non-polar amino acids, glycine, proline, alanine, and valine account for 80% of amino acids.

Serine and threonine account for less than 10%. Elastin contains only 1–2% hydroxyproline and hydroxylysine. The fibroblast is major site of synthesis, but this process may also take place in muscle cells. It is probable that a soluble precursor is formed intracellularly (similar to collagen formation) with extracellular transformation to elastic fibers, via formation of interchain cross-links-lysyl cross-links. There are data to suggest that the cross-linkage process may involve monoamine oxidase (MAO)-like enzymes. These enzymes are copper- and pyridoxal-dependent also. Lathyrism affects cross-linkage of elastin as well as that of collagen.

GLYCOPROTEINS

The essential characteristic of glycoproteins is the occurrence of carbohydrate units of similar structural features attached covalently to proteins or peptides. These compounds possess no unique amino acid composition, but there is a characteristic series of sugars which include D-galactose, D-mannose, D-glucose, L-fucose, D-xylose, N-acetyglucosamine, N-acetylgalactosamine, and various neuraminic acid (sialic acid) derivatives. There is a wide range in the content of carbohydrate per glycoprotein molecule, from $< 1\%$ to $> 80\%$ by weight; two to seven sugar types may be linked to a given amino acid core. The carbohydrates of glycoproteins range in size from molecular weight 3,500 (as in fetuin) to single residues of molecular weight 162. They range in carbohydration from high density carbohydrate units (as in mucin) to low density carbohydrate units (as in plasma proteins). Three major types of carbohydrate-peptide linkages have been described, the glucosylamine linkage, as in IgG and in α_1-acid glycoprotein, the O-glycosidic bond to serine or threonine, as in mucins and in blood group active glycoproteins, and the O-glycosidic linkage between a galactose residue and hydroxyl group of hydroxylysine, as in basement membrane and in collagen. Glycoproteins are of very wide occurrence in the body in both structural and functional groupings.

Synthesis of Glycoproteins

The liver is the major locus of glycoprotein synthesis, but connective tissues in several areas, as well as tumors, may also release glycoproteins, the synthetic process involving an extremely intricate system. Intrinsic to this system is the mechanism of heterogeneity of glycoprotein types, as well as of microheterogeneity in the specific glycoprotein molecules. The peptide core is synthesized on ribosomes by the usual method for protein synthesis. As the peptide moves through the tubular endoplasmic reticulum, membrane-bound transferases attach single sugar structures to the growing carbohydrate appendage. The carbohydrated protein may then be concentrated and packaged by the Golgi apparatus before storage or discharge, or, as with many glycoproteins, may be discharged through the cell membrane without packaging into concentrated units. Indeed, it has been suggested that the major purpose of carbohydration of the peptides is to provide a "passport" through the cell membrane (5). There are data which demonstrate, however, that the attached carbohydrate serves additional functions. While peptide synthesis is ribosomal, the carbohydration steps are postribosomal and not under direct genetic control, even though synthesis of the carbohydration enzymes (glycosyltransferases) may be under genetic control one or several stages removed. These postribosomal steps will depend on substrate and cofactor availability, as well as on other environmental influences. It is at this postribosomal level that physiological regulation of synthesis and release of these substances and alterations by pathological process may largely influence the type of glycoprotein released.

Functions of Glycoproteins

Several glycoprotein molecules function as structural substances (e.g., collagen, ground substance, and basement membrane), while others are released into the circulating plasma. The mechanisms of release after packaging or by trans-membrane passport have been alluded to. Glycoproteins may function as: 1) hormones—thyroglobulin, follicle-stimulating hormone, thyroid-stimulating hormone; 2) enzymes—ribonuclease, deoxyribonuclease, amylase, glucose oxidase, serum cholinesterase, plasma esterase, β-glucuronidase, N-acetylglucosamidase; 3) substances with blood group activity; 4) mucous secretions in respiratory, gastrointestinal, and genitourinary tracts to increase viscosity of the secretions and to serve as a protective coat and lubricant; 5) transport factors—transferrin, ceruloplasmin, haptoglobin, thyroxin-binding globulin, cortisol-binding globulin; 6) brain glucoproteins; 7) part of cell membranes as in erythrocytes, lymphocytes, and other mammalian cells; 8) structural proteins—insoluble fibrous proteins, collagen, elastin, basement membranes; and 9) clotting factors—fibrinogen. Several of these functions are related to the presence of carbohydrate in the molecules, whereas others are not dependent on carbohydration. For example, there is a correlation between the biological activity of some of the hormones and the carbohydrate content. Similarly, the viscosity of mucous secretion is carbohydrate dependent, as is the blood group type activity of the MN system. On the other hand, the blood group activities of the ABH and Lewis systems are not affected by changes in carbohydration, nor are the activities of plasma esterase, or cholinesterase.

Catabolism of Glycoproteins

Intracellular organelles, lysosomes, contain glycosidases which hydrolyze the appropriate carbohydrate structures from the protein core (e.g., galactosidase, α-N-acetylgalactosaminidase, α-mannosidase, and neuramini-dase). In addition, these lysosomes also contain enzymes which disrupt the carbohydrate-peptide linkages (e.g., N-acetylgalactosaminyl serine linkage). The lysosomal glycosidases, along with proteases, degrade the glyco-proteins in a stepwise manner.

Classification of Glycoproteins

Based largely on the chemical properties of the various glycoproteins, Meyer (6) presented a classification of compounds with protein-carbo-hydrate linkage which has been employed quite extensively. In this classification, there is a major division of compounds into mucopoly-saccharides, mucoproteins, and glycoproteins.

Mucopolysaccharides were defined as high molecular weight poly-saccharides containing hexosamine. This group was further divided into neutral mucopolysaccharides containing neutral monosaccharides and acid mucopolysaccharides containing uronic acid and/or sulfuric acid.

Mucoproteins were defined as protein combined with acid mucopoly-saccharides in polar or other easily split type of linkage.

Glycoproteins were defined as substances with the properties of proteins which contain 0.5% of hexosamine firmly bound to protein. A distinction was made between glycoids containing 0.5–4% of hexosamine and mucoids which contain greater than 4% hexosamine. Unfortunately, the term "mucoprotein" has been used to refer both to seromucoid and to acid glycoprotein, with considerable confusion resulting. A more biolog-ically oriented classification (e.g., into hormones, enzymes, transport substances, and structural substances), while attractive, is probably not advisable because of the fact that the carbohydrate component is not a constant determinant of the measured biological activity of the substances.

ACID MUCOPOLYSACCHARIDES

Acid mucopolysaccharides (glycosaminoglycans) constitute the major component in the ground substance of connective tissues. The synthesis of these substances takes place in the fibroblast and its derivatives. A protein core is synthesized by the ribosomes, and sugars of varied chemical structures, modifications, and substituents are added to the protein core by glucosyltransferases which are associated with the membrane of the tubular endoplasmic reticulum. The chemical steps in acid mucopoly-saccharide synthesis are depicted in Figure 6.4. Acid mucopolysaccharides are macromolecules made up of many saccharide units, alike or different, but only a few different kinds in any one acid mucopolysaccharide. The molecular weights range from 15,000–10,000,000, with 40,000–50,000 saccharide units/molecule. The most common saccharide in the world is glucose, and the most common polysaccharide is cellulose which is made up of glucose in unbranched chains. Saccharide units are united by either link between OH on C_1 and another OH on a second saccharide unit. Each polysaccharide is composed of two different saccharide units which alternate regularly along a chain in which there is no branching demonstrated. In all cases, one of the saccharide units is a hexosamine (glucosamine or galactosamine). The other saccharide unit is a uronic acid (glucuronic or iduronic acid), but in keratan it is galactose. The amino group seems never to be free as it is either acetylated or sulfated. Mucopolysaccharides possess several features in common, such as production by connective tissue cells, possession of similar chemical structures, and their activity as regularly repeating polyanions. Table 6.2 presents a classification of acid mucopolysaccharides.

The mucopolysaccharides are located mainly in the space between cells and fibers and are called ground substance. In this location they are water-soluble and exist in solution as compounds with (rather than compact) molecules which extend throughout the volume of the solution (called the domain). That is, the domain is large in comparison to the size of the molecule, 1–10 liters/g. As an example, the spaces occupied by equal weights of tropocollagen and hyaluronate are different. The hyaluronate molecule (molecular weight 10^6) occupies a sphere of diameter 4,000 Å or $330,000 \times 10^{-19}$ ml, whereas a molecule of soluble collagen (molecular weight 345,000) occupies a rigid cylinder of diameter 14 Å and length 2,500 Å or 4.3×10^{-19} ml. This domain occupied by the diffused molecule in solution has different degrees of porosity to molecules of different sizes and offers different degrees of resistance to passage of other molecules. Some studies reveal that the mucopolysaccharide may exclude large solutes from part of the solution it occupies. As a clinical example of this principle, normal serum contains 7% protein, whereas synovial fluid contains 2%. In arthritis fluid, where the hyaluronate is roughly one-half normal, the protein content is doubled (to 4%).

The linkage region between protein and polysaccharide has been shown (7) to have the structure glucuronic acid-galactose-galactose-xylose-serine in many polysaccharides, including chondroitin-4-sulfate, dermatan sulfate, heparin, and probably heparan sulfate. The xylosyl group is linked to the hydroxyl of serine by an O-glycosidic bond. Physicochemical properties of acid mucopolysaccharide include the following: 1) viscosity which is especially marked in hyaluronate; and 2) polyelectrolyte activity which implies that all carry a large number of negative groups and, therefore, are always associated with an equal number of cations. The most common cation in extracel is Na, hence, the mucopolysaccharides occur mainly as sodium salts, but under certain conditions may be salts of potassium, calcium, or magnesium. Cations of higher valence are bound to a higher degree; hence, cobalt precipitates

Table 6.2. Glycosaminoglycans Acid Mucopolysaccharides

Old terminology	New terminology	Amino sugar	Uronic acid	Sulfate	Distribution
Hyaluronic acid[a]		Glucosamine	Glucuronic acid	0	Viteous, synovial, umbilical cord, skin
Chondroitin sulfate A[b]	Chondroitin-4-sulfate	Galactosamine	Glucuronic acid	1	Cartilage, bone, aorta
Chondroitin sulfate B[b]	Dermatan sulfate	Galactosamine	Iduronic acid	1	Skin, heart valves, lung, tendon
Chondroitin sulfate C[b]	Chondroitin-6-sulfate	Galactosamine	Glucuronic acid	1	Cartilage, aorta, heart valves
Heparitin sulfate[b]	Heparan sulfate	Glucosamine	Glucuronic iduronic	1	Aorta, liver, lung
Heparin		Glucosamine	Glucuronic iduronic	3	Liver, mast cells
Chondroitin[a]		Galactosamine	Glucuronic	0	Cartilage, bone, vessels
Keratosulfate[c]	Keratan sulfate	Glucosamine	Galactose	1	Cornea, cartilage, nucleus pulposus

[a]Polycarboxylate mucopolysaccharides (glycosaminoglycans).

[b]Polycarboxysulfates glycosaminoglycans.

[c]Polysulfate glycosaminoglycan (keratan sulfate contains no uronic acid).

chondroitin sulfate and heparin directly from aqueous solution. These polyanionic properties are employed in precipitation and quantitation of mucopolysaccharides and in histochemical detection, e.g., metachromatic staining. Another example of this physical property becomes apparent when albumin (present in synovial fluid) in an acid medium becomes cationic and precipitates with anionic hyaluronate.

Biological Functions of Acid Mucopolysaccharides

The functions of these substances are caused by the physicochemical properties described above: 1) molecular transport of substances is affected by the polyelectrolyte properties of acid mucopolysaccharides; 2) resiliency of cartilage is attributed to the ability of protein-polysaccharides to water and exclude large molecules; and 3) lubrication of joints and in tissue plasma is facilitated by the acid mucopolysaccharide hyaluronic acid.

In their native state, the mucopolysaccharides are bound to protein, but there is some evidence that very small amounts of polysaccharide in connective tissue may be free of protein; estimates have shown the half-life of this free mucopolysaccharide is about 7 days. It is not known whether this free component may represent a first step in the breakdown of native protein-polysaccharide. Two types of protein-polysaccharide (PP) are distinguished (PP-L and PP-H) based on their sedimentability. It is suggested that more specific names, e.g., protein-chondroitin-4-sulfate, protein-hyaluronate, be used instead of mucoproteins or similar terms. It is likely that the properties of the mucopolysaccharide dominate those of the protein-polysaccharide, and partial digestion of the protein with protease does not alter the viscosity properties of PP.

Degradation of Mucopolysaccharides

Lysosomes present in various tissues are responsible for degradation of acid mucopolysaccharides. The entire processes are not clearly known, but several studies have demonstrated the presence of lysosomal hyaluronidases, β-N-acetylhexosaminidases, β-glucuronidases, cathepsins, carboxypeptidases, and sulfatases. More recently an L-iduronidase has been reported in fibroblast preparations. There are data which demonstrate that the protein core of the mucopolysaccharide is fragmented, with various degrees of fragmentation of the polysaccharide substitutents. Fragments of the protein core with intact linkage regions have also been found (Figure 6.5). Acid hydrolysases present in lysosomes function mainly at weakly acid pH and depolymerize protein-polysaccharides (Figure 6.6). Rheumatoid synovial membrane contains high proteolytic activity and lysosomal granules. The molecular properties of hyaluronic acid from rheumatoid

NORMAL

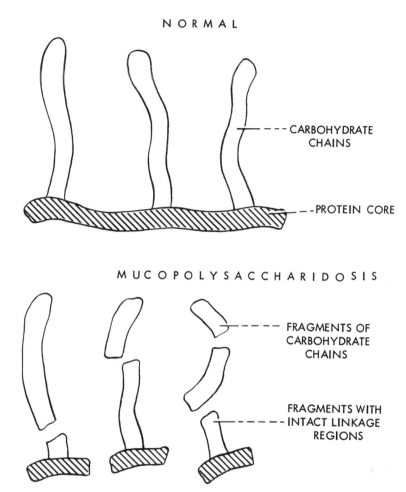

CARBOHYDRATE CHAINS

-PROTEIN CORE

MUCOPOLYSACCHARIDOSIS

FRAGMENTS OF CARBOHYDRATE CHAINS

FRAGMENTS WITH INTACT LINKAGE REGIONS

Figure 6.5. Degradation of protein-polysaccharide complex. The end products vary in chemical composition depending on the area of fragmentation. Note the presence of linkage-region fragments containing portions of the protein core and carbohydrate. Errors in specific steps in the degradative pathways are found in the clinical mucopolysaccharidoses and in other clinical diseases.

synovial fluid are consistent with partial enzymatic degradation of this macromolecule. Similar lytic properties are found in cultured fibroblasts from rheumatoid synovial membranes. Substances which labilize lysosomes (e.g., streptolysins, endotoxin, large doses of vitamin A) increase or exacerbate arthritis in animals, whereas substances which stabilize lysosomes (e.g., glucocorticoids, acetylsalicylic acid) probably inhibit release of lysosomal hydrolases. Chloroquine, ϵ-aminocaproic acid, and gold salts

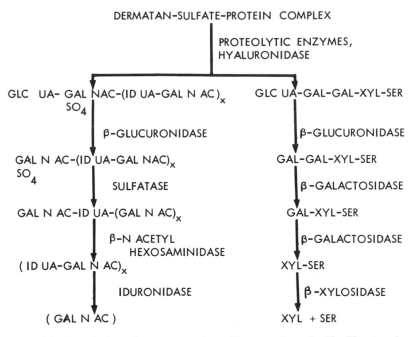

DERMATAN-SULFATE-PROTEIN COMPLEX

PROTEOLYTIC ENZYMES,
HYALURONIDASE

GLC UA- GAL NAC-(ID UA-GAL N AC)$_x$ GLC UA-GAL-GAL-XYL-SER
        SO$_4$

            β-GLUCURONIDASE   β-GLUCURONIDASE

GAL N AC-(ID UA-GAL NAC)$_x$ GAL-GAL-XYL-SER
SO$_4$
            SULFATASE   β-GALACTOSIDASE

GAL N AC-ID UA-(GAL N AC)$_x$ GAL-XYL-SER

            β-N ACETYL   β-GALACTOSIDASE
            HEXOSAMINIDASE
(ID UA-GAL N AC)$_x$ XYL-SER

            IDURONIDASE   β-XYLOSIDASE

(GAL N AC)   XYL + SER

Figure 6.6. Degradation of a representative acid mucopolysaccharide. The stepwise enzymatic degradation of dermatan sulfate is depicted. Absence or deficiencies of specific enzymes in the mucopolysaccharide degradation pathways have been demonstrated in the clinical mucopolysaccharidoses.

inhibit the activity of the lysosomal hydrolases. Colchicine does not appear to have a direct effect on lysosomal enzymes, but interferes with the formation of phagolysosomes by inhibiting release of lysosomal enzymes into endocytic vacuoles. A lysosomal hyaluronidase from synovia and synovial fluid may contribute to changes in the osteoarthritis articular cartilage. Studies have shown a decreased staining of cartilage matrix for polysaccharides and a reduction of chondroitin sulfate concentration, as well as a shortening of polysaccharide chain length. Collagen and non-fibrous protein in osteoarthritis cartilage are unchanged.

The metabolic turnover of acid mucopolysaccharides is more rapid than that of fibrous proteins. Acid mucopolysaccharide synthesis is known to be decreased in insulin deficiency, apparently at some stage beyond the formation of precursor nucleotide sugars. Estrogens, as well as androgens, affect acid mucopolysaccharide synthesis, with androgens generally stimulating synthesis. Estrogens have a variable effect, but acid mucopolysaccharide synthesis at target organs is stimulated by these hormones. Corticosteroids have a variable effect on acid mucopolysaccharide synthesis depending on several factors.

GENETIC MUCOPOLYSACCHARIDOSES

Mucopolysaccharidoses constitute a group of disorders characterized by varying degrees of skeletal changes, mental retardation, visceral involvement, and corneal clouding. The defects are caused by accumulations of mucopolysaccharides in various tissues; in all types, there is an increased excretion of acid mucopolysaccharides or its fractions in the urine. The original description of this type of disorder was made by Thompson in the early 1900's. At least 400 cases of mucopolysaccharidoses have been reported. These disorders have no specific racial predominance. With the exception of the Hunter syndrome, these disorders are inherited as autosomal recessive characteristics. The Hunter syndrome is inherited as an X-linked recessive disorder.

The clinical and laboratory features of the various mucopolysaccharidoses are listed in Table 6.3 which presents the classification devised by McKusick et al. (8). Alternative classifications have been suggested by van Hoof and Hers (9) based on the enzyme defects and by Kaplan (10) based on the type of mucopolysacchariduria so that mucopolysaccharidosis III is termed heparansulfaturia, type II mucopolysaccharidosis is called mixed mucopolysaccharidosis type A, types I and V mucopolysaccharidoses are included in mixed mucopolysaccharidosis type B, and mucopolysaccharidosis VI is called dermatansulfaturia.

There is a wide spectrum of organ involvement in the mucopolysaccharidoses. Morphological changes in the Hurler syndrome encompass almost all organs and tissues; the most severe changes take place in the brain, heart, liver, and spleen. A patchy and nodular thickening of the epicardium, endocardium, valvular leaflets, and chordae tendinae is seen. The coronary arteries are occluded by intimal deposits and may "stand out like cords." Microscopic examination of the heart, blood vessels, meninges, cornea, periosteum, and tendons reveals the presence of large cells distended with a material containing acid mucopolysaccharides (clear cells, gargoyle cells, Hurler cells, balloon cells). These cells are probably derivatives of fibroblasts. Metachromatic granules in fibroblasts and lymphocytes are a characteristic finding in several patients with mucopolysaccharidoses. Metachromatic granules also occur in polymorphonuclear leukocytes (Reilly or Alder bodies) and in bone marrow cells.

Nature of Metabolic Defect

Early studies suggested a defect in the linkage region of protein-polysaccharide as responsible for the synthesis of abnormal amounts of mucopolysaccharide. More recent data are consistent with the concept that the accumulation of mucopolysaccharide in urine and tissues is caused by an inability of mechanisms for degradation of protein-polysaccharides to cope

Table 6.3. Genetic Mucopolysaccharidoses[a]

Syndrome	Clinical manifestations					Predominant AMPS[b] and enzymes involved
	Somatic and skeletal	Mental retardation	Cardiopulmonary	Hepato-splenomegaly	Eyes and ears	
Hurler (I)	Appear in early childhood lumbar gibbus, chest deformity, dwarfism, stubby fingers, shoe-shaped sella, saddle-shaped nose	Severe	Valvular and coronary disease → cardiac failure; valve defect, mitral aortic tricuspid pulmonic	Marked	Corneal clouding; retinal degeneration; deafness	Dermatan sulfate and heparan sulfate; decreased β-galactosidase in tissues; metachromasia in lymphocytes, and occasionally in neutrophils; decreased fibroblast iduronidase
Hunter (II)	Moderate to marked; stiff joints; claw hands; dwarfing; no lumbar gibbus; nodular skin lesions hypertrichosis, premature osteoarthritis	Progress more slowly than in Hurler's	Valvular disease; pulmonary hypertension; impaired ventilation	Marked	Corneal clouding is infrequent; deafness of early onset	Dermatan sulfate and heparan sulfate; decreased β-galactosidase in tissues; metachromasia in lymphocytes, fibroblasts, and occasionally in neutrophils; decreased L-iduronidase in fibroblasts
Sanfilippo (III)	Mild changes; moderate dwarfism	Marked		Moderate	No corneal clouding; hearing loss is present	Heparan sulfate metachromasia in lymphocyte, γ in PMNs
Morquio (IV)	Strikingly dwarfed; beaking of lumbar spine; crouching stance, spinal cord compression from skeletal deformity	Absent or slight	Aortic regurgitation	Slight	Cornea is diffusely opacified; mild deafness	Keratan sulfate; no metachromasia in lymphocytes; atypical in PMNs
Scheie (V)	Stiff joints; claw hands; genu valgum; broad mouth; coarse skin; Carpal Tunnel Syndrome, hypertrichosis	Absent	Aortic valvular disease	Variable	Marked corneal clouding; variable hearing loss	Dermatan sulfate and heparan sulfate; metachromasia

Maroteaux-Lamy (VI)	Growth retardation from 2–3 years genu valgum; anterior sternal protrusion; dwarfism: trunk and limbs[c]	Absent	Moderate	Cardiac murmurs	Corneal opacities develop early recurrent otitis media	Dermatan sulfate; metachromasia
"I" cell disease	Features similar to Hurler's	Severe				Dermatan sulfate in fibroblasts; urine AMPS variable; increased lipids in fibroblasts
Lipomucopolysaccharidosgal + disease (inheritance ?)	Similar to Hurler's	Severe			Corneal clouding	Urine AMPS normal; increased mucopolysaccharides and lipids in tissues
Mucopolysaccharidosis (VII) (inheritance ?)	Similar to Morquio's					
GM1-gangliosidosis neuro-visceral lipodosis	Marked skeletal changes	Marked				Keratan sulfate-like material in urine; very low galactosidase in tissues

[a] All are inherited as autosomal recessive characteristics except in Hunter (type II) which is inherited as an X-linked recessive disorder. Kaplan (10) has suggested nomenclature based on acid mucopolysaccharides in urine, e.g., heparansulfaturia, type III; mixed mucopolysacchariduria, type A: to include type B: types I and V; dermatansulfaturia, type VI. In all types, there are "clear cells" with lysosomal vacuoles. There may also be a glycolipid abnormality. Pathology is similar in all mucopolysaccharidoses. In Hunter-Hurler, almost all organs, especially brain, heart (patchy, nodular thickening of epi- and endo-cardium, valves, and chordae tendinae, intimal deposits in coronary A), liver, and spleen (hard, gray).

[b] AMPS, acid mucopolysaccharides.

[c] A distinctive myelopathy caused by compression of the cervical spinal cord by thickened dura was recently described in the Maroteaux-Lamy syndrome (12).

with excessive production. Selected deficiencies of various lysosomal hydrolytic enzymes explain the varied patterns of urinary mucopolysaccharide.

Methods of Laboratory Diagnosis of Mucopolysaccharidoses

Screening methods for the detection of increased urinary excretion of acid mucopolysaccharides are based largely on their polyanionic properties. Acid mucopolysaccharides are precipitated by compounds such as cetylpyridinium chloride, cetyltrimethylammonium bromide, and 5-aminoacridine. The component moieties of the precipitate can then be estimated (e.g., uronic acid, sulfate, and hexosamine), or the individual fractions separated by chromatographic methods before quantitation. These latter methods are too complex for routine clinical measurements. The most widely used tests employed for clinical detection of excess acid mucopolysaccharide include: 1) metachromatic spot test in which filter paper impregnated with excess acid mucopolysaccharides reacts with toluidine blue to produce a purple color against a blue background; 2) acid albumin turbidity test which is based on the principle that acid mucopolysaccharides at an acid pH react with albumin to form a precipitate. A large scale survey employing this test revealed no false positives, but only one false negative result; 3) the precipitate acid mucopolysaccharide is quantitated by the orcinol or carbazole reactions; and 4) chromatographic fractionation, as well as determination of the orcinol/carbazol reactions, has been used for identification of individual acid mucopolysaccharides (Table 6.4). It should be noted that the above tests are not reliable for the detection of excessive keratosulfate which is found in Morquio's syndrome. Keratosulfate contains no uronic acids.

Table 6.4. Normal Total Acid Mucopolysaccharides Excretion in Urine

Age (years)	Acid mucopolysaccharides (mg/24 hr)
0–1	3.8
2–8	10.1
9–12	15.6
22–40 (male)	6.8
22–40 (female)	4.8
40–64	6.5

Taken from Dorfman.

There is no definitive treatment for the mucopolysaccharidoses at the present time. Thyroid hormone, growth hormone, and salicylates failed to affect acid mucopolysaccharide excretion in Hurler syndrome patients. Prednisone (2 mg/kg/day) resulted in a decreased acid mucopolysaccharide excretion, whereas hydroxyquinoline administration (20 mg/kg/day) was followed by increased urinary acid mucopolysaccharide. Retinol has been shown to increase the excretion of acid mucopolysaccharide in the Hunter and Hurler syndromes. Recent studies suggest the efficacy of infusions of L-iduronidase from lymphocytes or of normal plasma (containing the enzyme) in reducing the excretion of acid mucopolysaccharide.

INHERITED DISORDERS OF CONNECTIVE TISSUES

A common feature of the inherited disorders of connective tissues is in the formation of elastic or collagen fibers (Table 6.5). The mechanisms of the errors may differ in the various entities, but many of the contributory factors may be similar. Various degrees of disturbances in the vascular, skeletal, pulmonary, ocular, and auditory systems characterize this group of disorders.

Marfan Syndrome

The Marfan syndrome is an autosomal dominant inherited disorder which is characterized by skeletal, cardiovascular, and ocular abnormalities. The patient with this abiotrophic disorder exhibits arachnodactyly, long spider-like fingers, dolichostenomelia or long, slender extremities, dolicho-cephaly, an overgrowth of the bones of the skull, pectus excavatum, or

Table 6.5. Mechanisms of Errors in Formation of Connective Tissue Complex

Nature of defect	Diseases
Defective cross-linkage of collagen monomer	Osteogenesis imperfecta and Ehlers-Danlos syndrome
Defective cross-linkage of elastin	Pseudoxanthoma elasticum
Defective cross-linkage of both collagen and elastin	Homocystinuria, Marfan syndrome, and alcaptonuria
Defective degradation of protein-polysaccharide linkages	Mucopolysaccharidoses
Depolymerization of glycoproteins	Tumors, inflammation, rheumatoid arthritis, epidermolysis bullosa, etc.

carinatum caused by growth of the rib cage. The disturbed growth of the bones of the skull is also responsible for the presence of the gothic arched palate. The patients also have weak joint capsules, ligaments, and tendons, resulting in joint hyperextensibility. This may result in dislocations, pes planus, and kyphoscoliosis. A decrease in muscle mass and tissue of subcutaneous fat is also evident. The upper skeletal measurement (U = symphysis to crown) to lower (L = symphysis to floor) measurement is lower (0.85) than normal (0.93).

The cardiovascular manifestations in the Marfan syndrome include arterial dilation with dissecting aneurysm of the ascending aorta being the most common abnormality. Aneurysms of the sinus of Valsalva and of the pulmonary artery are also prevalent, these disorders occurring early or late in life. Aortic regurgitation results from dilation and stretching of the cusps and from myxomatous changes in the valves. Mitral regurgitation caused by redundant valve cusps and chordae tendinae may also occur. Similar processes may occur in the tricuspid valve. These patients may suffer from chest pain caused by coronary insufficiency. Dilation and aneurysms of the descending aorta, as well as cystic disease of the lungs complicated by pneumohemothorax, may occur in patients with this disorder.

The most common ocular defects seen in these patients are ectopia lentis and subluxation of the lens. These changes are caused by weakness of the suspensory ligaments and hypoplasia of the ciliary processes. The patients exhibit severe myopia, retinal detachment, iridonesis, and nystagmus. (Ectopia lentis may occur as an isolated finding in the Weil-Marchesani syndrome and should be differentiated from that in the Marfan syndrome.) Hernia formation (umbilical and inguinal) and cutaneous atrophic striae are also seen occasionally in patients with the Marfan syndrome.

The pathogenesis of the above findings is related to the disruption, fragmentation, and sparsity of the elastic fibers associated with decrease in the vascularity of the media and adventitia and an increase in collagen and smooth muscle fibers. Deposition of acid mucopolysaccharide in amorphous intercellular masses and in cystic areas or lacunae is responsible for metachromatic staining pattern seen in many tissues. The involved elastic and collagen fibers are more likely to occur in areas where functional hemodynamic pressures are higher, and, despite intrinsic defects in the fibers in the trachea and lung, they are not as apparent because of absence of this factor of pressure phenomena. Defects in the steps of cross-linkage involving both collagen and elastin synthesis are the most likely metabolic basis of the Marfan syndrome. This cross-linkage step requires formation and condensation of lysyl-derived aldehydes. It is possible that glycoproteins and glycolipids may participate in this step. No definitive therapeutic method to reverse or delay the various manifestations of the Marfan syndrome is yet available.

Homocystinuria

Homocystinuria was considered in Chapter 4. In this disorder, several of the characteristics seen in the Marfan syndrome are present, and the differential diagnosis is often difficult. Homocystinuria is inherited as an autosomal recessive disorder. Arachmodactyly, kyphoscoliosis, rib cage deformities, joint laxity, and genu valgum are prominent skeletal abnormalities. The U:L ratio lower than normal is similar to that in the Marfan syndrome. Osteoporosis is a prominent feature in homocystinuric patients but is not found in Marfan patients.

The cardiovascular abnormalities in homocystinuria include thrombosis in the intermediate sized arteries, including the coronary, renal, cerebral, and peripheral arteries. These patients may, therefore, suffer from coronary occlusive disease, hypertension, strokes, intermittent claudication, and, when vessels to the gastrointestinal tract are involved, gastrointestinal hemorrhage. Venous thrombosis and pulmonary embolic phenomena occur, probably related to the presence of intimal fibrosis. Patients with this disorder are not subject to aortic aneurysms as found in patients with the Marfan syndrome. Hernias are common in patients with homocystinuria.

The ocular changes are quite similar to those in the Marfan syndrome and 60% of patients with homocystinuria exhibit ectopia lentis. Mental retardation, sometimes of a severe degree, may be present in approximately 50% of homocystinurics, and is not a sine qua non for this diagnosis. This manifestation is ascribed to a low level of cystathione in the brain. The metabolic defect in homocystinuria is an absence or deficiency of the enzyme cystathionase, a result of which defect is the accumulation of methionine and serine. It is likely also that there are blocks or reverses in lysyl-derived linkages. Diagnostic and possible therapeutic methods for this disorder are discussed in Chapter 4.

Alcaptonuria

The clinical manifestations and disturbed biochemistry in alcaptonuria were discussed in Chapter 4. This disorder which exhibits defects in the skeletal system as well as in the genitourinary and ocular systems is inherited as an autosomal recessive characteristic. It is essentially asymptomatic during childhood. The most serious skeletal manifestation is ochronotic arthropathy, which involves the spine and large diarthrodial joints but spares the small joints of the hands and feet. This disorder is more severe in male patients, who most frequently suffer from knee joint problems. Occasionally, ochronotic spondylitis may result in rupture of the intervertebral disc. Patients with alcaptonuria may have synovial effusions after minimal trauma.

Patients with alcaptonuria may suffer from uremia caused by obstructive uropathy caused by calculus disease and prostatitis. Ocular defects may result from the accumulation of homogentisic acid in the sclera. The accumulation of homogentisic acid in the tympanic membrane and auditory ossicles results in hearing impairment in these patients. The connective tissue defects are caused by an error in elastin and collagen cross-linkages which are more easily degraded. The accumulation of homogentisic acid and polymerization of benzoquinone acetic acid results in the formation of a melanin-like pigment irreversibly bound to collagen.

Ehlers-Danlos Syndrome

The Ehlers-Danlos syndrome is inherited as an autosomal dominant disorder which is characterized by skeletal, cutaneous, and vascular manifestations. Hyperextensibility of the joints is associated with habitual dislocations and kyphoscoliosis. The patients exhibit papyraceous (cigarette-paper) scars over the elbows, knees, and shins. Subcutaneous nodules include fatty or calcified cysts or hematomas, or collections of cystic tissue (molluscoid pseudotumors) over pressure points. Increased friability of the skin and underlying blood vessels render the patients highly susceptible to large gaping wounds and to formation of ecchymoses even after minor trauma. The patients are also subject to spontaneous rupture of the cerebral and other blood vessels. Rupture of pulmonary structure because of connective tissue weakness may result in pneumothorax and pneumomediastinum. Patients with the Ehlers-Danlos syndrome have a high incidence of hernias, diverticuli of the small intestine, stomach, and colon, and spontaneous bowel perforation with bleeding is not uncommon.

The cutaneous manifestations include hyperelasticity of the skin on stretching, with return to the original state when tension is released. Ocular changes include the presence of microcoria, keratocornea, and blue sclerae. Epicanthal folds are characteristically seen. The metabolic defect underlying this disorder is a decrease in collagen fibrogenesis, and it is possible that defects in glycoproteins and protein-polysaccharides may contribute to the problem. The tissues of patients with the Ehlers-Danlos syndrome show decreased collagen fibers and increased elastic fibers. There is no definitive therapy for the disorder, but supportive and protective measures may prevent severe trauma which leads to poor scar formation. The use of knee pads and similar measures is recommended in patients with this disorder who are quite active.

Osteogenesis Imperfecta

Osteogenesis imperfecta (OI) evolves in two major forms, OI-congenita and OI-tarda, both of which are inherited as autosomal dominant characteristics with variable expressivity. Osseous involvement is a major feature in this syndrome, and the patients may have auditory and occular manifestations. In OI-congenita, the osseous involvement is severe and in utero deaths are common; the bony involvement occurs much later in OI-tarda. Because of the very severe skeletal and vessel problems in the congenita form, the babies may suffer from intracranial or other hemorrhage at the time of delivery. These babies may exhibit a caput membranaceum reminiscent of that seen in achondroplasia. In the OI-tarda form, the lower extremities are shorter because of bowing and deformities of the femora, microfractures at the epiphyseal plate, and decreased growth. The bone disorder results in a rounded back and codfish or hourglass deformity of the vertebra. Herniation of the nucleus pulposus may result in nerve compression. Platybasia of the skull may also be the basis of neurological problems because of nerve compression. Joint dislocations and rupture of the patellar ligament are also seen in OI-tarda.

In both forms of the disorder, subcutaneous hemorrhages caused by laxity of the subcutaneous supportive structures are seen frequently. Auditory manifestations include otosclerosis with conductive and nerve deafness, and the patients often have tinnitus and vertigo. Blue sclerae are also present caused by the thinness of the sclerae and visualization of the underlying choroid. The skin is atrophic and thin, and surgical incisions or trauma may lead to wide hypertrophic scars and elastosis perforans. Histological examination of involved tissues reveals absence of normal collagen, and there is replacement by argyrophilic collagen caused by mucopolysaccharide. Disruption of the macromolecular organization of collagen results from the excess polysaccharide. No definitive therapy is available, and the prognosis depends on the severity of bleeding and the neurological problems.

Pseudoxanthoma Elasticum

Pseudoxanthoma elasticum (PXE) is a clinical disorder characterized by cutaneous, vascular, skeletal, and ocular problems. It is inherited as an autosomal recessive characteristic. The cutaneous manifestations appear in childhood and include yellowish coloration of the skin with crepe paper appearance especially noted over areas subject to stress, such as the penoral area, neck, axilla, marginal folds, penis, antecubital fossa, and waist. The skin becomes lax, inelastic, and redundant. Similar changes are seen in the buccal mucosa, soft palate, inner aspects of the eyes, rectal, and vaginal mucosa. Elastosis perforans and calcification of the dermis are also seen. The skeletal problems are mainly caused by hemarthroses.

Manifestations of vascular involvement include peripheral and coronary arterial insufficiency, intermittent claudication, and hypertension. There is medial calcification of the peripheral arteries with angiographic evidence of arterial narrowing. As a result of the vascular problems combined with weakness in mucosa, these patients may have bleeding in the gastrointestinal and genitourinary tracts; hemorrhage into the subarachnoid space is not unusual. Ocular manifestations include severe diminution of vision associated with the presence of angioid streaks in the retina, as well as retinitis proliferans. A frequent presenting complex in patients with PXE includes severe diminution of vision, hematemesis, and cutaneous changes.

A disturbance in the process of elastinogenesis associated with an increase of mucopolysaccharide is considered to be of pathogenetic significance in PXE. No definitive therapy is available for PXE.

OTHER DISORDERS OF CONNECTIVE TISSUE METABOLISM

The content and physical properties of collagen in tissues alter with the aging process. In the aorta, skin, cartilage, and other tissues, the collagen concentration increased as a result of a decreased mucopolysaccharide and water content. The susceptibility to collagenase and solubility of collagen have been noted to diminish with age. Acid mucopolysaccharide concentration in various tissues varies with age, with a rapid diminution in the concentration during growth and a slower decrease thereafter. The relative concentrations of different acid mucopolysaccharides also vary with age.

Rheumatoid Arthritis

Abnormal lysosomal activity in rheumatoid arthritis is suggested by the finding that rheumatoid synovial membrane exhibits high proteolytic activity and increased lysosomal granules. The physical properties of synovial hyaluronic acid in this disorder are consistent with partial enzymatic degradation of the macromolecule. Further support for this concept comes from the observations that agents which labilize lysosomes (streptolysins O and S, endotoxin, large doses of vitamin A) induce or exacerbate rheumatoid arthritis. Agents which stabilize lysosomes and inhibit release of lysosomal hydrolases (corticosteroids, salicylates) are often effective in rheumatoid arthritis. The activity of lysosomal hydrolases is inhibited by drugs such as aminocaproic acid, chloroquine, and gold salts. Colchicine does not have a direct effect on lysosomal enzymes, but may interfere with the formation of phagolysosomes by inhibiting release of lysosomal enzymes into endocytic vacuoles. Bollet (11) has suggested that a lysosomal hyaluronidase originating in synovia and synovial fluid may contribute to the changes observed in osteoarthritis articular cartilage.

Effects of Drugs and Other Factors on Connective Tissue Metabolism

Several drugs, chemicals, and nutritional agents affect the synthetic and degradation pathways of the connective tissue complex. These factors are discussed in the following section according to the classification of the constituents of the complex (depicted in Figure 6.1) affected, namely, collagen, elastin, glycoprotein, and protein-polysaccharides.

Collagen Synthesis Ascorbic acid affects the conversion of protocollagen to collagen monomer by increasing the hydroxylation of prolyl and lysyl side chains. Glucoascorbic acid and glucocorticoids depress this step in collagen synthesis. Covalent cross-linking of collagen monomer to form fibrillar collagen is inhibited by β-aminoproprionitrile (BAPN) from lathyrus odoratus and vicia sativa. Isonicotinic acid hydrazide (INH) and hydrazines, as well as penicillamine, also inhibit this step in the formation of collagen fibrils.

Elastin Synthesis The covalent cross-linking of soluble elastin precursor to form elastin fibers is inhibited by β-aminoproprioitrile, vicia sativa, lathyrus odoratus factor, INH, hydrazines, and penicillamine.

Glycoproteins Corticosteroids may inhibit the synthesis of the protein core of glycoproteins, as well as enhance depolymerization of the glycoprotein ground substance. Similar depolymerization results from dietary deficiency of ascorbic acid.

Protein-Polysaccharides The normal turnover of these complexes is inhibited by corticosteroids and salicylates. Gold salts, chloroquine, and ϵ-aminocaproic acid may inhibit the degradation of protein-polysaccharide by inhibition of the release of lysosomal hydrolases. Streptolysins, endotoxin, and vitamin A enhance the normal turnover of protein-polysaccharide complexes.

LITERATURE CITED

1. Bornstein, P. 1969. Disorders of connective tissues. *In* P. K. Bondy (ed.), Diseases of Metabolism, pp. 654–710. W. B. Saunders Co., Philadelphia.
2. Robertson, W. V. B. 1964. Metabolism of collagen in mammalian tissues *In* Connective Tissues: Intercellular Macromolecules, pp. 93–114. Little, Brown & Co., Boston.
3. Bacchus, H. 1971. Clinical significance of serum glycoproteins. Int. Med. Digest 22–23.
4. Stetten, M. 1955. Metabolic relationship between glutamic acid proline, hydroxyproline and ornithine. *In* W. McElroy and B. Glass (eds.), Amino Acid Metabolism, p. 277. The Johns Hopkins Press, Baltimore.
5. Eylar, E. H. 1965. On the biological role of glycoproteins. J. Theor. Biol. 10:89–113.
6. Meyer, K. 1953. *In* W. H. Cole (ed.), Some Conjugated Proteins, p. 64. Rutgers University Press, New Brunswick, N.J.
7. Roden, L. 1968. Linkage of acid mucopolysaccharides to protein. *In* E. Rossi and E. Stoll (eds.), Biochemistry of Glycoproteins and Related Substances, p. 185. S. Karger, New York.

8. McKusick, V. A., D. Kaplan, D. Wise, W. B. Hanley, S. B. Suddarth, M. E. Sevick, and A. E. Maumance. 1965. The genetic mucopolysaccharidoses. Medicine 44:445—483.

9. van Hoof, F., and H. G. Hers. 1968. The abnormalities of lysosomal enzymes in mucopolysaccharidoses. Eur. Biochem. J. 7:34—48.

10. Kaplan, D. 1969. Classification of mucopolysaccharidoses based on pattern of mucopolysacchariduria. Am. J. Med. 47:721—729.

11. Bollet, A. J. 1967. Connective tissue polysaccharide metabolism and the pathogenesis of osteoarthritis. Adv. Intern. Med. 13:33—60.

12. Peterson, D. I., H. Bacchus, J. L. Seaich, and T. E. Kelly. 1975. Myelopathy associated with Maroteaux-Lamy syndrome. Arch. Neurol. 32:127—129.

7

Clinical Disorders of Porphyrin Metabolism

Disorders of porphyrin metabolism present an unusual variety of clinical and laboratory findings which may be encountered in many clinical specialties. It has been stated that "recent progress in the biochemistry and physiology of the porphyrias is an excellent example of how basic science can be combined with clinical medicine in a comprehensive approach to complicated medical problems" (1). The study of porphyrin metabolism is of fundamental importance as a model of defects in enzyme regulation.

The basic structure in all porphyrins is the compound porphyrin consisting of four rings (tetrapyrrole) joined together by methene bridges. Because of resonance from the conjugated double bond system, the ring possesses high chemical stability. Porphyrins are classified as: 1) etioporphyrins, each pyrrole having one methyl and one ethyl substituent; and 2) mesoporphyrins, each of two adjacent pyrrole rings having one methyl and one ethyl substituent, and each of the two remaining pyrrole rings having one methyl and one propionic acid substituent. All naturally occurring porphyrins when converted to etioporphyrins are of the I or III type depending on the order of the methyl and ethyl groups substituents on the rings. Only type III isomers have functional activity as components of hemoglobin and enzymes. There are 15 forms of mesoporphyrins. When the protoporphyrin of certain hemoproteins is converted to mesoporphyrins by reduction of two vinyl groups, isomer type 9 is obtained.

PHYSICAL AND CHEMICAL PROPERTIES

Solubility characteristics of the various porphyrins influence their pathways of excretion, the water solubility increasing with numbers of carboxyl- or hydroxyl-containing substituents. Protoporphyrin (dicarboxylic) is normally excreted exclusively in the bile, coproporphyrin (tetracarboxylic) mainly in bile but also in urine as coproporphyrinogen, and uroporphyrin (octacarboxylic) primarily in the urine. All porphyrins possess a characteristic type of absorption spectrum caused by the conjugated double bond system of the tetrapyrrole ring. These characteristics are important in physicochemical identification as well as some of the clinical effects (photosensitivity) of the compounds. All porphyrins have an intense absorption band near 400 nm, the Soret band.

HEME STRUCTURE AND FUNCTION

Porphyrins function in living systems only as metal chelates-iron porphyrins (hemes) and magnesium di- or tetrahydroporphyrins (chlorophylls). These compounds serve as prosthetic groups involved in catalysis of energy reactions on which life is dependent:

$$2 H_2O \underset{\text{heme}}{\overset{\text{chlorophyll}}{\rightleftharpoons}} 4 H + O_2 + 4e$$

in which radiant energy is used by chlorophyll.

The development of porphyrins and hemoproteins provides a means of iron being utilized for the following five types of biochemical functions: 1) transport of molecular O_2 (hemoglobins); 2) transport of electrons (mitochondrial cytochromes); 3) activation of oxygen (cytochrome oxidase, tryptophan pyrrolase, and mixed function oxidases such as microsomal cytochromes); 4) activation of H_2O_2 (peroxidases); and 5) decomposition of H_2O_2 (catalases).

These functions are dependent on the state of oxidation of the chelated iron, the nature of the ring substituents, and the structure of the protein to which heme is bound. The heme of hemoglobin is the ferrous chelate of protoporphyrin 9. (Vitamin B_{12} contains a tetrapyrrole moiety (corrin) which functions as a cobalt chelate. This corrin ring is not a porphyrin, but is closely related, being synthesized from porphyrin precursors.)

BIOSYNTHESIS OF HEME AND PORPHYRINS

The biosynthesis of these compounds (Figure 7.1) is dependent on the substrates glycine and succinyl-CoA in the presence of pyridoxal phosphate and the enzyme δ-aminolevulinic acid synthetase (ALA synthetase). This first step takes place in the mitochondria wherein the tricarboxylic acid cycle provides the substrate succinyl-CoA. This synthesis is dependent

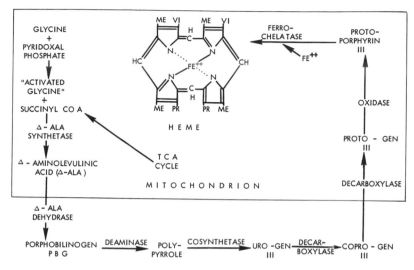

Figure 7.1. Biosynthesis of porphobilinogen, porphyrins, and heme. Note compartmentalization of the various steps in this synthesis. *Broken lines* refer to inhibitory mechanisms. *TCA,* tricarboxylic acid.

on pantothenic acid for CoA. Glycine is activated by pyridoxal phosphate ("activated glycine"), then condenses with succinyl-CoA. The presumed intermediate α-amino-β-ketoadipic acid is unstable and is rapidly converted to δ-aminolevulinic acid (δ-ALA). It has been suggested that α-amino-β-ketoadipic acid may not be an obligatory intermediate and that the decarboxylation of activated glycine and condensation with succinyl-CoA may occur simultaneously.

The immediate subsequent steps in porphyrin synthesis take place extramitochondrially; the δ-ALA diffuses through the mitochondrial membrane where it is acted upon by an enzyme in the cytosol, δ-ALA dehydrase. This results in the condensation of 2 molecules of δ-ALA to form porphobilinogen (PBG). This reaction requires GSH for activation of δ-ALA dehydrase.

ALA and PBG are obligatory intermediates in the synthesis of porphyrins, heme, and hemoproteins. δ-ALA dehydrase is present in relatively high concentrations in liver and marrow cells; its ability to utilize ALA for PBG production exceeds the ability of ALA synthetase to produce ALA by a ratio of 80:1 in normal human liver.

The biosynthetic intermediates between PBG and protoporphyrin are not porphyrins but are reduced porphyrins called porphyrinogens or hexahydroporphyrins. These compounds are readily oxidized to porphyrins by weak oxidizing agents.

PBG Deaminase and Uroporphyrinogen III Cosynthetase

The conversion of PBG to uroporphyrinogen III requires two enzymes. The first, PBG deaminase ("uroporphyrinogen I synthetase"), converts PBG to a polypyrrole of unclear structure, probably open ringed. The second enzyme, uroporphyrinogen III cosynthetase (also called isomerase), is thought to close the polypyrrole ring to form uroporphyrinogen III. If the polypyrrole is not acted upon by cosynthetase, it can spontaneously cyclize to uroporphyrinogen I.

Uroporphyrinogen Decarboxylase

The uroporphyrinogen III is converted to coproporphyrinogen III by decarboxylation of the four acetic acid side chains to form methyl groups. This enzyme is located in the cytosol and can act on the I isomer, but at a slower rate.

Coproporphyrinogen Oxidation

Coproporphyrinogen III enters the mitochondria and is converted to protoporphyrin by decarboxylation and oxidation reactions. The oxidation steps require molecular oxygen.

Ferrochelatase

The last step in heme biosynthesis involves chelation of ferrous iron by protoporphyrin to form heme. The reaction is catalyzed by ferrochelatase (heme synthetase). This reaction does not utilize ferric iron and is inhibited by aerobic conditions.

In summary, ALA and PBG are obligatory intermediates for porphyrin synthesis. The early steps, as well as the late steps, occur in the mitochondrial compartment and, therefore, do not take place in non-nucleated erythrocytes. However, the steps from ALA to coproporphyrinogen III are possible in mammalian erythrocytes. The synthesis of heme requires 8 moles of glycine and 8 moles of succinyl-CoA. Catabolism of heme and heme proteins does not lead to porphyrins but rather to the formation of bile pigments.

The bone marrow of the human adult forms 300 mg of heme daily for replacement of senescent erythrocytes and heme proteins. It is estimated that heme proteins synthesized in loco in all aerobic cells exceed the amount produced in the marrow; the liver and bone marrow sources are major contributors to the total heme pool.

CONTROL OF HEME BIOSYNTHESIS

Consideration of control of heme biosynthesis (Figure 7.2) is important because many of these factors operate in the clinical patterns of por-

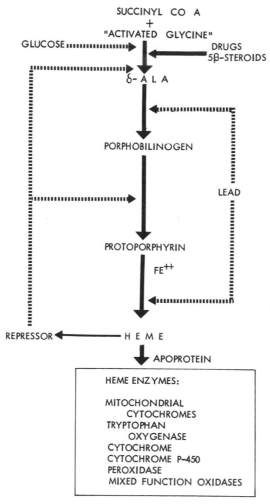

Figure 7.2. Control of heme synthesis. Negative feedback controls are represented by *broken lines*. Note the importance of δ-aminolevulinic acid synthetase, and secondarily of δ-ALA dehydrase in the regulatory mechanisms.

phrias. The mechanism in this regulation involves: induction—repression phenomena; feedback inhibition; possibly mitochondrial permeability; and partial pressure of oxygen.

The first and last several enzymes in heme synthesis are located in the mitochondria, and intermediate steps are located in the cytosol. The intramitochondrial steps involve oxidation and utilize oxidatively generated substrates, whereas the cytosol steps require self-condensations and decarboxylations. The following facts are known:

1. Heme inhibits the activity of δ-ALA synthetase, δ-ALA dehydrase, and ferrochelatase.

2. Lead is an inhibitor of δ-ALA dehydrase and ferrochelatase; hence, in lead poisoning, these are marked effects in porphyrin metabolism and in the excretion of porphyrins.

3. Relatively low levels of heme repress the synthesis of δ-ALA synthetase.

4. Oxygen inhibits some steps in heme synthesis, while other steps are oxygen dependent.

5. Hepatic δ-ALA synthetase is an inducible enzyme. Several drugs have been found to cause a severalfold increase in hepatic δ-ALA synthetase, probably by increased synthesis. The control of production of this synthetase is most likely through repression in which heme (or a derivative) serves as co-repressor.

6. Estrogens in minute doses intravenously cause oscillation of hepatic δ-ALA synthetase and δ-ALA dehydrase levels lasting for several days, suggesting an involvement in biological clock mechanism.

7. Cortisol exerts a permissive effect on induction of δ-ALA synthetase.

8. Studies by Tschudy et al. (2) showed that the induction of hepatic δ-ALA synthetase in animals is blocked by sufficient carbohydrate intake. (A similar effect of glucose to block the induction of enzymes in microorganisms was previously described.) This "glucose effect" (or catabolite repression phenomenon) on the genetically mediated induction of hepatic ALA synthetase in acute intermittent porphyria presumably underlies the reciprocal relationship between carbohydrate intake and porphyrin excretion seen in that disorder.

DESCRIPTIONS OF CLINICAL
DISORDERS OF PORPHYRIN METABOLISM

Hepatic Porphyrias

Acute Intermittent Porphyria Acute intermittent porphyria (AIP) is also called Swedish genetic porphyria and pyrroloporphyria (dominant). Clinical manifestations of this disorder begin at puberty or thereafter and are extremely rare prepubertally. The major symptoms occur during the early part of the reproductive period. This disorder is seen more frequently in subjects of Scandinavian and English ancestry, and it is estimated that the incidence is 1 in 13,000.

Clinical attacks of AIP may be precipitated by various drugs, including barbiturates, sulfonamides, griseofulvin, and estrogens. The clinical pattern is characterized by marked neurological involvement including autonomic neuropathy and intermittent abdominal pain which is often colicky. The abdominal pain may be localized or generalized; the abdomen is soft and there is no tenderness. Acute attacks may last several days to several months, with intervening asymptomatic periods. The gastrointestinal manifestations may lead to anorexia and weight loss. Vomiting may predispose to oliguria and azotemia. Neurological manifestations may also involve peripheral nerves, the brain stem, cranial nerves, and cerebral function. Patients may have hypertension and sinus tachycardia during attacks of AIP and the sinus tachycardia is often a reliable index of disease activity. During an attack, the patient may rarely exhibit fever and leukocytosis. Medullary paralysis is often a cause of death in patients with acute attacks of AIP, but uremia and cachexia may also contribute.

Several additional interesting features seen in patients during attacks of AIP are as follows: 1) increased protein-bound iodine (PBI) and thyroxin-binding globulin (TBG), and prolonged biological half-life of T4 (despite these findings, the patients are euthyroid); 2) hyponatremia secondary to inappropriate secretion of ADH (Tschudy et al. (2) demonstrated a hypo-thalamic lesion involving the supraoptic and paraventricular nuclei as the basis of this observation); 3) abnormalities of GH and ACTH secretion, possibly caused by associated hypothalamic lesions; 4) a probable relationship to gonadal activity with exacerbations often correlated with the menstrual cycle or following the use of oral contraceptive agents; 5) abnormalities in carbohydrate tolerance and an elevation of serum cholesterol; 6) bromsulfalein retention despite otherwise overtly normal liver function; 7) a striking response to the "glucose effect" phenomenon, in which glucose infusions may be of therapeutic value by affecting enzyme induction and repression processes.

The metabolic defect (3) in AIP is a decrease in uroporphyrinogen I synthetase (PBG deaminase) with a secondary increase in δ-ALA synthetase caused by decreased heme repression of δ-ALA synthetase (Figure 7.3). The defect is obviously only partial since complete absence of enzymatic activity would be incompatible with life.

Chemical findings in AIP include the excretion of large amounts of urinary porphobilinogen indicated by a positive Ehrlich's aldehyde reaction which is not extractable with chloroform or butanol. Excretion of PBG in normal subjects is less than 3 mg/24 hr, and it is markedly increased during an acute attack of AIP. During latent periods, the PBG value is above 3 mg/24 hr, but is close to normal. Excretion of δ-ALA is also marked during an acute attack; normal values are less than 3 mg/24 hr, but may approach 180 mg/24 hr during an attack of AIP. Urinary amino acids and indolic acids may also be elevated during an attack. A slight to moderate increase in fecal excretion of porphyrins also occurs under these conditions.

Treatment of AIP includes prophylaxis by avoiding the inducing drugs,

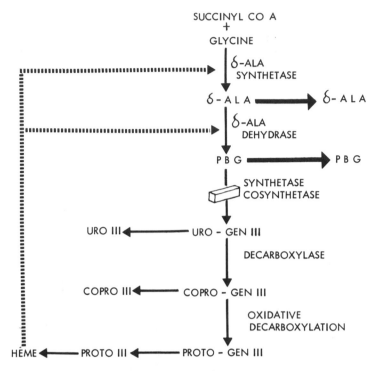

Figure 7.3. Metabolic defect in acute intermittent porphyria. The metabolites in the urine of diagnostic value are also identified.

and the use of chlorpromazine for symptoms during an attack. The infusion of glucose intravenously to inhibit induction of δ-ALA synthetase ("glucose effect" phenomenon) has been successful in management of an attack. More recently, the intravenous infusion of heme has been successfully tried in patients who failed to respond to glucose. The usefulness of hematin infusion has also been demonstrated recently (4).

Porphyria Variegata Porphyria variegata (PV) is also called South African genetic porphyria and is a disorder of porphyrin metabolism which is probably of autosomal dominant inheritance. It is estimated to be present in 3 in 1,000 of descendants of the early Dutch settlers in South Africa. The disorder rarely becomes manifest before puberty, and it exhibits many features similar to AIP. The significant clinical features include the following:

1. A positive family history of a chronic skin disorder, occasionally associated with acute abdominal and neurological symptoms. These latter symptoms may be preceded by the cutaneous manifestations for years. Most, or all, of the abdominal and neurological manifestations may be

precipitated by drugs such as barbiturates, sulfonamides, and other porphyrinogenic drugs, and by hepatotoxic drugs such as alcohol and general anesthetics. Abdominal pain and anorexia and vomiting may lead to oliguria and azotemia. Hyponatremia, hypochloremia, and hypokalemia are often found during an acute attack.

2. Increased sensitivity of the skin to light and minor mechanical trauma resulting in bullae, erosions, scarring, pigmentation, and thickening of the skin, as well as occasionally hypertrichosis, are often present.

3. Continuous fecal excretion of large amounts of proto- and coproporphyrins, and of peptide conjugates of dicarboxylic prophyrins.

The metabolic defect in PV is considered to be an exaggerated responsiveness of δ-ALA synthetase. It is assumed that a defect before ferrochelatase is unlikely (Figure 7.4). Treatment of PV includes the avoidance of inducing drugs, the use of sun screens on the skin, and other therapy as outlined for AIP.

Hereditary Coproporphyria Hereditary coproporphyria (HC) is similar clinically to PV, but the pattern of urinary end products is different. One review of 30 cases revealed an almost equal distribution among the sexes.

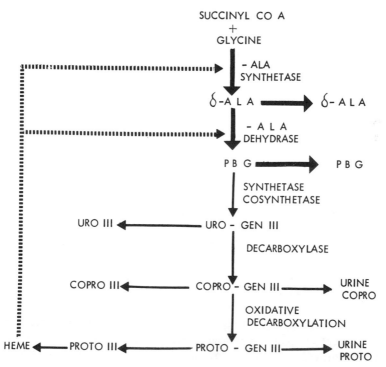

Figure 7.4. Metabolic defect in porphyria variegata.

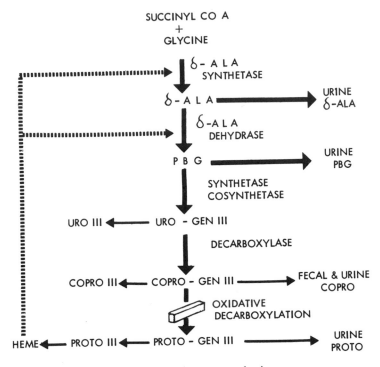

Figure 7.5. Metabolic defect in hereditary coproporphyria.

There is a familial occurrence of dominant characteristics. Patients with this disorder may be asymptomatic or may have mild, intermittent abdominal, neurological, and psychiatric manifestations. Photosensitivity is a minor manifestation. Attacks may be precipitated as in AIP and PV by drugs, including barbiturates, anticonvulsants, and tranquilizers. Some studies suggest a primary metabolic defect in the enzymatic conversion of coproporphyrinogen III to protoporphyrin by the enzyme coproporphyrinogen oxidase. The hepatic levels of δ-ALA are markedly elevated (Figure 7.5).

Chemical findings in HC include an unremitting excretion of large amounts of coproporphyrin III in the feces. Urinary coproporphyrin is frequently increased, especially during attacks. δ-ALA and PBG in the urine are elevated and may approach the levels seen in AIP. Treatment of HC includes the avoidance of inducing drugs, the use of chlorpromazine for abdominal and neurological problems, and glucose infusion for the "glucose effect" phenomenon on enzyme induction.

Porphyria Cutanea Tarda Porphyria cutanea tarda (PCT) is also known as symptomatic, constitutional, or idiopathic porphyria. It is assumed to be an acquired abnormality of porphyrin metabolism. Most of the affected patients consume large amounts of alcohol with especially high iron content. In Johannesburg, the incidence among the hospital population is 5 in 1,000 and, in the outpatient population, is 13 in 1,000. The disorder is assumed to be an occult genetic problem which is activated by ethanolism.

Clinical features include major findings which are limited to the skin, frequently associated with evidence of liver dysfunction. This disorder is reported in many parts of the world, with the highest incidence in South African Bantus of middle age. Vesicular and ulcerative lesions on exposed surfaces of the skin of face, hands, and feet are found, and depigmented scars may accompany healing. Hypertrichosis of the forehead and hyperpigmentation of the exposed skin are almost constant features. Hepatomegaly with abnormal liver function tests is present in almost all patients. Acute neurological and abdominal attacks do not usually occur in these patients.

It is probable that there is a genetic predisposition for this type of

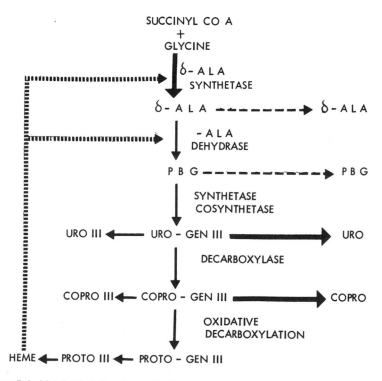

Figure 7.6. Metabolic defect in porphyria cutanea tarda.

porphyria. A remarkably high incidence of liver disease suggested that alterations in liver enzymes may be the responsible precipitating mechanism. Hepatic levels of δ-ALA synthetase are normal. Rimington suggests that there occurs formation of porphyrins in the liver because of increased oxidation of porphyrinogens. As a result of this, there is decreased heme synthesis (Figure 7.6).

Chemical findings include increased urinary excretion of uroporphyrins and other ether insoluble porphyrins, but excess ALA and PBG are not usually seen in patients with PCT. Treatment consists of repeated phlebotomy for removal of excess iron and chloroquine therapy to bind uroporphyrin in the liver.

Several thousand cases of porphyria in Turkey resulted from ingestion of wheat treated with the fungicide hexachlorobenzene. This form was seen more frequently in males and in children. Clinical manifestation included blistering and epidermolysis on exposed areas, hyperpigmentation, hypertrichosis, and red urine. The cutaneous manifestations and red urine were worse in summer and improved in winter. A large number of patients exhibited hepatomegaly, 30% had thyromegaly, and others had anorexia, emaciation, and suppurative lymphadenopathy.

Erythropoietic Porphyrias

Congenital Erythropoietic Porphyria Congenital erythropoietic porphyria is also known as Günther's disease, erythropoietic uroporphyria (recessive), and is a rare autosomal recessive disease which is characterized by urinary excretion of large amounts of uroporphyrin I, mutilating skin lesions, and hemolytic anemia. It is rarer than any other form of porphyria. Approximately 60 authenticated cases are described in world literature, showing essentially equal sex distribution, with patients of several different racial backgrounds.

The major clinical manifestations are skin lesions caused by photosensitivity and hemolytic anemia. Photosensitivity may become apparent early in life with the infant crying after exposure to sunlight. Onset of symptoms occurs between birth and 5 years of age, but one patient is described with onset at age 50. The first sign suggesting this disorder is red or pink urine.

Vesicles or bullae appear on skin exposed to sunlight. These lesions may ulcerate and heal with scarring. Severe deformity of the nose, ears, eyelids, and fingers may follow repeated infections in the lesions. Nails and terminal phalanges may be lost. Conjunctivitis, keratitis, and ectropion are often found. Areas of pigmentation and depigmentation are common, and areas of scalp alopecia may occur as result of scarring.

Hypertrichosis consisting of fine lanugo hair may occur on face and limbs and is ascribed to increased porphyrins, but the mechanism is not known. The skin lesions are worse during months of increased light exposure; hence, the term *hydroa estivale.*

Light exposure causes porphyrin oxidation and possibly also causes release of porphyrin from the skin. Porphyrin deposition in teeth and bones causes a brown or pink discoloration, viz., erythrodontia. Such tissues fluoresce under ultraviolet light. The porphyrin deposition is caused by chemical binding to calcium phosphate.

Hemolysis is seen in most patients, but, rarely, bone marrow hyperplasia may prevent the usually normochromic anemia. In patients with the hemolytic disorder, increased reticulocytes, increased fecal urobilinogen, normoblastic hyperplasia of the bone marrow, and circulating normoblasts may be found. Erythrocyte life span is normal or reduced. Splenomegaly is found in 75% of the patients, and a few patients have thrombocytopenia ascribed to hypersplenism. Overt jaundice is rarely found, but slight bilirubin elevations are found in some patients. The processes responsible for anemia are hemolysis and ineffective erythropoiesis. The mechanism of the hemolysis is not clear (studies on osmotic fragility of red cells being normal), and the Coombs test is negative (except in one described patient). Possible causes of hemolysis are either sensitization of red cells by high contents of porphyrins or an intracorpuscular defect. All manifestations, hemolytic and cutaneous, vary from time to time.

Normoblastic hyperplasia in the marrow is the source of excess porphyrins, and 70% of the cells show ultraviolet fluorescence. Basophilic stippling occurs in the cytoplasm of fluorescent normoblasts. The peripheral blood may show anisocytosis, poikilocytosis, and polychromatophilia. Reticulocytosis is often present, and some erythrocytes may exhibit fluorescence. There are follicular hyperplasia in the spleen and increased melanin and fibroblast proliferation in the skin. Hemosiderin infiltration may cause moderate hepatomegaly.

The metabolic defect must account for increased levels of uroporphyrin I isomers with increased type III isomers sufficient to maintain heme synthesis. Normally, when PBG deaminase acts in the absence of sufficient uroporphyrinogen III cosynthetase, there is an increase of uroporphyrinogen I. A primary defect in uroporphyrinogen III cosynthetase is considered as the most likely metabolic defect so that channeling of tetrapyrrole substrate to the I isomer series depletes the substrate for the III pathway relative to normal (Figure 7.7).

The urine may vary in color from pink to burgundy red to dark red-brown depending on the concentration of porphyrins. Uroporphyrin excretion in the urine may be as high as 500 mg/24 hr. Increased coproporphyrinuria is not as great. Porphyrins of greater polarity are also found. Most of the porphyrins are of the I series, although III isomers are also found. PBG and ALA excretion in the urine are not increased. Fecal

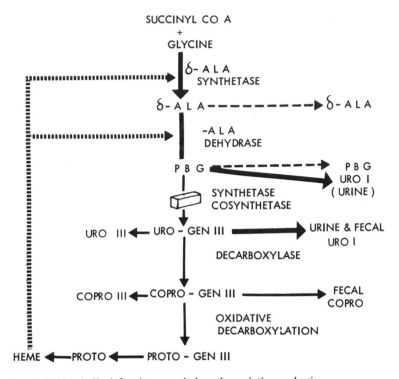

Figure 7.7. Metabolic defect in congenital erythropoietic porphyria.

coproporphyrin is increased, with lower increase of fecal uroporphyrins. High levels of uroporphyrin I may also be found in the circulating plasma. Treatment consists of the following measures: the use of protective clothing to protect the skin, as most creams do not absorb the Soret band (a sunscreen filter induced in normal skin has been promising); the systemic use of steroids may occasionally be helpful, especially if Coombs test is positive; and splenectomy may reduce hemolysis and may also aid in reducing photosensitivity. Urine and fecal porphyrin excretion usually decreases after splenectomy. Few patients survive beyond middle age.

Erythropoietic Protoporphyria Erythropoietic protoporphyria is more common than congenital erythropoietic porphyria. It is the one form of porphyria in which there is no increase of urinary porphyrin or porphyrin precursors. The disorder is inherited as an autosomal dominant characteristic; there are data to suggest equal incidence in both sexes.

The most common clinical manifestation of photosensitivity is a burning and stinging of the skin exposed to sunlight; exposure of a few minutes or hours may cause symptoms which may last for days. In most patients, erythema develops soon after exposure, and edema after a few hours; the latter may be persistent for weeks. Vesicles, bullae, and purpura may be seen in children and adults. Scabs and crusts may form and heal with scars. The skin lesions are not of the severity of congenital erythropoietic porphyria. Thickening and scarring of skin of nose, cheeks, back of hands, and fingers may occur. A cobblestone appearance of the skin is seen in patients in tropical areas. In some patients, absence of lunulae was seen. Cholelithiasis at a relatively early age may be found and is ascribed to precipitated protoporphyrin. Hirsutism and hyperpigmentation are rarely found in these patients. The photosensitivity is secondary to increased plasma porphyrin levels. Some narrow nomoblasts may show the occurrence of an amorphous material in and around capillary walls. Recent studies reveal disordered heme synthesis in various tissues—the most important being the maturing erythrocytes and the liver. A possible defect in ferrochelatase has been suggested. This probably results in increased ALA synthetase activity (Figure 7.8). Chemical studies show no increase of porphyrins or porphyrin precursors in the urine. Three patterns have been described: 1) increase in free erythrocyte, plasma, and fecal protoporphyrin; 2) increased free erythrocyte protoporphyrin with no increase of

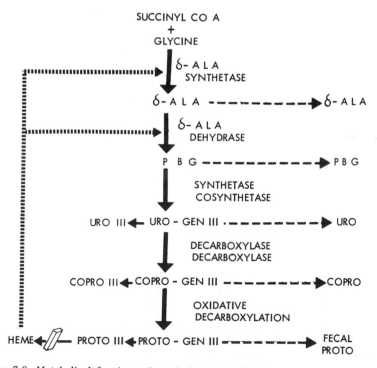

Figure 7.8. Metabolic defect in erythropoietic protoporphyria.

the plasma or fecal protoporphyrin; and 3) increased fecal protoporphyrin with no increase of fecal or erythrocyte protoporphyrin (rare).
Treatment consists of avoidance of sunlight and use of antihistamines for
solar urticaria. Sytemic use of quinacrine may be helpful, and chloroquine
is occasionally helpful. This disorder does not overtly reduce longevity,
and the skin lesions decrease with age. Cholelithiasis is often clinically
significant. Tables 7.1, 7.2, and 7.3 summarize diagnostic, clinical, and
laboratory features of the various porphyrias.

Drugs Affecting Porphyrin Synthesis

The drugs which affect the induction or progress of the hepatic porphyrias
(AIP, PV, HC, but not PCT) have been classified by Tschudy as follows:
1) drugs implicated in precipitating attacks including barbiturates, sulfonamides, griseofulvin (Fulvicin, Grifulvin), chlordiazepoxide (Librium),
meprobamate (Miltown, Equanil), isopropylmeprobamate (Soma), di-
phenylhydantoin (Dilantin), methsuximide (Celontin), tolbutamide
(Orinase), and possibly ergot derivatives; 2) drugs which produce significant "porphyria" in liver cells in vitro, such as glutethimide (Doriden),

Table 7.1. Clinical Disorders of Porphyrin Metabolism

I. Hepatic porphyrias
  A. Acute intermittent porphyria, Swedish genetic porphyria, pyrrolo-
    porphyria (dominant)
    1. Manifest
    2. Latent
  B. Porphyria variegata, mixed porphyria, South Africa genetic por-
    phyria, protocoproporphyria (dominant)
    1. Cutaneous with little or no acute manifestations
    2. Acute intermittent without cutaneous symptoms
    3. Various combinations
    4. Latent
  C. Hereditary coproporphyria
    1. Manifest
    2. Latent
  D. Porphyria cutanea tarda, symptomatic porphyria, urocopropor-
    phyria, constitutional porphyria
    1. With familial evidence of the disease
    2. Without familial incidence of the disease
      a) "Idiosyncratic"—associated with alcohol, liver disease, etc.
      b) Acquired, hexachlorobenzene-induced porphyria, hepatoma
II. Erythropoietic porphyrias
  A. Congenital erythropoietic porphyria, Gunther's disease, erythro-
    poietic uroporphyria (recessive)
  B. Erythropoietic protoporphyria (dominant)
  C. Erythropoietic coproporphyria

Table 7.2. Differential Diagnostic Points in Disorders of Porphyrin Metabolism

Disorder	Neurological disorder	Abdominal and gastrointestinal disorder	Photosensitivity and skin lesions	Hemolysis	Hypertrichosis	Hypertension
Erythropoietic porphyria	0	0	+++	+++	++	0
Erythropoietic protoporphyria	0	0	+	0	0	0
Acute intermittent porphyria	+++	+++	0	0	+	±
Porphyria variegata	+++	+++	++	0	+	±
Hereditary coproporphyria	++	+++	+	0	+	±
Porphyria cutanea tarda	0	0	++	0	+	0

Table 7.3. Laboratory Features of Disorders of Porphyrin Metabolism

Disorder	Urinary				Fecal			Erythrocyte		
	ALA	PBG	URO	COPRO	URO	COPRO	PROTO	URO	COPRO	PROTO
Erythropoietic porphyria	N[a]	N	(I)+++ (III)±	(I)++	+	(I)++	(I)+++	+++	++	+
Erythropoietic protoporphyria	N	N	N	N	N	N	++	N	+	+++
Acute intermittent porphyria	+++	+++	+;N	++	+;N	++		N	N	N
Porphyria variegata	++	++	+	++		+++	++++	N	N	N
Hereditary coproporphyria	++	++ (During crisis)		++		Constant		N	N	N
Porphyria cutanea tarda	N	N	+++	++				N	N	N
Lead poisoning	++	N		(I)++						+++
Factors which decrease Fe incorporation into heme, e.g., Fe deficiency, lead poisoning; also hemolysis, leukemias, azotemia; infectious hepatitis and obstructive jaundice										+++

[a] N, normal.

mephenytoin (Mesantoin), methprylon (Noludar), and chloramphenicol (Chloromycetin); and 3) drugs which are known to be safe in these disorders, including meperidine (Demerol), chlorpromazine (Thorazine), aspirin, penicillin, and probably propoxyphene (Darvon).

LITERATURE CITED

1. Tschudy, D. P. 1974. Porphyrin metabolism and the porphyrias. *In* P. K. Bondy and L. E. Rosenberg (eds.), Diseases of Metabolism, pp. 775–824. W. B. Saunders Co., Philadelphia.
2. Tschudy, D. P., F. H. Welland, A. Collins, and G. Hunter. 1964. The effect of carbohydrate feeding on the induction of amino levulinic acid synthetase. Metabolism 13:396–406.
3. Meyer, U. A., L. J. Strand, M. Doss, A. C. Rees, and H. Marver. 1972. Intermittent acute porphyria genetic defect in porphobilinogen metabolism. N. Engl. J. Med. 286:1277–1282.
4. Watson, C. J. 1975. Hematin and porphyria. N. Engl. J. Med. 293:605–606.

8
Clinical Disorders of Bilirubin Metabolism

HEME DEGRADATION AND BILIRUBIN METABOLISM

In the previous chapter, it was shown that the porphyrin of naturally occurring heme is protoporphyrin IXa (ferroprotoporphyrin IXa). This structure is the prosthetic group of hemoglobin and other hemoproteins. The heme group of hemoglobin is the major source of bilirubin in man; this source accounts for about 80% of the 250–300 g of pigment formed in 24 hr. Senescent red cells are sequestered in the reticuloendothelial cells of the spleen, bone marrow, and liver, and their heme (from hemoglobin) is converted to bilirubin (1). Bile pigment formation from subcutaneous hematomas occurs in macrophages.

The catabolism of other hemoproteins (myoglobin, cytochromes, catalases, and peroxidases), under physiological conditions, accounts for approximately 20% of all bile pigments formed in man. Because the liver contains an abundance of heme enzymes, it plays an important role in bile pigment metabolism. The hepatic microsomal cytochrome P-450 and cytochrome b_5 are involved in the metabolism of many hormones, drugs, and toxins. These enzymes are present in hepatic cells in high concentration which may be further increased by drugs whose metabolism is dependent on such enzymes, viz., enzyme induction. These hepatic cytochromes have considerably shorter biological half-life than hemoglobin, and account for the "early labeled" fraction of bilirubin fraction after administration of labeled glycine or 5-ALA.

255

ENZYMATIC DEGRADATION OF HEME TO BILIRUBIN

The initial step in this process involves the cleavage of the ferroprotopor-phyrin ring at its α-methene bridge by microsomal heme oxygenase, yielding 1 mole each of biliverdin, iron, and carbon monoxide (CO). The heme oxygenase system contains cytochrome P-450 as a terminal oxygenase, and requires NADPH and O_2 as cofactors (Figure 8.1). In the second step, biliverdin is reduced to bilirubin by the soluble enzyme biliverdin reductase, which is linked to the previous enzyme and also has a requirement for NADPH.

Heme oxygenase is most active in tissues involved in heme degradation, the spleen and liver, with lower activities in the kidneys, macrophages, and

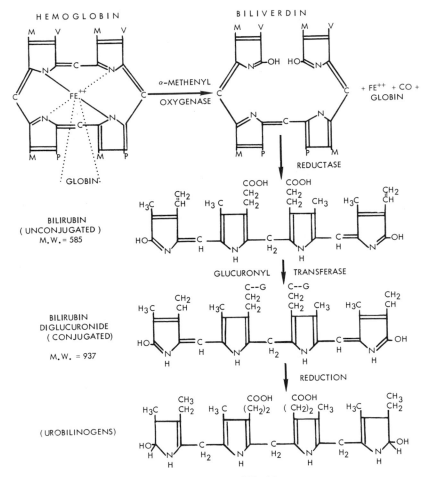

Figure 8.1. Enzymatic degradation of heme to bilirubin.

brain. It is of interest, however, that the substrate heme stimulates the induction of the oxygenase. For example, in hemoglobinuria, the hemoglobin absorbed by the renal tubules induces increased heme oxygenase activity in these cells. This might explain the finding that, in hemolytic states, the plasma contains unconjugated bilirubin rather than unreacted heme (methemalbumin). The heme oxygenase system does not attack porphyrins that lack a centrally located metal atom. Therefore in porphyric states, in the absence of hemolysis, defects in heme synthesis result in increased porphyrin excretion, but normal excretion of bile pigments. In hemolytic states, the breakdown of hemoglobin results in increased bile pigments, but normal porphyrin excretion.

BILIRUBIN TRANSPORT IN PLASMA

The pigment bilirubin is quite lipid soluble and, therefore, diffuses freely across cell membranes of various tissues. The intracellular occurrence of this substance has been shown to disturb various vital metabolic functions, culminating, for example, in the encephalopathy which occurs in severe unconjugated hyperbilirubinemia of neonates. Physiological mechanisms have evolved, tending to limit the access of bilirubin to tissues. These mechanisms are binding of bilirubin to albumin (and other proteins) and conjugation mechanisms.

In the circulating plasma, virtually all bilirubin is bound tightly to albumin; 1 molecule of human albumin binds at least 2 moles of bilirubin. This complex cannot freely diffuse across cell membranes; hence, potentially dangerous accumulations of bilirubin in cells are prevented. Certain drugs, e.g., sulfonamides, thyroxin, fatty acids, and acetylsalicylate, may displace bilirubin from albumin, permitting rapid diffusion of bilirubin into tissues. In neonates in whom the bilirubin levels have saturated the total binding capacity of plasma, such compounds may induce bilirubin encephalopathy by releasing bilirubin into the central nervous system.

The hepatic transformation of bilirubin is presented in Figure 8.2. For this process, bilirubin carried in the plasma to the hepatic sinusoids is mainly albumin-bound, with only a small unbound fraction. The unbound fraction is freely diffusible through the hepatocyte membrane. The bilirubin entering the cell becomes attached to acceptor proteins. Two such acceptor proteins of low molecular weight, termed Y and Z proteins, have been characterized (2). The protein acceptors may also bind other organic anions which are excreted in bile, and may compete with bilirubin for available binding sites in the liver.

The uptake of bilirubin by the hepatocyte is described as composed of two compartments, one extracellular (plasma) and one intracellular (hepatocyte) separated by a membrane permeable to free (unbound) bilirubin,

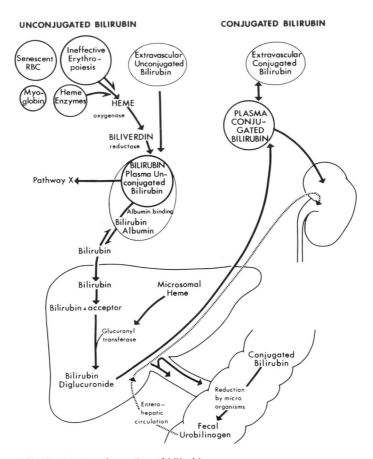

Figure 8.2. Hepatic transformation of bilirubin.

but not bound bilirubin. The ultimate equilibrium between the two compartments depends on relative binding forces on either side of the membrane. A concentration gradient across the membrane would tend to increase the flow of pigment from liver sinusoid to intracel. Such a process is facilitated by the ability of the hepatocyte to convert bilirubin to bilirubin diglucuronide which is readily excreted into the biliary tract.

The conjugation of bilirubin in the liver is catalyzed by enzymes located in the smooth endoplasmic reticulum of the hepatocyte. Glucuronyltransferase in the smooth endoplasmic reticulum transfers glucuronic acid from uridine diphosphoglucuronic acid to the two propionic groups of bilirubin, forming an ester glucuronide. The diglucuronide is the major excretion product, but some monoglucuronide may also be excreted. This conjugation process is essential for excretion of bilirubin. The secretory mechanism by which the bilirubin diglucuronide leaves the cell probably involves packaging by the Golgi apparatus and extrusion against a concentration gradient; it is probable that this process is carrier mediated and energy consuming.

The processes of hepatic uptake, conjugation, and excretion of bilirubin are very efficient, so that, in normal subjects, the serum bilirubin level is usually 1 mg/100 ml or less. These three steps may be regarded as a single operational unit, and the effect of drugs, such as phenobarbital, which increase transfer of bilirubin from plasma by a coordinate increase in each of these steps, appears to confirm this concept.

Bilirubin glucuronide which is discharged into the intestinal tract is converted by bacterial flora in the lower tract to a group of chromogens called urobilinogen. In this process, most of the carbohydrate moiety is cleaved off, but there may be small amounts of urobilinogen conjugates. Most of the urobilinogen is excreted in the feces, but a small portion undergoes reabsorption and re-excretion in the bile. This is the source of small amounts of urobilinogen in bile and in the urine. In complete extrahepatic obstruction of the bile ducts, there is a disappearance of urine urobilinogen because no conjugated bilirubin reaches the gastrointestinal tract. Similarly, broad-spectrum antibiotics, which suppress the intestinal flora, reduce the conversion of bilirubin in the colon. While under normal conditions bilirubin elimination is almost exclusively by hepatic conjugation, there are, nevertheless, alternative mechanisms which are quantitatively less efficient. In certain situations where there is an accumulation of unconjugated bilirubin because of defective conjugation (Crigler-Najjar syndrome), gradual degradation of bilirubin may occur. The end products exhibit a progressively decreased yellow color and are more water soluble. A similar phenomenon occurs when bilirubin is exposed to intense white or blue light. The process is oxygen dependent; the chemical nature of the derivatives is not known.

CLINICAL DISORDERS OF BILIRUBIN METABOLISM

Hyperbilirubinemia is usually the result of two distinct phenomena which may, nevertheless, be associated. "Retention" of unconjugated bilirubin may be caused by 1) overproduction of the pigment such as in overt hemolysis, ineffective erythropoiesis, 2) decreased hepatic uptake, or 3) failure of conjugation mechanisms.

"Regurgitation" of conjugated bilirubin into the plasma may result from extrahepatic obstruction of the biliary tract, interruption of the hepatic architecture, or cholestasis. Jaundice caused by primary hepatocellular disease is associated with increased concentrations of both conjugated and unconjugated bilirubin, with the relative proportions being quite

Table 8.1. Summary of Hyperbilirubinemias

Disorders	Defects and clinical features
Unconjugated hyperbilirubinemias	
Overproduction of bilirubin	Hemolysis, ineffective erythropoiesis, degradation of heme enzymes
Gilbert's syndrome	Decreased membrane transport and/or decreased carrier proteins. Autosomal recessive disorder with decreased transport of organic anions and mild icterus. Similar defect in Southdown sheep, and may be induced by flavaspidic acid.
Crigler-Najjar syndrome	Decreased glucuronyltransferase activity with severe icterus and bilirubin encephalopathy. Rapidly fatal.
Chronic unconjugated hyperbilirubinemia	Dominant inheritance with icteric skin, sclerae, and mucous membranes. Enzyme induction with phenobarbital may be helpful.
Neonatal hyperbilirubinemia	Immaturity of hepatic glucuronyltransferase may lead to bilirubin encephalopathy. Displacement of bilirubin binding may also precipitate this complication.
Transient familial neonatal hyperbilirubinemia (Lucey-Driscoll)	Probably caused by steroid metabolites associated with pregnancy. Similar defect is found in the Gunn rat.
Breast-feeding hyperbilirubinemia	Ascribed to pregnanediol in mother's milk. Inhibition of glucuronyltransferase.

Conjugated hyperbilirubinemias Idiopathic recurrent cholestasis	Onset in childhood usually with jaundice, pruritus, malaise, and irritability. Steatorrhea may occur. Alkaline phosphatase and transaminase are increased. Corticosteroid therapy may be helpful.
Recurrent intrahepatic cholestasis of pregnancy	May be found in last 4 months of pregnancy and characterized by conjugated and unconjugated hyperbilirubinemia and pruritus. Possibly related to steroid metabolites in pregnancy.
Drug-induced intrahepatic obstruction	May be induced by phenothiazines, C-17 alkylsteroids. Ascribed to cholestasis.
Dubin-Johnson syndrome	Decreased membrane transport of organic anions out of hepatocyte results in syndrome of jaundice with abdominal pain, fatigue, dark urine, and hepatosplenomegaly. Pigment deposition in liver is found. Prognosis is excellent.
Rotor syndrome	Decreased membrane transport of organic anions out of hepatocyte results in early and lifelong jaundice. BSP excretion is decreased. No pigment accumulation is found in liver.
Extrahepatic biliary obstruction	Obstruction of bile duct or other parts of excretory system by calculus, inflammation, neoplasm results in decreased excretion of bilirubin diglucuronide. Serum levels of conjugated and unconjugated bilirubin are elevated. Deconjugation of bilirubin diglucuronide may also occur. Urine urobilinogen is decreased.

variable. Often there may also be an associated defect in erythrocyte life span associated with liver disease.

Clinical disorders of bilirubin metabolism are classified as: 1) unconjugated hyperbilirubinemia and 2) conjugated hyperbilirubinemias; in certain clinical situations both types may be found (Table 8.1).

Unconjugated Hyperbilirubinemias

The hepatic excretory mechanism operates at such a degree of efficiency that the normal level of total bilirubin is usually below 1.0 mg/100 ml. Even in the presence of low grade hemolysis, the excretory mechanisms may compensate in clearing the plasma of excess bilirubin in most individuals.

Neonatal hyperbilirubinemia is a benign condition occurring in most newborn infants and characterized by a low grade elevation of plasma bilirubin. The hyperbilirubinemia reaches peak levels by the 7th day of life and returns to normal by 2 weeks of age. This "physiological" jaundice is caused by immaturity of the hepatic excretory mechanisms. There are data to show that fetal bilirubin excretion is dependent on placental transfer and after delivery this mechanism is lost. The demonstration that certain other excretory functions of the liver are intact indicates that the failure to excrete bilirubin is not caused by complete failure of excretory function or anatomic block. The defect is ascribed to a decreased glucuronyltransferase level in the fetal liver. It is probable that there is also a decreased level of uridine diphosphoglucuronic acid in the fetal liver. Glucuronyltransferase activity increases slowly toward the end of gestation and reaches normal adult levels by 14 days after birth. There are data in other species which indicate a decreased Y protein level in fetal liver tissue; this defect might be related to a possible decreased hepatic uptake of unconjugated bilirubin. It is of some interest that this phase of BSP uptake is also decreased in newborns. It might be suggested that an accumulation of bilirubin may induce maturation of the excretory mechanisms.

Plasma unconjugated bilirubin levels greater than 20 mg/100 ml may lead to kernicterus whereby bilirubin uptake by the central nervous system results in ataxia, convulsions, and death. There is an equilibrium between albumin-bound unconjugated bilirubin and unbound bilirubin in the plasma. At high levels of bilirubin, there is diffusion of unbound bilirubin across the blood brain barrier. The threat of such transfer is greater in the presence of hypoalbuminemia and in the presence of excess free fatty acids, in acidotic states, and also in the presence of certain drugs, e.g., salicylates and sulfa drugs. It has been suggested that the neonatal central nervous system is more susceptible to the toxic effects of bilirubin. The actual mechanism of the toxicity of this pigment is not known.

Unconjugated hyperbilirubinemia associated with breast feeding is a form of hyperbilirubinemia that has been reported repeatedly in certain infants who were breast fed. This form of jaundice, often seen in successive breast-fed siblings, becomes maximally manifest by 10–20 days postpartum, and gradually disappears 1–2 months after birth, despite continued breast feeding. This form of jaundice is ascribed to the presence of pregnanediol (pregnane 3α,20β-diol) in the mother's milk. There are data which prove an inhibition of hepatic glucuronyltransferase activity by pregnanediol and related steroids.

Studies by Lucey et al. (3) showed that normal maternal serum may inhibit bilirubin conjugation in vitro. Exaggeration of this process results in a rare, transient, familial neonatal hyperbilirubinemia (Lucey-Driscoll enzyme inhibition) which develops during the first 48 hr of life.

Gilbert's syndrome (constitutional hepatic dysfunction; low grade chronic hyperbilirubinemia) is presumed to be an autosomal dominant inherited disorder which is characterized by a chronic mild unconjugated hyperbilirubinemia, normal erythropoiesis and red cell survival, and absence of overt histological or functional disorder of the liver and biliary tract. Mild icterus may be seen shortly after birth, but often is not recognized until later in life, often in an incidental laboratory study. Serum bilirubin levels vary considerably ranging from 1.6–3 mg/100 ml. These levels seem to be inversely related to dietary caloric intake, suggesting participation of enzyme induction and repression phenomena. Bilirubinuria is absent, and urobilinogen is usually normal or low, both of these observations a reflection of the absence of any elevation of conjugated bilirubin. There is no hepatosplenomegaly, and liver function tests are essentially normal except for occasional decreased BSP excretion. Histological studies reveal no hepatic abnormality, but recent electron microscopic studies suggest presence of minor alteration of hepatocyte membrane adjacent to the sinusoidal lumen. There are no major clinical subjective manifestations.

The pathogenesis of the defect is not clear, but the best working hypothesis is that there is a defect in the transport of organic anions from the plasma into the liver. The possibility of competition with other anions at this site is to be considered.

Chronic unconjugated hyperbilirubinemia of adolescents and adults is an autosomal dominant disorder with incomplete penetrance and varied expressivity. These patients exhibit variable degrees of icterus with serum bilirubin ranging from 6–25 mg/100 ml. The patients range in age from infancy to adulthood. The levels of conjugated bilirubin (measured as "direct reacting") are normal. Erythrocyte generation and survival are normal. Jaundice may be noted in the 1st year of life. Icterus of skin, sclera, and mucous membranes may be the only overt abnormality, but neurological problems caused by bilirubin encephalopathy have been described. Several studies suggest that this disorder is caused by a defect in the glucuronyltransferase system responsible for bilirubin conjugation. The findings that large doses of phenobarbital, as well as the oral administration of dichlorodiphenyltrichlorethane (DDT), are followed by a progressive decrease of serum bilirubin to nearly normal levels in 2–3 weeks suggest that microsomal glucuronyltransferase may be induced by these drugs.

Crigler-Najjar syndrome (congenital non-hemolytic jaundice; severe icterus caused by defective conjugation of bilirubin) is a genetically transmitted disorder which is the result of a double dose of a rare, non-X-linked allele. The original report by Crigler and Najjar (4) described six infants in three related families. Severe icterus was observed in all of the patients starting from 1st to 3rd day of birth and persisting throughout their lives. These patients exhibited no evidence of blood group incompatibility or of hemolysis. The bilirubin was virtually all of the "indirect reacting" type, and there was no bilirubinuria. Liver function tests and histology were described as normal. Five of the six infants developed a neurological disorder resembling kernicterus, and they died by the age of 15 months. Examination of the brain at autopsy revealed intense staining of the cerebral cortex and basal ganglia with bile pigment. The sixth child of this group escaped neurological disability up to age 15.5 years, but had persistent jaundice. At this time, without overt precipitating causes, he developed the neurological disorders and died within 6 months. The brain showed neuronal loss and gliosis of the thalamus with moderate changes in the basal ganglia. Approximately 20 additional patients have been described with this disorder, most of them dying of nervous system damage. Four are known to be neurologically normal in their teens.

The patients exhibited no evidence of hemolysis, erythropoiesis was normal, and there was no hepatosplenomegaly. Liver histology only showed occasional presence of bile thrombi in hepatic canaliculi. Electron microscopy studies revealed minor changes at the sinusoidal pole of the hepatocytes. Bilirubin concentrations ranged from 15–48 g/100 ml of serum.

The metabolic defect in this disorder is now known to be in the glucuronyltransferase system, involving bilirubin conjugation as well as the other glucuronidation mechanisms. However, certain other glucuronyltransferase activities are present. It is presumed that the glucuronyltransferase system consists of several distinct related microsomal enzymes with overlapping substrate specificity, and, in this syndrome, the major abnormality is in the mechanism of bilirubin conjugation.

The goal of therapy is to decrease the unconjugated bilirubin levels and prevent bilirubin encephalopathy. The methods employed are phenobarbital therapy and phototherapy.

Administration of large doses of this phenobarbital has not resulted in significant improvement in patients who are hemozygous for this disorder. Heterozygotes do respond, and it has been suggested that a phenobarbital challenge may be used for identifying heterozygotes.

On exposure to visible light, bilirubin decomposes to more polar compounds. This principle was applied in the management of these patients by Cremer, Perryman, and Richards (5), as well as by others, with significant degrees of success.

Animal Models for Unconjugated Hyperbilirubinemias An hereditary acholuric jaundice occurring in a strain of Wistar rats caused by a defect in formation of conjugated bilirubin has been described (the Gunn rat). Rats with bilirubin levels over 12–15 mg/100 ml exhibited signs resembling kernicterus and ataxia. An associated abnormality is a polyuria which may result in dehydration. This renal defect is ascribed to interference by bilirubin with sodium and urea transport in the renal medulla. Metabolic studies demonstrated that the primary defect in these animals involves the glucuronyltransferase system of the liver microsomes.

Southdown mutant sheep have an autosomal recessive disorder characterized by congenital hyperbilirubinemia. These sheep also exhibit a facial photosensitivity caused by accumulation of phylloerythrin derived from chlorophyll. The disorder is caused by a defect in hepatic uptake of organic anion; a similar defect may be present in renal excretory apparatus.

Conjugated Hyperbilirubinemias

Chronic idiopathic jaundice (Dubin-Johnson syndrome) is a syndrome of chronic idiopathic jaundice with unidentified pigment in liver cells independently described by Dubin and Johnson (6) and by Sprinz and Nelson (7) in 1954. This disorder is inherited as an autosomal dominant with variable expressivity. The disorder is characterized by jaundice associated with abdominal pain, fatigue, dark urine, and hepatosplenomegaly of onset usually before 25 years of age. Three modes of onset have been described: insidious, acute, or following some other major disease. Pregnancy may be a precipitating factor in some cases. The jaundice is characteristically variable, and this life-long disorder has a good prognosis. Osmotic fragility and Coombs tests are normal, and red cell survival studies have revealed no abnormality. The serum bilirubin ranges from 2.4–19.0 mg/100 ml, of which the bulk is conjugated. Bromsulfalein retention is found in many of the patients. There is an interesting pattern of greater retention at 60–90 min than at 45 min. This is attributed to reflux of BSP from the liver. In many of these patients, it is difficult to visualize the gallbladder either after oral contrast media or by intravenous cholangiogram. The liver is darkly pigmented but otherwise normal. Microscopic examination reveals the presence of a lipofuscin-like pigment in liver cells; recent studies suggest the pigment may be melanin.

The basic defect is an inability to transport organic anions from the liver. The excretion of organic cations is normal, however. The absence of pruritus in these patients is consistent with normal bile acid metabolism. There is no therapy for this disorder, and the prognosis is excellent.

Rotor syndrome is a disorder which was originally described by Rotor (referred to in Ref. 1) as a "familial non-hemolytic jaundice with direct Van den Bergh reaction." It is thought to be transmitted as an autosomal recessive characteristic. The clinical features include mild and fluctuating icterus originating shortly after birth, or in early childhood, and persisting throughout life. There is usually a moderate elevation of serum bilirubin with mainly conjugated bilirubin, but there is no bilirubinuria. Patients may have intermittent abdominal pain and fever, and BSP excretion is markedly impaired. Microscopic examination of liver biopsy specimens reveals no pigment accumulation. The basic defect is similar to that in the Dubin-Johnson syndrome, i.e., defective transport of organic anions from liver cells. It has been suggested that this disorder is probably a variant of the Dubin-Johnson syndrome.

Idiopathic recurrent cholestasis is a rare form of hyperbilirubinemia found mainly, but not exclusively, in male patients. The clinical features include onset from age 9–27 years, with frequent recurrent attacks of pruritus followed by jaundice, malaise, and irritability. Steatorrhea, weight loss, and dark urine may follow. Some patients may have hepatomegaly. Significant negative findings include lack of fever, chills, and upper abdominal pain. The serum bilirubin may exceed 20 mg/100 ml and is predominantly conjugated. Serum alkaline phosphatase and transaminase are elevated. Prothrombin may be decreased, but responds to vitamin K therapy. The basic defect is revealed by liver biopsy as a cholestasis. This disorder responds to corticosteroid therapy.

Recurrent intrahepatic cholestasis of pregnancy is a disorder found in the last 4 months of pregnancy and is considered to be more common in Sweden. Pruritus is usually the first symptom, followed by dark urine, clay-colored stools, and jaundice. The jaundice disappears within 2 weeks after delivery. Elevated levels of both conjugated and unconjugated bilirubin are found. Prothrombin activity is decreased, but is responsive to vitamin K therapy. Microscopic studies on liver biopsy reveal cholestasis. The disorder may recur with subsequent pregnancies. The participation of estrogens in the pathogenesis has been suggested.

Drug-induced intrahepatic cholestasis results from the ingestion of certain drugs, such as phenothiazines and C-17 alkyl substituted steroids. The cholestasis is clinically manifested by jaundice without pain or fever, pruritus, and clay-colored, bulky fatty stools. The serum conjugated bilirubin, alkaline phosphatase, and cholesterol are elevated. Bilirubinuria is present, and fecal urobilinogen is decreased. These drug effects are thought to be caused by depression of excretion of bilirubin diglucuronide by an unknown mechanism.

Extrahepatic bile duct obstruction is a frequent cause of hyperbilirubinemia, the rise in bilirubin mainly caused by an increase in the bilirubin diglucuronide, but significant elevations in unconjugated bilirubin may also occur. It has been demonstrated recently that the rise in the unconjugated fraction is caused by deconjugation of bilirubin diglucuronide.

Animal Model of Conjugated Hyperbilirubinemia A hyperbilirubinemic syndrome was described in mutant Corriedale sheep and has been compared to the Dubin-Johnson syndrome in man. There is a defect in the hepatic secretion of organic anions. The sheep exhibit a facial photosensitivity caused by retention of phylloerythrin, a porphyrin which is formed in the rumen by bacterial degradation of chlorophyll. The disorder is transmitted as an autosomal dominant trait.

DRUG EFFECTS IN BILIRUBIN METABOLISM

Several chemical agents may affect the formation and degradation of bilirubin at several levels. These are discussed under the following categories of drug effects on: 1) hemolysis, 2) displacement of bilirubin from albumin, 3) competition for acceptor proteins in the liver, 4) enzyme induction, 5) cholestasis, and 6) intestinal flora activity.

Hemolysis

Several drugs may induce hemolysis by decreasing erythrocyte GSH. These include sulfonamides and primaquine. Immune mechanisms which induce hemolysis may be activated by drugs such as *p*-aminosalicylic acid, quinine, quinidine, phenacetin, penicillin, and α-methyldopa. Hemolysis by other mechanisms may be induced by amphetamines, barbiturates, mesantoin, and methylene blue.

Displacement of Bilirubin from Albumin

Drugs such as caffeine and sulfonimides may displace unconjugated bilirubin from albumin binding sites with resulting increased potential for bilirubin deposition in tissues, e.g., bilirubin encephalopathy in newborns.

Competition for Hepatic Acceptor Proteins

Organic anions, indocyanine green, and flavaspidic acid compete for the hepatic acceptor proteins and may thereby induce unconjugated hyperbilirubinemia.

Enzyme Induction and Repression Phenomena

Drugs such as phenobarbital and DDT may induce synthesis of glucuronyl-transferase and, thereby, increase bilirubin conjugation. Other chemicals such as novobiocin and pregnanediol may repress or inhibit enzyme action. Pregnant women may produce the Lucey-Driscoll factor which inhibits conjugation of bilirubin.

Cholestasis

Drugs such as methyltestosterone, estrogens, anabolic agents, and oral contraceptive agents may induce cholestasis in susceptible individuals leading to conjugated hyperbilirubinemia.

Intestinal Flora Activity

Destruction of intestinal flora by certain antibiotics decreases the production of urobilinogen from bilirubin.

LITERATURE CITED

1. Berlin, N. I., P. D. Berk, and R. B. Howe. 1974. Disorders of bilirubin metabolism. In P. K. Bondy and L. E. Rosenberg (eds.), Diseases of Metabolism, pp. 825–880A. W. B. Saunders Co., Philadelphia.
2. Levi, A. J., Z. Gatmaitan, and I. M. Arias. 1969. Two hepatic cytoplasmic protein fractions, Y and Z, and their possible role in the hepatic uptake of bilirubin, bromsulfalien, and other anions. J. Clin. Invest. 48:2156–2167.
3. Arias, I. M., S. Wolfson, J. F. Lucey, and R. J. MacKay. 1965. Transient familial neonatal hyperbilirubinemia. J. Clin. Invest. 44:1442–1450.
4. Crigler, J. F., and V. A. Najjar. 1952. Congenital familial non-hemolytic jaundice with kernicterus. Pediatrics 10:169–174.
5. Cremer, R. J., P. W. Perryman, and D. W. Richards. 1958. Influence of light on hyperbilirubinemia of infants. Lancet 1:1094.
6. Dubin, I. N., and F. B. Johnson. 1954. Chronic idiopathic jaundice with unidentified pigment in liver cells: New clinic pathologic entity with report of 12 cases. Medicine 33:155–165.
7. Sprinz, H., and R. S. Nelson. 1954. Persistent non-hemolytic hyperbilirubinemia associated with lipochrome like pigment in liver cells: Report of 4 cases. Ann. Intern. Med. 41:952–958.

9
The
Vitamins

VITAMIN A

The chemical structure of vitamin A is presented in Figure 9.1. Plants are the major source of this fat-soluble vitamin. There are over 100 carotenoids, of which 10 are converted to vitamin A in the mammalian organism. Lutein and lycopene among the carotenoids are inactive, but carotene and cryptoxanthin are actively converted to vitamin A. Highest contents of the precursors are found in green leafy vegetables, spinach, turnip greens, and carrots among the plant sources. Animal sources with high vitamin A content include liver, kidneys, milk, fish liver, cheeses, and egg yolk. The minimum requirements for this vitamin vary with age as follows: 6 months–3 years, 250 μg of retinol/day; beyond 3 years into adulthood, approximately 750 μg/day. The requirement may reach 1,200 μg/day in pregnant women (0.3 μg of retinol is equivalent to 1.0 IU of vitamin; this is equivalent to 0.6 μg of carotene) (1).

Deficiency of vitamin A may be caused by decreased dietary intake, malabsorption, or decreased storage. Secondary causes of deficiency include celiac disease, sprue, cirrhosis, mucoviscidosis, and obstructive jaundice. The deficiency state is characterized by keratinizing metaplasia and xerophthalmia. Keratinizing metaplasia affects the ducts of the exocrine glands of the respiratory, genitourinary, and upper part of the gastrointestinal systems. Xerophthalmia is a major cause of blindness in Africa, Middle East, Near East, Latin America, and certain parts of Asia. Epidemics of conjunctival xerosis and nyctalopia have occurred when crops fail in certain geographical areas. Occasional sporadic cases are caused by malabsorption or hepatocellular disease. The eye involvement includes nyctalopia, in which the posterior segment is affected and rod function is impaired. This alteration is the basis of several tests for vitamin A deficiency, viz., dark adaptometry, rod scotometry, and electroretinography. Enlargement of the blind spot, greater at the lower pole of the

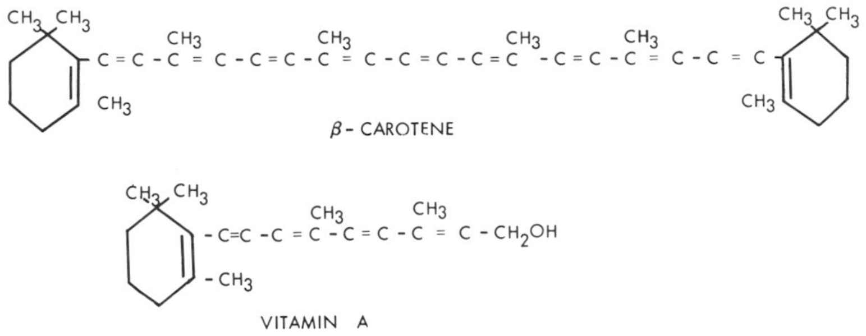

Habeeb Bacchus

Figure 9.1. Chemical structure of vitamin A.

nerve head, a reduction in sensitivity of the rod area to the limit of the visual field is later followed by concentric contraction of the peripheral fields. These changes respond quite well to vitamin A therapy. Bitot's spots, localized heaping up of keratinized cells, occur most commonly on the temporal areas of the interpalpebral fissure near the limbus. These silvery grey spots may be removed by wiping.

Changes in the anterior segment of the eye appear later and involve the conjunctiva and cornea. Dryness, thickness, wrinkling, pigmentation, and loss of wetability of the bulbar part of the conjunctiva and interpalpebral fissures occur bilaterally. These changes are described by the term xerosis. Keratomalacia, a softening of the cornea, follows rapidly, with the cornea melting into a gelatinous mass. Extrusion of the lens and loss of vitreous humor follow. If the cornea stays intact sufficiently long, then ectasia corneae and anterior staphyloma may occur.

Plasma levels of vitamin A or its metabolites are not reliable in the diagnosis of the deficiency state, but therapeutic responsiveness is a reasonably good criterion. The disorders described above must be distinguished from infection and other causes of surface irritation. Therapy with vitamin A in the form of fish oil at the dosage of 30,000 IU daily for 7–14 days is followed by reversal of nyctalopia and the conjunctival changes. It is essential in all cases that corneal involvement should be regarded as a medical emergency.

Clinical manifestations of vitamin A excess may occur as this vitamin is fat-soluble and is stored in tissues. Excess of vitamin A in animals leads to congenital malformations, eye defects, anencephaly, hydrocephalus, macroglossia, hare-lip, and cleft palate. Acute and chronic types of vitamin A excess are observed in man. Acute excess is seen in infants given excessive amounts of vitamin A. The clinical effects include increased intracranial pressure, bulging anterior fontanelles, and vomiting. Spontaneous recovery follows removal of sources of the excess vitamin, and there are no sequelae. Adults may become drowsy, irritable, and may suffer headaches, vomiting, and desquamation of the skin. Chronic vitamin

A excess is occasionally seen in children and is associated with anorexia, painful extremities, dry skin, sparse hair, hepatosplenomegaly, hypoplastic anemia, leukopenia, hydrocephalus, and periosteal thickening of the long bones. Hypercarotenosis occurs when the serum carotene level exceeds 120 μg/100 ml. This is usually caused by prolonged excessive intake of carrots and dark green leafy vegetables. Secondary hypercarotenemia may occur in hypothyroidism, diabetes mellitus, and hyperlipidemic states. There are no major clinical abnormalities associated with this state.

VITAMIN D

The structure of the fat-soluble vitamin D is presented in Chapter 19 (Figure 19.1). Sources of this vitamin include the preformed vitamin in fish liver oils, irradiated yeast added to milk, cereals, and candy. Metabolically inadequate precursors in the skin are converted to vitamin D by ultraviolet irradiation to the skin. The dietary requirements of this vitamin vary with age, diet, pregnancy, and lactation. The dose of 400 units daily is antirachitic, and osteomalacia is prevented by 5,000 units daily (1).

Biosynthesis of Vitamin D

This vitamin is derived from ergosterol from plant sources and 7-dehydrocholesterol from animal sources. Ultraviolet irradiation cleaves the steroid ring between C-9 and C-10 to produce tachysterol and calciferol, respectively, from the precursors listed above. The various synthetic steps are presented in Figure 19.2. Formation of 25-hydroxycholecalciferol in the liver confers biological activity to the vitamin. Optimal activity is provided by the formation of 1,25-dihydroxycholecalciferol from 25-hydroxycholecalciferol in the kidneys. This conversion is stimulated by parathyroid hormone. There are data to suggest that the substrate 25-hydroxycholecalciferol may be converted to the compound 24,25-dihydroxycholecalciferol by renal tissue under the influence of calcitonin.

The biological properties of vitamin D_2 and D_3 are equal in man, but they differ in their potencies for correction of hypocalcemia in hypoparathyroidism. The active vitamin D principle increases intestinal transport of calcium, and secondarily of phosphate, in the absence of parathyroid hormone and calcitonin. The vitamin is also capable of sustenance of increased levels of bone absorption and of providing calcium and phosphorus for the skeleton, as well as of maintenance of extracel calcium and phosphorus.

Vitamin D Deficiency

Four major types of vitamin D deficiency are recognized: 1) rickets or simple vitamin D deficiency; 2) vitamin D deficiency associated with malabsorption; 3) vitamin D deficiency caused by abnormal vitamin D metabolism in chronic renal disease; and 4) phosphate diabetes.

Rickets or Simple Vitamin D Deficiency   The clinical features in this disorder include osteomalacia in children before epiphyseal closure. In infants, craniostosis, flattening of the skull and pelvis and incomplete microfractures of the lower extremities may occur. The primary sites of involvement in children are the sites of active endochondreal bone formation, such as the ends of long bones. Costochondral swelling is the basis of the rachitic rosary. Deformity of the ribs at their junctions with the diaphragm causes Harrison's grooves, and protuberance of the sternum (pigeon breast) is also found in this deficiency. Growth retardation, hypocalcemic tetany, and proximal muscle weakness may also be found.

In adult osteomalacia the cortical and trabecular areas of the diaphyses of the long bones are involved, but gross deformities are uncommon. Pain in the areas of skeletal involvement is common in both osteomalacia and rickets. X-ray findings in this condition include generalized rarefaction and increased trabecular markings and specific bone deformities. Laboratory findings in both forms of osteomalacia include hypophosphatemia, increased serum alkaline phosphatase, and low or normal serum calcium.

Vitamin D Deficiency Associated with Malabsorption   As vitamin D absorption requires micelle formation in the intestinal lumen, biliary and pancreatic diseases may lead to malabsorption of the vitamin. Absorption may also be decreased in decompensated heart disease and after gastrectomy. Treatment of the vitamin deficiency includes the parenteral administration of 10,000 units of vitamin D weekly.

Vitamin D Deficiency Caused by Chronic Renal Disease   The disturbance in vitamin D metabolism in this state is caused by a decreased conversion of vitamin D_3 to the active principle 1,25-dihydroxycholecalciferol (see Chapter 20).

Phosphate Diabetes   This disorder may be of two types: 1) a familial sex-linked disorder which is seen more frequently and with greater severity in males; and 2) adult sporadic cases which are non-familial and often associated with tumors and proximal muscle weakness. The primary defect in both forms is in the renal transport of phosphate leading to a phosphate leak. There is probably an abnormal conversion of D_3 to the active metabolite, or an increased degradation thereof, underlying these disorders. Treatment consists of administration of 10,000 units of vitamin D daily.

VITAMIN E

Vitamin E (α-tocopherol) (Figure 9.2) is a fat-soluble vitamin which is found in vegetable oils in which the content correlates with the content of

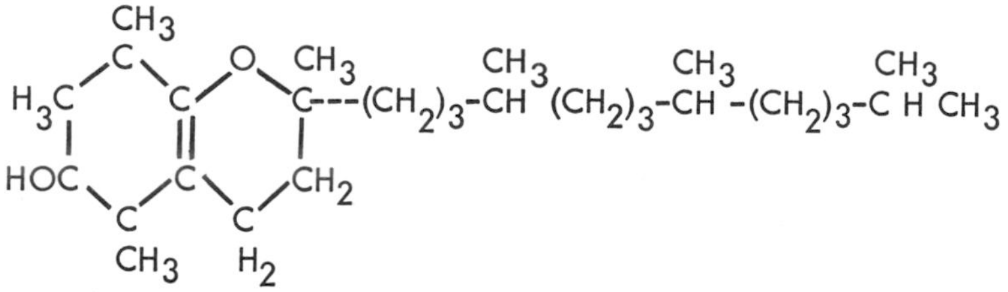

VITAMIN E
(α-TOCOPHEROL)

Figure 9.2. Chemical structure of vitamin E.

unsaturated fatty acids. Dietary requirement of this vitamin is related to the tissue content of polyunsaturated fatty acids. In adults, the requirement is 10–30 mg/day, while children require 0.5 mg/kg/day and more in newborn and premature infants. The vitamin is distributed widely in tissues with wide variations in plasma and tissue contents. In adults, the plasma vitamin E level ranges from 0.8 mg–1.4 mg/100 ml and, in infants, 0.05 mg–0.4 mg/100 ml. Highest tissue contents are in the pituitary, testes, and adrenal. The vitamin functions as an antioxidant of lipids by preventing the formation of peroxides of polyunsaturated fatty acids and in maintenance of stability of biological membranes as in lysosomes in liver, muscle, and erythrocytes.

Human vitamin E deficiency is not known to occur. Occasionally increased erythrocyte fragility and decreased erythrocyte associated with high dietary polyunsaturated fatty acids may be improved with this vitamin. A megaloblastic anemia of starved children is reported to respond to vitamin E. In various malabsorption states, cystic fibrosis, biliary disease, nontropical sprue, chronic pancreatitis, and xanthomatous biliary cirrhosis, there may be a secondary vitamin E deficiency. This disorder is characterized by increased erythrocyte fragility, decreased erythrocyte life span, decreased serum α-tocopherol, increased creatine phosphokinase, ceroid deposits, and creatinuria. In these states, therapy with 100 mg–600 mg of vitamin E daily may be helpful.

VITAMIN K

Vitamin K (Figure 9.3) is a fat-soluble vitamin which is found in dark green leafy vegetables, some fruits, tubers, and seeds, occurring in association with chlorophyll in chloroplasts. The vitamin may also be synthesized in the bacterial flora present in the gastrointestinal tract after about the 3rd to 4th day of life. The daily requirement of vitamin K in adults is estimated to be 30 mg/kg, and between 1–5 mg in newborns. This vitamin

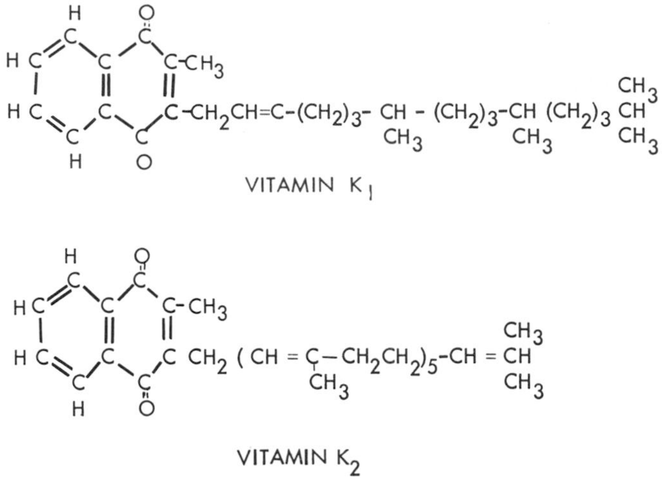

VITAMIN K$_1$

VITAMIN K$_2$

Figure 9.3. Chemical structure of vitamin K.

is involved in the formation of prothrombin in the liver, probably by activating protein synthesis at the step of DNA-dependent RNA synthesis or at the ribosomal level.

Vitamin K deficiency is rare except in the presence of defects in its absorption. The deficiency is characterized by decreased coagulability of the blood caused by deficiency of prothrombin. This state is also recognized occasionally in newborns as the hemorrhagic disease of newborns, which is probably ascribable to the absence of bacterial flora in the gastrointestinal tract in the first few days of life and to breast feeding without receiving vitamin K. Chronic antibiotic therapy may cause hypoprothrombinemia by eliminating or decreasing the gastrointestinal bacterial flora. Vitamin K absorption is decreased in patients with chronic intestinal disease or with biliary obstruction. In the presence of hepatocellular disease, the synthesis of prothrombin is decreased. Hemorrhagic disorders caused by vitamin K deficiency are treated with 100 μg–5 mg of the synthetic analogue menadione. Icterus neonatorum and kernicterus may follow the excessive dosage of water-soluble vitamin K analogues, perhaps through increased hemolysis or hepatocellular damage.

THIAMIN

Thiamin or vitamin B$_1$ is also known as the antineuritic vitamin (Figure 9.4). The sources of this water-soluble vitamin in the average American diet are cereals which provide one-third, fish and poultry which provide one-fourth, and milk products which supply one-eighth of the requirement. Thiamin from animal sources exists as thiamin pyrophosphate which requires hydrolysis in the gastrointestinal tract before absorption. The vitamin is in the nonphosphorylated form in plant sources. Enriched bread is fortified with thiamin. The requirements are estimated at 0.33–0.44 mg/1,000 cal in the diet. This requirement is increased in childhood, in pregnancy, and in lactation. Free thiamin is absorbed in the gastrointestinal tract and circulates in the plasma bound to α- and β-globulins.

The vitamin is involved in decarboxylation reactions involved in carbohydrate metabolism. This activity is dependent on the formation of thiamin pyrophosphate, and the reactions mediated by this factor include the conversion of pyruvate to acetyl-CoA and of α-ketoglutarate to succinate. The vitamin also activates the transketolase reaction which converts ribulose to sedoheptulose in the pentose phosphate pathway.

Thiamin Deficiency

Experimental thiamin deficiency is characterized by anorexia, psychiatric disturbances, paresthesias, aching in the calf muscles, impaired pinprick, vibratory, and light touch sensations. Deep tendon reflexes may be increased early and are absent later. Additional findings include conduction defects, cardiac arrhythmias, decreased voltage on the electrocardiogram, and decreased blood pressure.

Childhood beriberi is a form of thiamin deficiency found in children breast fed by thiamin-deficient mothers. Clinical features include a characteristic cry, aphonia, heart failure, and decreased deep tendon reflexes. Otherwise, the child appears normal. This clinical disorder is rapidly responsive to the administration of 10–50 mg of thiamin.

Beriberi heart disease accompanies the deficiency of thiamin. The mechanism of this disorder is related to abnormal myocardial metabolism of pyruvate and lactate, as well as to a defect in the peripheral vessels. Clinical features include low peripheral vascular resistance, increased oxygen comsuption, high output failure with increased left and right ventricular filling pressure leading to congestive heart failure and pulmonary congestion. There is a narrow arteriovenous oxygen difference. The high output failure is associated with increased blood pressure and increased

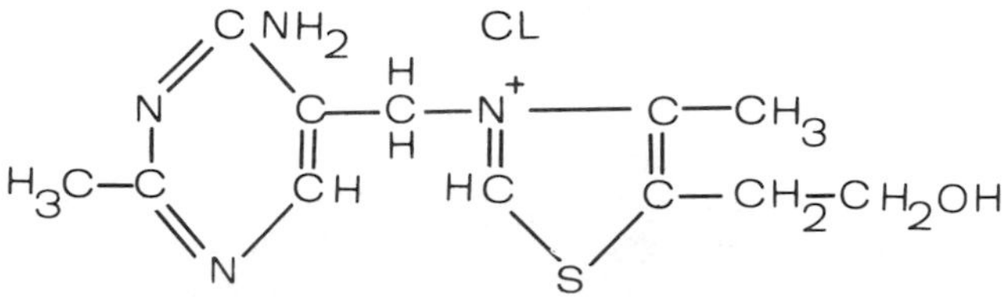

Figure 9.4. Chemical structure of thiamin.

blood volume. The pulmonary wedge pressure is increased. Anasarca may be an associated problem, perhaps secondary to decreased renal blood flow and glomerular filtration rate. The clinical manifestations of this disorder improve dramatically with the intravenous infusion of 100 mg of thiamin, the response often noted within minutes to hours.

Neurological manifestations may accompany the pattern described above. They are characterized by symmetrical foot drop, muscle tenderness, paresthesias and altered sensation over the legs, thighs, chest, and forearms. Ataxia and amblyopia may occasionally be found. Wernicke's encephalopathy and polyneuropathy often accompany severe dietary deficiency associated with alcoholism, especially after vomiting. The most prominent clinical finding is mental confusion leading to coma; sixth nerve weakness is also found occasionally. Korsakoff's syndrome is a milder degree of confusional state found in this deficiency. The mechanism of the above neurological findings involves decreased cerebral oxygen and glucose metabolism. Wallerian degeneration and demyelination may occur.

Laboratory findings associated with the above clinical states include increased pyruvate and decreased transketolase activity. These disorders are treated with the intravenous injection of 100 mg of thiamin, followed by 10–20 mg of thiamin orally three to four times daily. Treatment should be continued for several weeks or months.

NIACIN

Niacin, also known as nicotinic acid, exists as the acid and as the amide (Figure 9.5). This water-soluble vitamin is present in yeast, liver, meat, poultry, peanuts, and legumes. Milk and eggs are high in tryptophan which contributes to niacin nutrition, 60 mg of tryptophan being equivalent to 1 mg of niacin.

Requirement of this vitamin is 6.6 niacin equivalents/1,000 cal in the diet. This requirement is increased in children and in lactating women. The circulating level of this vitamin is 0.3–0.8 mg/100 ml of blood, most of which is present in erythrocytes as NAD or NADP.

Biological Functions of Niacin

The vitamin is involved in oxidation-reduction reactions through NAD and NADP. These reactions include synthesis of high energy phosphate compounds, the glycolysis cycle, pyruvate metabolism, pentose synthesis (hexose monophosphate shunt), glycerol and fatty acid metabolism, and protein catabolism.

Tryptophan metabolism is related to niacin availability (see Chapter 4).

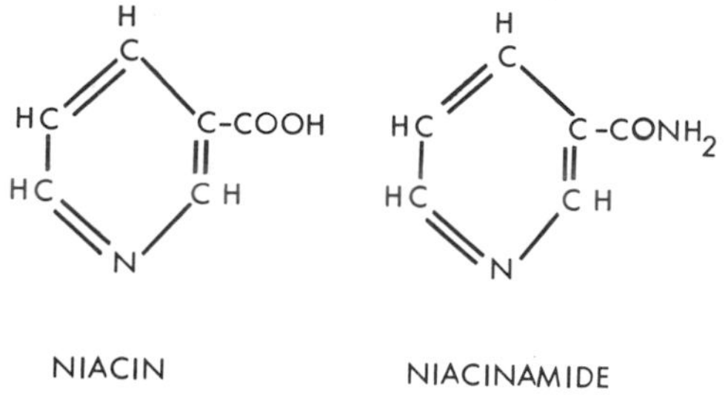

NIACIN   NIACINAMIDE

Figure 9.5. Chemical structure of niacin.

Niacin Deficiency

The clinical features of niacin deficiency evolve through a chronic and relapsing course, the peak incidence of this disorder occurring at the end of winter. Prodromal symptoms include weight loss, anorexia, stomatitis, indigestion, diarrhea, insomnia, and confusion. Severe deficiency is characterized by skin, gastrointestinal, and neurological manifestions termed the 3 D's, viz., dermatitis, diarrhea, and dementia.

There are characteristic and pathognomonic skin manifestations in this deficiency disease. The areas involved are determined by exposure to the sun and to pressure. The earliest finding is an erythema on the dorsum of the hands with pruritus and burning and edema. Blebs appear and may coalesce and burst after which dry scales may form. The dermatosis then becomes cracked, brownish, and brittle. The epidermis of the fingers thickens, the articular folds disappear, and painful fissures may occur in arms and hands. The usual sites of appearance are the face, neck, hands, and feet (glove or gauntlet, and boot distribution). There is often a butterfly lesion on the face, and Casal's necklace, a necklace distribution of dermatitis, is occasionally seen. Scrotal dermatitis is seen in male patients, and pellagrous vulvitis in female patients.

The gastrointestinal manifestations include glossitis and stomatitis which appear early. The tip and margins of the tongue appear red and swollen at first, with the tongue showing a raw beef appearance. Penetrating ulcers with considerable debris are found in the mouth. These changes spread to lower parts of the gastrointestinal tract, with indigestion and diarrhea being the major manifestations. Achylia gastrica is observed in 60% of patients with niacin deficiency.

Neurological manifestations evolve in the early stages as depression, apprehension, insomnia, headaches, dizziness, tremulous movements, or rigidity of the limbs. A loss of deep tendon reflexes and numbness and paresis of the extremities incapacitate the patient. An encephalopathy resembling Wernicke's syndrome may be seen in severe cases.

The major laboratory finding in patients with niacin deficiency is a low range of N'-methylnicotinamide in the urine.

Treatment with 500 mg of niacinamide is followed by improvement in glossitis, stomatitis, and mental state within 24 hr. Daily treatment with 500 mg of niacinamide is followed by healing of the skin lesions within 5 days.

RIBOFLAVIN

Riboflavin is also known as vitamin B_2 or lactoflavin. This water-soluble vitamin has the chemical structure 6,7-dimethyl-9-(D-ribityl)isoalloxazine (Figure 9.6). The major sources include animal and vegetable foods, germinating cereals, and milk. A diet high in starch, cellose, and lactose stimulates intestinal synthesis of riboflavin. The recommended intake of this vitamin is 0.55 mg/1,000 cal intake, with increased needs in children, and pregnant or lactating women. This vitamin is not stored to any significant extent in the body. The liver has 16 μg/g, the kidney 25 μg/g, and muscle 2–3 μg/g.

Biological Functions of Riboflavin

Riboflavin functions as a coenzyme for several reactions. All flavoproteins consist of specific proteins (apoenzymes) containing either flavin mononucleotide (FMN) or flavin adenine dinucleotide (FAD) as prosthetic group. Three flavoproteins with enzyme activity, Warburg's yellow enzyme, cytochrome c reductase, and L-amino acid reductase, contain FMN. The riboflavin enzymes are involved in oxidoreduction reactions passing hydrogen atoms from 1 molecule to another to be taken up by oxygen. They also function as dehydrogenase for L-amino acids, xanthine, and

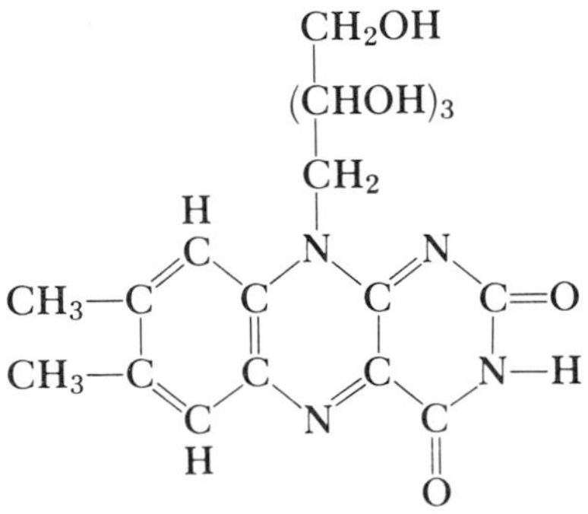

Riboflavin

Figure 9.6. Chemical structure of riboflavin.

hypoxanthine. Hydrogen is accepted from NADH and NADPH to be passed to the cytochrome system to oxygen (respiratory chain). Flavoproteins are unstable, especially when tissue proteins are depleted by stress, dietary deficiency, or disease.

Riboflavin Deficiency

The clinical pattern of riboflavin deficiency is characterized by pallor and maceration of the mucosa in the angles of the mouth followed by crusted fissures. The skin of the nasolabial folds, alae nasi, ears, and eyelids become mildly edematous, scaly, and greasy. Magenta tongue, epithelial keratitis, nutritional amblyopia, scrotal dermatitis, and, occasionally, corneal vascularization, may appear. This deficiency is occasionally precipitated in patients with malignant neoplasms treated with galactoflavin and a riboflavin-deficient diet. An additional finding in patients exposed to this pharmacological agent is a severe normocytic normochromic anemia with reticulocytopenia. This selective erythroid hypoplasia suggests that riboflavin may function as a coenzyme for erythroporetin activity.

The deficiency state responds promptly to therapy with 6 mg of riboflavin daily.

PANTOTHENIC ACID

Pantothenic acid is a water-soluble vitamin which is present in all cells in the form of coenzyme A (Figure 9.7). The vitamin is obtained from all food groups, organ meats and whole grain cereals being the richest sources. The vitamin is destroyed by processing in dry heat. The human requirement is estimated to be 10 mg daily. Human blood contains 18–35 μg/100 ml, mostly in the cellular elements. The urinary excretion depends on the intake, but averages 3 mg/24 hr.

This vitamin, because of its presence in coenzyme A, serves important functions in intermediary metabolism. Coenzyme A activates acetate by converting it to acetyl-CoA which is important in synthesis of acetoacetic acid, fatty acids, cholesterol, and steroids, in oxidation of pyruvate, and in the acetylation of choline, aromatic amines, and other substances which are acetylated for excretion.

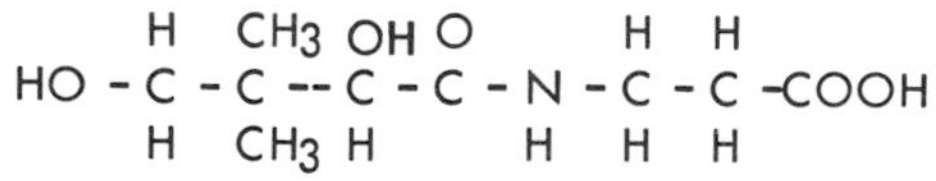

$$\begin{array}{ccccccc} \text{H} & \text{CH}_3 & \text{OH} & \text{O} & & \text{H} & \text{H} \\ \text{HO} - \text{C} - \text{C} -- \text{C} - \text{C} - \text{N} - \text{C} - \text{C} - \text{COOH} \\ \text{H} & \text{CH}_3 & \text{H} & & & \text{H} & \text{H} & \text{H} \end{array}$$

PANTOTHENIC ACID

Figure 9.7. Chemical structure of pantothenic acid.

No syndrome ascribable to pantothenic acid deficiency is known, but decreased antibody formation and a peripheral neuropathy have been found. Claims of a beneficial effect of this vitamin in rheumatoid arthritis, paralytic ileus, diabetic neuropathy, and psychoses have not been substantiated. Experimental pantothenic acid deficiency has induced adrenocortical insufficiency not correctible by pantothenic acid, but responsive to multiple vitamins.

PYRIDOXINE

Pyridoxine or pyridoxin is a water-soluble vitamin which is one of the forms of vitamin B_6. Other biologically active forms are pyridoxal and pyridoxamine (Figure 9.8). The sources of this vitamin are meats, liver, vegetables, whole grain cereals, and egg yolk. An intake of 2.2–2.9 mg daily is adequate for body needs, but, in certain pathological or dependency states, the requirements are higher. Approximately 0.4 mg is excreted daily. The biological activity of this vitamin is caused by the conversion to the active form pyridoxal phosphate. The conversion to the active form is decreased in the deficiency of pyridoxine kinase or antagonism to the enzyme by drugs, such as isonicotinic acid hydrazine (INH), hydralazine, and penicillamine. These agents may also block pyridoxal phosphate effect.

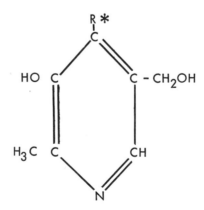

$*R = CH_2OH$ IN PYRIDOXINE

$R = CHO$ IN PYRIDOXAL

$R = CH_2NH_2$ IN PYRIDOXAMINE

Figure 9.8. Chemical structure of pyridoxine.

The functions of this vitamin include the following: 1) transamination reactions, for example, the conversion of α-ketoglutarate to glutamate and a ketoacid; 2) decarboxylation of amino acids to amines, e.g., histidine to histamine, 5-hydroxytryptophan to serotonin, aspartic acid to alanine, cysteic acid to taurine, and glutamic acid to γ-aminobutyric acid; 3) formation of melanin from tyrosine; 4) metabolism of tryptophan (in addition to the usual transamination and decarboxylation reactions, tryptophan is metabolized by pyridoxine enzymes in three ways, including conversion to indoles, pyruvate, and ammonia, the conversion to kynurenine, as well as the formation of tryptophan from serine and indole); 5) contributing to the trans-sulfuration activity of cystathionase; 6) affecting the activity of phosphorylase to release glucose from glycogen; 7) functioning as a cofactor for the activity of δ-aminolevulinic acid synthetase, the rate-limiting enzyme in porphyrin synthesis; and 8) involvement in metabolism of cholesterol and fatty acids in the central nervous system.

Deficiency of Pyridoxine

General clinical features of experimental pyridoxine deficiency include irritability, depression, and seborrheic dermatitis in the nasolabial folds, eyebrows, cheeks, neck, and the perineum. Glossitis, angular stomatitis, blepharitis, peripheral neuropathy, and lymphopenia have also been found.

Deficiency of the vitamin may follow starvation, associated with alcoholism, malabsorption, decreased cellular transport, drug antagonism to pyridoxine kinase, or antagonism to pyridoxal phosphate. A pyridoxine responsive anemia which may be normoblastic or megaloblastic has been described. It is likely that, in some of these patients, an increased dependency of the erythropoietic tissues pyridoxine may be present. Drug antagonism to pyridoxal phosphate action caused by INH or hydrazaline is responsible for a syndrome of hypochromic anemia, paresthesias, and neuropathy.

Four forms of pyridoxine dependency disorders have been described. These include the following:

1. Convulsive disorder of infancy which is caused by a defect in the decarboxylation of glutamic acid to form γ-aminobutyric acid. This disorder should respond within several minutes to parenteral administration of 5–100 mg of pyridoxine.
2. Mental deficiency associated with cystathionuria. Pyridoxal phosphate contributes to the trans-sulfuration activity of the enzyme cystathionase. This disorder is transmitted as an autosomal recessive characteristic.
3. "Iron loading" anemia, an X-linked disorder wherein there is a defect in the activity of δ-ALA synthetase activity, with resulting decreased heme synthesis.

4. Urticaria and asthma is probably a recessive disorder which is associated with xanthurenic aciduria. It is ascribed to decreased activity of the enzyme kynureninase which is pyridoxal dependent.

In the pyridoxine dependency disorders, the dietary requirement of the vitamin is 2–11 mg daily.

BIOTIN

Biotin (2-keto-3,4-imidazolido-2-tetrahydrothiopene-*n*-valeric acid) (Figure 9.9) is a water-soluble vitamin which is found in a protein-bound form in liver, kidney, egg yolk, and yeast. The best plant sources of this vitamin are cauliflower, legumes, and nuts. Most diets contain 150–300 μg of biotin which is probably sufficient for the needs of the average individual. The vitamin is also synthesized by intestinal bacteria. Avidin in egg white may bind biotin and contribute to a deficiency.

The vitamin is involved in the activities of the biotin enzymes which include acetyl-CoA carboxylase, methylcrotonyl-CoA carboxylase, propionyl-CoA carboxylase, methylmalonyl oxalacetic acid CoA carboxylase, and pyruvate carboxylase. The vitamin is also involved in the metabolism of the amino acids serine, threonine, and citrulline. The formation of *cis*-unsaturated fatty acids is dependent on biotin. The vitamin may also be involved in carbamylation reactions.

Biotin deficiency may be induced in subjects on minimal biotin intake plus 30% protein as egg white. The clinical manifestations include an exfoliative dermatitis of the neck, arms, and legs which may lead to desquamation. A mild depression, extreme lassitude, somnolence, muscle pains, and hyperesthesia have also been found in these patients. Treatment with 75–300 μg of biotin/day by injection leads to prompt relief within 3–5 days.

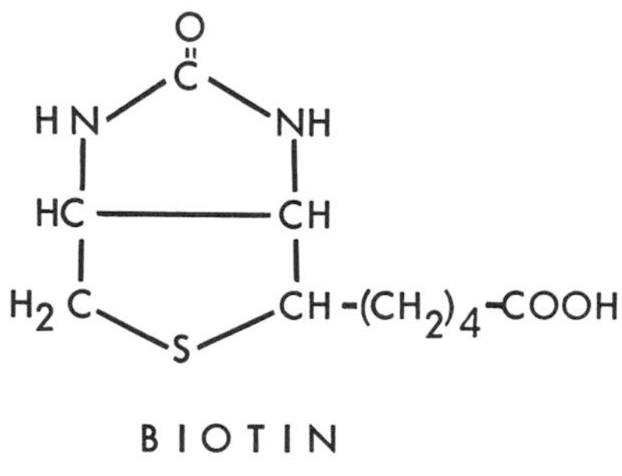

B I O T I N

Figure 9.9. Chemical structure of biotin.

FOLIC ACID

Folic acid (pteroylglutamic acid) (Figure 9.10) is a water-soluble vitamin found in liver, kidney, mushrooms, asparagus, lemons, strawberries, broccoli, spinach, lima beans, bananas, and cantaloupes. Pteroylmonoglutamic acid is the parent form of the vitamin, but the natural forms found in foods are conjugated with 2–6 molecules of glutamic acid. The monoglutamate is released by conjugates during absorption. The vitamin is eventually reduced to 5,6,7,8-tetrahydrofolic acid (THF) which is the physiologically active form. The oxidoreduction potential of the system ascorbic acid$\leftrightarrow$dehydroascorbic acid helps to maintain the folic acid coenzymes in the reduced form. The physiologically active form of the vitamin is linked in the N^5 or N^{10} or N^5-N^{10} positions with formyl hydroxymethyl, methyl, or formimino groups. The form present in liver, serum, and other tissues is probably the N^5-methyl-THF.

The vitamin is involved in several aspects of intermediary metabolism of nucleoproteins, especially thymine and uracil, as well as in 1-carbon transfer in the synthesis of DNA, RNA, methionine, and serine. The conversion of serine to glycine and of histidine to glutamic acid contributes largely to the 1-carbon pool. This finding is the basis of a test of folate deficiency which depends on quantitation of products of 1-carbon transfer after a loading dose of a precursor such as histidine. The minimum daily requirement is about 150 μg/day, but this may increase in pregnancy and in certain disease states.

Folic Acid Deficiency

Experimental folic acid deficiency has been produced in human subjects on 5 μg of folic acid daily. Hematological effects of this deficiency correlate with decreased levels of the vitamin in plasma. Hypersegmentation of polymorphonuclear neutrophils is a prominent hematological finding. Increased excretion of formiminoglutamic acid (a reflection of defective 1-carbon transfer) also results from the deficiency state. After 4 months on the deficient diet, decreased folic acid levels are noted in the erythro-

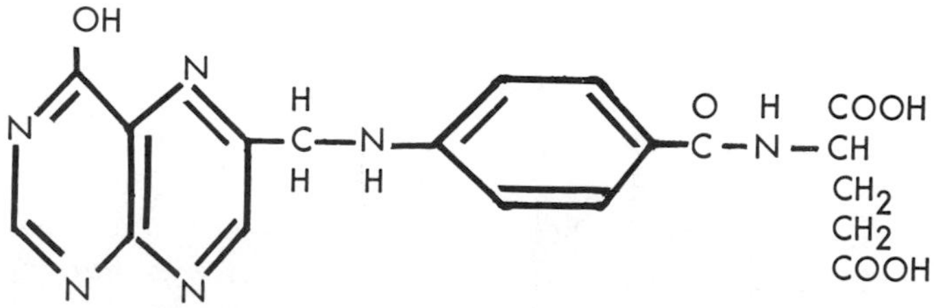

Figure 9.10. Chemical structure of folic acid (pteroylglutamic acid).

cytes, with resultant macrocytosis, megaloblastosis, ovalocytosis, and anemia. Similar features are seen in patients on antifolic drugs, such as amethopterin where thrombocytopenia and leukopenia are also found.

In spontaneous folic acid deficiency, the major clinical features include myopathy and neuropathy. Abruptio placenta, abortion, and fetal abnormalities have also been ascribed to this vitamin deficiency. Hematological features are megaloblastic anemia with effects on the thrombocyte and leukocyte series. Macrocytosis and ovalocytosis occur early; hypersegmentation of polymorphonuclear leukocytes with increased interlobular strands and lobules preceded the anemia. Erythrocyte precursors in the bone marrow show stippled appearance of nuclear elements. Morphologically, the hematological features are indistinguishable from those of B_{12} deficiency. Folate deficiency is prevalent in neonates in patients with alcoholism, hookworm infestation, pregnancy, malignant neoplasms, sprue, and nontropical sprue. Diagnosis is based on the hematological pattern and on folic acid determination in the plasma. The increased excretion of FIGLU after histidine loading is characteristic, but may also be found in pregnancy and in patients with tuberculosis. Treatment of folic acid deficiency requires 5 mg of folic acid three times daily. Infantile megaloblastic anemia is treated with 5 mg of folic acid/day.

VITAMIN C

The chemical structures of vitamin C (ascorbic acid) and its oxidation products are presented in Figure 9.11. This water-soluble vitamin is obtained mainly from vegetables, citrus fruits, guava, turnips, broccoli, brussel sprouts, and lettuce. It is also present in kidney, liver, roe, and, to some extent, in milk. The requirements have been established as 75–100 mg/day, with increased requirement in stress, illness, and during corticosteroid therapy. The largest amount of this vitamin in the human body is in the adrenal, liver, and spleen. In blood, it is distributed as follows: 25–32 mg/100 ml in the buffy coat and 1.4 mg/100 ml in plasma. The metabolic pool is 2–3 g, and the biological half-life is 20 days. A biosynthetic pathway is present in most animal species, but a key step is missing in primates, the fruit bat, and the guinea pig.

Ascorbic Acid Deficiency

Deficiency of this vitamin is associated with the following general findings: weakness, fatiguability, listlessness, dyspnea, bone pain, arthralgia, and myalgia especially at night. There are significant cutaneous changes which are quite characteristic. Keratosis of the hair follicles with the occurrence of a horny material in the follicles results in coiled or looped hairs on the arms, back, buttocks, and shins. Furuncles over previous acne scars may

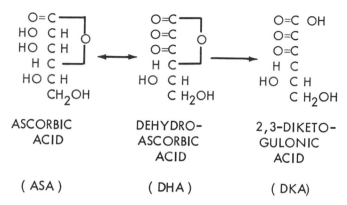

ASCORBIC ACID (ASA) — DEHYDROASCORBIC ACID (DHA) — 2,3-DIKETOGULONIC ACID (DKA)

Figure 9.11. Chemical structures and interconversion of the forms of vitamin C. Ascorbic acid and dehydroascorbic acid are known to be biologically active; diketogulonic acid is not active as a vitamin. Note the potential for participation in oxidation-reduction mechanisms. For example, the system ASA ↔ DKA is involved in glutathione oxidation and reduction, as well as in corticosteroid biosynthetic and degradation pathways.

lead to hemorrhage. Gingivitis and peridontal disease lead to bleeding gums. The disorder is rare in most countries now, but may still be seen in slum dwellers, recluses, and in babies fed processed milk formulas.

Infantile scurvy is seen after age 6 months. The infants are irritable, exhibit a "pseudoparalysis" caused by tenderness of the legs, and fail to use arms and legs. There is cessation of sitting and standing because of pain. Pain in the costochondral junctions leads to respiratory difficulty. Bleeding, except around the erupting teeth, is not a major manifestation in infantile scurvy. The patients assume a pithed frog appearance with legs flexed at the knees, legs partly flexed and externally rotated. The costochondral rosary is tender, and subperiosteal hemorrhages occur at the distal end of the femur and proximal end of the tibia. Retrobulbar hemorrhage and exophthalmos may be seen occasionally.

There are some characteristic radiological findings in infantile scurvy. These are seen mainly at the sites of active bone growth and include the "corner fracture sign," a ground glass appearance caused by decreased trabecular markings, cortical atrophy, and the absence of the cortical shaft junction. The white line of Frankel representing a zone of provisional calcification is seen. The "penciled effect" is best seen at the periphery of centers of ossification, especially in the knees. Fractures and displaced epiphyses may also be seen.

The basic pathology involves the failure of deposition of intercellular cement, leading to a defect in the capillaries and resultant bleeding. Decreased fibroblast activity leads to defective collagen formation (see Chapter 6). Defective osteoid leads to defective dentin formation. Treat-

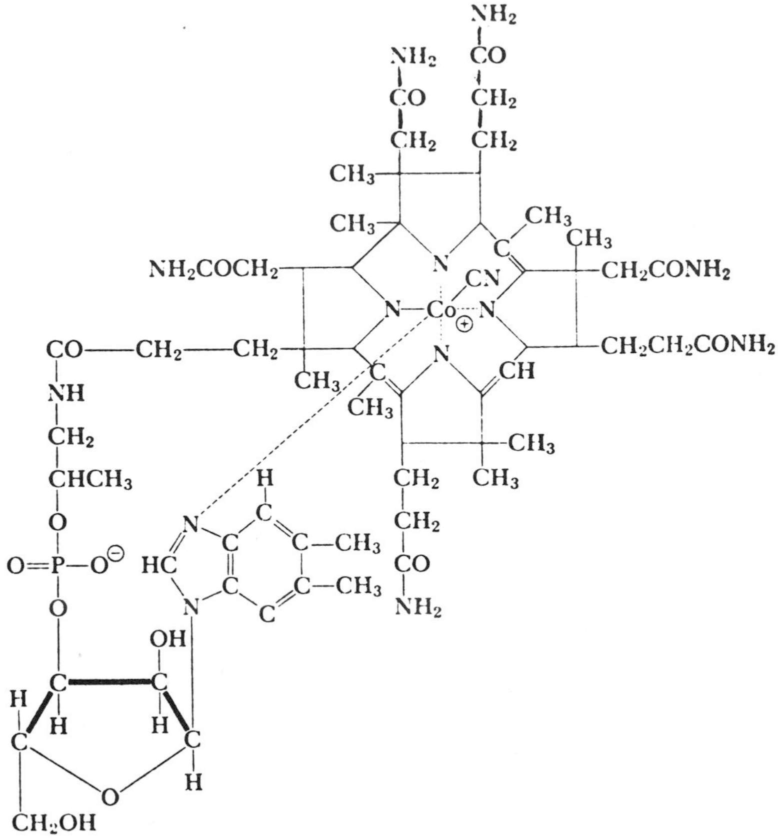

Figure 9.12. Chemical structure of vitamin B_{12} (cyanocobalamin).

ment of infantile scurvy requires the oral administration of 200 mg of ascorbic acid daily for at least 10 days. This is followed by regression of several of the clinical features described.

Adult scurvy is characterized by hemorrhage into joints and muscles, splinter hemorrhages, spongy gums, and loss of teeth. Occasionally the various cutaneous manifestations described above may also be seen. Treatment requires 10 mg of ascorbic acid five times daily for at least 10 days.

VITAMIN B_{12}

Vitamin B_{12} is a water-soluble vitamin which exists in the three forms of cyanocobalamin, hydroxycobalamin, and nitritocobalamin. The structure of cyanocobalamin is presented in Figure 9.12.

This vitamin is synthesized by microorganisms and is present in all animal tissues including liver, kidney, meat, and fish. Negligible amounts are found in plants and vegetables. The minimum daily requirement of the vitamin is 0.1 μg/day, but because only 10% is absorbed, the recommended intake is 10–15 μg daily. The molecular weight of the compound is 1,500, but it cannot diffuse through the plasma membrane of the intestinal mucosal cell. The process of absorption requires attachment to the glycoprotein intrinsic factor of molecular weight 50,000, which is produced in the gastric mucosal cells. The site of absorption of the vitamin-intrinsic factor complex is the ileum, the complex entering the columnar epithelial cells by pinocytosis. The vitamin is stored in the liver, and this storage form is depleted very slowly. Massive oral doses of the vitamin may permit some absorption by diffusion. The normal serum level of B_{12} is 320 pg/ml. This level drops before the body stores are depleted; hence, serum levels do not necessarily reflect available stored vitamin.

The metabolic actions of vitamin B_{12} include the following: 1) 1-carbon transfer by folic acid enzymes; 2) reduction of ribose to deoxyribose, e.g., uracil ribotide to uracil deoxyribotide which in the presence of folic acid and 1 carbon forms thymine ribotide; 3) transmethylation reactions along with folic acid; 4) an effect on folic acid conjugase; and 5) the conversion of methylmalonic-CoA to succinyl-CoA.

Vitamin B_{12} deficiency is seen in vegetarians who have less than 120 pg of B_{12} /ml of serum. In patients with this deficiency, glossitis, paresthesias, and subacute combined degeneration of the spinal cord are observed. Similar clinical findings may be seen in patients who have metabolic defects in the handling of the vitamin. Pathological changes caused by the deficiency are most evident in areas of active cell production such as the hemopoietic, gastrointestinal, and nervous systems. The hematological disorder caused by the vitamin deficiency, pernicious anemia, is associated with the presence of antibodies against intrinsic factor. Patients with pernicious anemia also possess a complement-fixing system directed against gastric parietal cells. These facts suggest an autoimmune disorder in pernicious anemia. The hematological disorder is identical with folic acid deficiency, but, in pernicious anemia, the macrocytosis, megaloblastosis, hypersegmented neutrophils, and anemia take longer to appear.

Neurological manifestations of pernicious anemia often precede the hematological changes. The patients may also exhibit atrophic glossitis, nausea, vomiting, diarrhea, constipation, histamine-fast achlorhydria, and increased unconjugated bilirubin, leading to a lemon-yellow skin color.

Pernicious anemia of childhood is rare and is caused by a congenital lack of intrinsic factor production, without a loss of gastric acid production, and lacking abnormal gastric morphology. Juvenile pernicious anemia is similar to adult pernicious anemia, but is often associated with concurrent endocrine defects.

Subacute combined degeneration of the spinal cord is a complication of pernicious anemia. The clinical manifestations include dysesthesias, muscle tenderness, decreased deep tendon reflexes, decreased deep sensation, positive Romberg's sign, positive Babinski sign, ataxia, spasticity, occasional ankle clonus, histamine-fast achlorhydria, and megaloblastic anemia. These patients excrete increased amounts of methylmalonic acid.

Nutritional amblyopia is a retrobulbar neuropathy which is associated with cyanide-induced vitamin B_{12} deficiency, with tobacco or alcohol excess, and with tapeworm infestation. Visual acuity improves more satisfactorily after treatment with hydroxycobalamin than with cyanocobalamin.

Occasional psychiatric syndromes may be caused by vitamin B_{12} deficiency; these include cerebral arteriosclerosis, cerebral degeneration, dementia, and depression. In many of these patients, hyperpigmentation of the skin and palms may be seen.

Procedures for the diagnosis of vitamin B_{12} deficiency include the following: 1) the Schilling test for vitamin B_{12} absorption before and after administration of intrinsic factor (see Chapter 3 on malabsorption syndrome tests); and 2) the urinary excretion of methylmalonic acid. This metabolite is increased in the urine of patients with vitamin B_{12} deficiency. The hematological findings in this deficiency are not pathognomonic as stated above.

Pernicious anemia is treated with a starting dose of vitamin B_{12} of 30–60 μg intramuscularly daily for 2 weeks, followed by 30–60 μg intramuscularly at monthly intervals. Hydroxycobalamin is absorbed more slowly by parenteral injection, and higher levels are maintained in the serum than when cyanocobalamin is used.

LITERATURE CITED

1. MacLaren, D. S. 1969. The vitamins. *In* P. K. Bondy (ed.), Diseases of Metabolism, pp. 1280–1320. W. B. Saunders Co., Philadelphia.
2. Kodicek, E. 1972. Recent advances in vitamin D metabolism. 1,25-Dihydroxy cholecalciferol, a kidney hormone controlling calcium metabolism. *In* I. MacIntyre (ed.), Clinics in Endocrinology and Metabolism. Vol. 1, No. 1, pp. 305–323. W. B. Saunders Co., London.

10
Trace
Minerals

COPPER

Copper is an essential trace mineral for several metabolic processes, includ-ing myelination of nerves, pigmentation of skin, hair, ureal tract, mobiliza-tion and utilization of iron, taste, reproduction, and metabolism of bone and connective tissues, e.g., cross-linking of elastin and collagen (1). This mineral is widely present in foodstuffs and is especially high in oysters, liver, mushrooms, nuts, and chocolate. Approximately 60% of dietary intake is excreted in the feces. Copper is absorbed in the small intestine and is transported in the blood stream bound to albumin and amino acids. It is then deposited in the liver temporarily in the form of the copper-pro-teins namely, L-6D (molecular weight 10,000) which is colorless and contains cuprous ions; hepatocuprein (molecular weight 30,000), which is bluish green; and hepatomitochondrocuprein, which is found in mito-chondria of fetal and neonatal liver. The circulating copper proteins include the following: 1) ceruloplasmin, a blue protein of molecular weight 160,000 containing cuprous and cupric ions (it serves as an active catalyst in the oxidation of phenylethylenediamine, polyamines, and poly-phenols, and is increased in pregnancy and following estrogen therapy); 2) cytochrome oxidase, which is involved in electron transport; 3) tyrosinase in melanosomes of the skin and eyes; 4) erythrocuprein, which is present in erythrocytes, brain, liver, and kidney; 5) monoamine oxidase in which the cupric ion is the active metabolic center; and 6) cerebrocuprein 1 which is found in brain tissue. Copper deficiency in man is rare, but may be induced by diets low in copper, by inhibition of absorption, or by increased gastrointestinal loss in children suffering from kwashiorkor, and in malnourished infants fed milk exclusively. Diminished copper intake or malabsorption caused by sprue is reflected by hypocupremia. Infants with this deficiency may show anemia, neutropenia, and bone lesions. Copper loss is also seen in protein-losing gastroenteropathy, while patients with collagen disorders and Wilson's disease treated with penicillamine also show hypocuprinemia. A common complaint in patients with hypocupremia is decreased taste acuity.

Acute copper toxicity in man occurs after "bluestone" ingestion or application of copper to burned skin. Clinical manifestations include metallic taste, ptyalism, nausea, vomiting, epigastric burning, diarrhea, gastrointestinal bleeding, hemolytic and parenchymal jaundice, hemoglobinuria, proteinuria, oliguria, azotemia, hypotension, tachycardia, convulsions, and coma which may lead to death. Liver tissues in such toxicity usually show central lobular necrosis and bile stasis, and tubular necrosis is observed in the kidneys. The mechanism of the gastrointestinal toxicity is dependent on coagulation of mucus, mitochondrial swelling, decreased mitochondrial ATPase activity, increased hepatic lysomomal activity, decreased erythrocyte G-6-P dehydrogenase, denaturation of hemoglobin, and oxidation of glutathione.

Chronic copper toxicity in man is seen in Wilson's disease (hepatolenticular degeneration), which is an autosomal recessive disorder observed in 1 in 200,000 of the population. A persistent decrease in ceruloplasmin with increased hepatic copper is found. This sustained high hepatic level results in parenchymal damage and release of copper into the blood stream with accumulation in the central nervous system and with induced hemolysis. Accumulation of copper in Descemet's membrane produces the Kayser-Fleischer ring, but this is not associated with visual defects. Symptoms seldom appear at less than 6 years of age and may not be evident until age 40. Incoordination, tremors, drooling, open-mouthedness, dysarthria, rigidity and seizures, neurotic, psychotic, or other behavioral disorders, and parenchysmal and circulatory liver dysfunction are the usual manifestations, and death results from liver failure mainly. In Wilson's disease, the serum ceruloplasmin levels are less than 20 mg/100 ml. Hepatic copper is elevated. Treatment of Wilson's disease consists of lifelong use of penicillamine 1–3 g/day to enhance copper excretion. Pyridoxine supplements have been reported to be helpful in some patients.

ZINC

Zinc is widely distributed in foods such as meat, eggs, fish, cocoa, tea, nuts, grains, legumes, oysters, cow's milk, and water from galvanized pipes. The mineral is absorbed in the distal small intestine, and it is estimated that the total absorption is less than 10% of that in dietary intake. The absorption is increased with lowered pH. Phytic acid and calcium in the diet inhibit zinc absorption. Thirty-five percent of the absorbed zinc is stored in the liver, from which it is distributed to the plasma and to other organs. Plasma zinc level is estimated to be 120 μg/100 ml, and it is bound to albumin and several globulins, but there is no specific zinc-binding protein. Tissue stores of zinc are as follows: adrenal, 12 μg/g; prostate, 102 μg/100 g; semen, 3,000 μg/g; erythrocytes, 1.4 μg/100 ml; and leukocytes, 14 μg/100 ml. The estimated total body pool of zinc is 2 g, with a turnover of 6 mg/day, the urinary excretion is 0.5 mg/24 hr, and it is estimated that 63% of the bodily stores of zinc is in striated muscle. This metal is essential for the activity of the zinc protein enzymes which are carbonic anhydrase, pancreatic carboxypeptidases, alcohol dehydrogenase, alkaline phosphatases, tryptophan desmolase, malic dehydrogenase, and lactic dehydrogenase (1).

Decreased zinc is found in the serum and liver of patients with alcoholic cirrhosis and other hepatic diseases. Patients with alcoholic cirrhosis excrete 400 mg/24 hr despite the low serum levels. Increased zincuria is also found in posthepatitic cirrhosis, Wilson's disease, porphyria, and nephrotic syndrome, but only in alcoholic cirrhosis has zinc been implicated in the pathogenesis. A syndrome of dwarfism, hypogonadism, and iron deficiency anemia has been ascribed to zinc deficiency in patients in Iran and Egypt. These patients had decreased levels of zinc in the plasma, sweat, skin, and hair. The deficiency has been ascribed to increased levels of phytate in the diet, to geophagia, or to parasitism.

Zinc toxicity is seen in man following inhalation or ingestion of zinc, as, for example, after ingestion of acid foods from zinc containers. Ingestion of 200 mg is followed by vomiting, gastrointestinal distress, and diarrhea. A zinc content of over 20 mg/100 ml of water is associated with a metallic taste. Inhalation of fumes is followed by metal fume fever characterized by chills, malaise, cough, salivation, and headache. This disorder is also termed brass-founder's ague, zinc shakes, or salvo. Treatment consists in removal from the environment of high zinc levels and the use of ethambutol, which has occasionally been helpful.

MANGANESE

Manganese is widely distributed in foodstuffs, including meat and plants. Tea is estimated to contain 1.3 mg/cup. The average intake of this mineral in man is 3–9 mg/day, of which only 50% of ingested manganese is absorbed, and fecal excretion of the mineral is partly through bile. There is a relatively high concentration of manganese in bone, and it has been suggested that a manganese-binding protein probably exists. The requirement of this mineral in children is estimated to be 0.2–0.3 mg/day. Manganese functions mainly as an activator of enzymes, including phosphatases, mixed function oxidases such as hydroxylases for the aromatic ring, phosphoglucomutase, cholinesterase, intestinal peptidase, isocitric dehydrogenase, carboxylases, arginase, and adenosinetriphosphatase (1).

Deficiency of manganese has been demonstrated in cattle (ataxia, bowing of bones, reproductive defects), but not convincingly in man. Manganese toxicity has not been observed in lower animals, but may occur in man following inhalation of dusts in coal mines. The clinical features develop insidiously and include psychiatric abnormalities, neurological symptoms resembling Parkinsonism with weakness, spasticity, tremors, and gait disturbances. The disorder is not fatal, and treatment consists of decreasing exposure to dusts containing manganese.

LITERATURE CITED

1. Scheinberg, I. L. H., and I. Steinleib. 1969. Metabolism of trace minerals. *In* P. K. Bondy (ed.), Diseases of Metabolism, pp. 1321–1334. W. B. Saunders Co., Philadelphia.

11
Mechanisms of Hormone Actions

Hormones are released into the circulation in extremely low concentrations, for example, peptide hormones circulate at the concentration of 10^{-10} to 10^{-12} M, whereas glucose is present at the level of 10^{-2} M. These low concentrations, therefore, require specific receptor sites for recognition. There is indeed marked target organ specificity for many of the hormones, e.g., ACTH acts on adrenal cortical cells specifically. The product of adrenocortical secretion, cortisol, on the other hand, has several targets, but they are specific rather than general. Hormones do not take part in energy production; rather, they exert regulatory influences on growth, differentiation, and metabolic activity of their target tissues. The mechanisms of hormone actions (1–4) are classified into two general types: 1) processes propagated by involvement of cell membrane adenylate (or adenylyl) cyclase and 2) processes propagated by participation of specific cytosol and nuclear receptor molecules. Most of the peptide and glycoprotein hormones (insulin excluded) operate under mechanism 1, whereas the steroid hormones operate by method 2. In this discussion, the prototype type 1 is ACTH and type 2 is cortisol.

PROCESSES PROPAGATED BY
RELEASE OF MEMBRANE ADENYLATE CYCLASE (1, 2)

Release of cell membrane adenylate cyclase is a hormone action in many endocrine as well as non-endocrine tissues. ACTH specifically affects cells of the adrenal cortex. This peptide hormone is made up of 37 amino acids assembled in the anterior pituitary. Biological activity resides in peptide sequence 1–24. This peptide regulates: (a) differentiated function of the adrenal cortical cells, viz., steroidogenesis; (b) growth; and (c) replication of adrenocortical cells. The initial event in ACTH action is the stereospecific binding of ACTH to the outside outer cell membrane of the adrenocortical cells. This initiates the process that results in the release of adenylate cyclase from the inner aspect of the cell membrane. The first event is independent of calcium, but the receptor binding apparently activates an influx of calcium. The release of the enzyme adenylate cyclase from the inner membrane is calcium dependent. The remarkable specificity of the normal cell membrane for ACTH is revealed by the fact that minor molecular change alters this affinity. The Lys-Lys-Arg-Arg sequence is regarded as especially important in the hormone-receptor binding. This marked affinity is altered in tumor cell lines from the adrenal. Luteinizing hormone (LH), follicle-stimulating hormone (FSH), and thyroid-stimulating hormone (TSH) are capable of binding to the receptor of adrenocortical tumor cells but not of normal cells. ACTH is known to react with the plasma membrane of fat cells.

Release of adenylate cyclase results in a series of intracellular events depicted in Figure 11.1. Adenylate cyclase releases cyclic adenosine monophosphate (cAMP) from ATP. Each molecule of ACTH results in the intracellular accumulation of a minimum of 500 molecules of cAMP, an example of amplification (magnification). The release of cAMP precedes steroidogenesis, indicating the role of cAMP as intracellular mediator (second messenger) of ACTH action. cAMP release does not require protein synthesis.

Mechanism of cAMP Action

The released cAMP is firmly and specifically bound to a receptor protein. Certain closely related analogues with the $3':5'$-cyclic ring, e.g., guanosine monophosphate and inosine monophosphate, may weakly compete for the receptor site. The receptor protein is localized in the cytosol and endoplasmic reticulum (ER) of the cell. While cAMP itself may be degraded by phosphodiesterase, the cAMP-receptor complex is resistant to phosphodiesterase action.

The major action of cAMP in mammalian tissues is regulation of a cAMP-dependent protein kinase. This protein kinase transfers the γ-phosphate of ATP to serine and threonine residues in a variety of substrate proteins. The cAMP-dependent receptor protein kinase contains two components, viz., a regulatory receptor and a catalytic kinase unit. The cAMP receptor inhibits the kinase unit. Binding of cAMP to the receptor unit releases the protein kinase, i.e., dissociation of the receptor-catalytic complex (located in the ER):

$$\text{Receptor-kinase} + \text{cAMP} \rightarrow \text{kinase} + \text{receptor} - \text{cAMP}$$

The free kinase is the fully activated form and no longer binds cAMP or responds to it. It is likely that the receptor-cAMP complex may serve to maintain a protected pool of the nucleotide within the cell. cAMP-dependent kinases are known in several other cell systems.

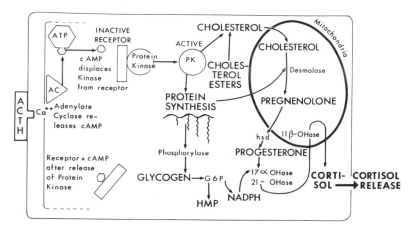

Figure 11.1. Mechanisms of action of a prototype peptide hormone. The action of ACTH (adrenocorticotropin) on the adrenocortical cell is depicted. The action of the tropic hormone on the outer cell membrane is not calcium dependent, but the release of adenylate cyclase from the inner membrane is. Adenylate cyclase releases cAMP from ATP. The cAMP displaces protein kinase from the receptor. Protein kinase *(PK)* then activates several steps as depicted, with the eventual production of cortisol from the adrenal cell.

In the adrenal cortical cell, the cAMP phosphokinase has the following actions: phosphorylation and activation of phosphorylase (via phosphorylase kinase (see Chapter 1), cholesterol esterase (release of free cholesterol), and ribosome phosphorylation (involved in regulation of protein synthesis at the level of translation).

Steroidogenic Pathway Biologically active corticosteroids are synthesized through a series of complex enzymatic reactions involving several intracellular organelles. Cholesterol synthesized from acetate is the precursor for corticosteroids. Cholesterol is esterified by fatty acids and stored in lipid droplets in the adrenocortical cells. The mitochondria contain the side chain cleaving enzyme (desmolase) which catalyzes the insertion of O_2 into the steroid molecule and cleavage of isocaproaldehyde, with the formation of pregnenolone. The following corticosteroidogenic steps take place in the soluble microsomal fractions of the cell: 1) Δ^5,3β-ol dehydrogenation (hydroxysteroid dehydrogenase); 2) 17α hydroxylation; and 3) 21-hydroxylation. The 11β hydroxylation step takes place in the mitochondrial compartment. The rate-limiting step is the initial desmolase reaction. The various steps listed above require NADPH and cytochrome P-450. NADPH is produced by the hexose monophosphate shunt which is stimulated by phosphorylase activation. Pregnenolone removal from the mitochondrial compartment permits continued synthesis. Accumulation of pregnenolone inhibits its synthesis. The actual details of activation of the desmolase reaction are not known, nor is the role of the cAMP-activated processes. Undoubtedly, the phosphorylase activation provides energy as well as cofactors for the desmolase reaction.

Role of Protein Synthesis in Control of Steroidogenesis

Steroidogenesis is dependent on protein synthesis. Apparently, a regulator protein with rapid turnover is stimulated by ACTH action.

Tropic Effects of ACTH on Adrenal Cortex ACTH administration induces in vitro protein synthesis caused by changes in the soluble fraction, microsomes, and polysomes. Increased RNA also occurs after ACTH stimulation. This RNA increase precedes stimulation of DNA synthesis.

ACTH Effects on Adrenocortical Replication The tropic effects of ACTH (and cAMP) include regulation of DNA synthesis. Hypophysectomy is followed by decreased adrenal DNA synthesis. Dibutyryl cAMP maintains adrenal weight, protein, RNA, and DNA after hypophysectomy. ACTH or cAMP stimulates differentiated (steroidogenic) function while inhibiting replication in adrenal tumor cell line.

PROCESSES PROPAGATED BY PARTICIPATION OF CYTOSOL AND NUCLEAR RECEPTORS (3, 4)

The steroid hormones act on several different types of tissue cells, e.g., in liver, kidneys, and adipose tissue, all essentially by similar steps. These are (Figure 11.2): permeation of cell membrane, binding to a cytosol receptor, transfer of steroid-receptor to nucleus (across nuclear membrane), binding of steroid-receptor complex to nuclear acceptor NAc (chromatin DNA), and synthesis of new RNA, protein synthesis, and cell function.

Permeation of Target Cell Membrane

There are relatively few reactive structures on the steroid molecule, and the specific factors responsible for transfer through the membrane are not known. It is well known that steroid hormones are transported in the plasma bound to carrier proteins, e.g., cortisol-binding globulin, sex hormone-binding globulin. It is likely that the complex is dissociated at the cell membrane.

Binding to Intracellular Cytosol Receptor

Glucocorticoid receptors have been studied in a variety of tissues including thymus, lymphocytes, hepatoma culture cells, fibroblasts, lungs, and mammary cells. The properties of these receptors are similar regardless of tissue of origin. Tomkins (5) classified glucocorticoid inducers as: 1) optimal inducers (glucocorticoids); 2) suboptimal inducers (e.g., 11-deoxycorticosterone and 11-deoxycortisol); 3) anti-inducers (e.g., testosterone and estradiol); and 4) inactive steroid inducers (e.g., epicortisol).

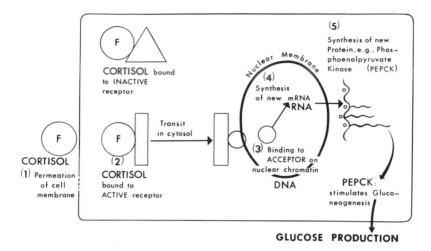

Figure 11.2. Mechanisms of action of a prototype steroid hormone. The action of cortisol on the hepatic cell is represented. Note the importance of the active protein receptor in the cytosol. Entrance of the steroid-receptor complex into the nuclear compartment permits attachment of the steroid to nuclear chromatin. New protein synthesis results in the production of, in this case, phosphoenolpyruvate carboxykinase. This enzyme stimulates gluconeogenesis, with resultant release of glucose from the hepatic cell.

It was concluded that cytosol receptor protein exists in two conformational states, an inactive and an active form. The uncomplexed aporeceptors are usually in the inactive form, and binding to optimal inducers pushes the equilibrium toward the active form. Type 2 inducers bind to both inactive and active receptors, while type 3 bind to the inactive receptor only. Based on these concepts, it became apparent that the affinity of the steroid for the specific binding site of the active aporeceptor is responsible for variations in glucocorticoid potency. Recent studies suggest some similarities between plasma glucocorticoid-binding proteins and the cytosol receptors. Biological potency of the glucocorticoid hormones correlates quite well with binding to cytosol receptor.

Transfer of Steroid-Receptor Complex to Nucleus

The active type 1-receptor complex moves from cytosol to nucleus, whereas types 2 or 3-receptor complexes do not. It is, therefore, likely that these suboptimal and anti-inducers may act as inhibitors at different stages of this process. The active receptor protein in the cytosol is probably not identical with that in the nucleus. Specific nuclear chromatin receptor sites bind the steroid-receptor complex.

The hormone-receptor complex interacts with the genome at specific DNA sites determined by the chromatin, acidic, non-histone proteins.

Synthesis of new mRNA

Steroid induction of protein synthesis involves enhancement of precursor incorporation into ribosomal mRNA. The mechanism involves increased nucleolar RNA polymerase activity. The specificity is dependent on the specific activation of mRNA synthesis by the steps described above. The current concept on action of the steroid-receptor complex on gene expression is that the steroid-receptor complex inhibits a repressor to a regulatory gene, thus permitting activity of a structural gene to stimulate RNA polymerase activity with resultant release of mRNA. It is likely that there is a post-transcriptional repressor which inhibits translation of specific mRNAs and increases degradation of the messenger. The steroid-receptor complex apparently inhibits this translational repressor (6).

Synthesis of New Proteins by Ribosomes

Glucocorticoids induce the production of several hepatic enzymes; these include tryptophan pyrrolase, tyrosine aminotransferase, as well as the enzymes regulating gluconeogenesis, viz., pyruvate carboxylase, phosphoenolpyruvate carboxykinase, and fructose-1,6-diphosphate phosphatase. There are data to suggest that secondary induction of these enzymes may occur during the process of gluconeogenesis. Nevertheless, the de novo synthesis of the gluconeogenic enzymes in hepatic cells is induced by glucocorticoid hormones.

LITERATURE CITED

1. Sutherland, E. W. 1972. Studies on the mechanism of hormone action. Science 177:401–408.
2. Gill, G. N. 1972. Mechanism of ACTH action. Metabolism 21:571–589.
3. Means, A. R., and B. W. O'Malley. 1972. Mechanism of estrogen action: Early transcriptional and translational events. Metabolism 21:357–371.
4. Feldman, D., J. W. Funder, and I. S. Edelman. 1972. Subcellular mechanisms in the action of adrenal steroids. Am. J. Med. 53:545–560.
5. Samuels, H. H., and G. M. Tomkins. 1970. Relation of steroid structure to enzyme induction in hepatoma tissues culture cells. J. Mol. Biol. 52:57–74.
6. Tomkins, G. M., T. D. Gelehrter, D. K. Granner, D. W. Martin, H. H. Samuels, and E. B. Thompson. 1969. Control of specific gene expression in higher organisms. Science 166:1474–1478.

12 Hypothalamic-Hypophysiotropic-Neurohypophysial System

HYPOTHALAMIC-NEUROHYPOPHYSIAL SYSTEM

The term hypothalamic-neurohypophysial system is employed in this discussion to refer to the neurosecretory system including the hypothalamic paraventricular and supraoptic nuclei, the neurohypophysial axons to these nuclei to the median eminence, the pituitary stalk, the posterior pituitary gland, the hypophysiotropic area of the hypothalamus, and the portal system supplying the anterior pituitary gland. The endocrinologic functions of this system are: 1) the formation and release of vasopressin, the antidiuretic hormone (ADH); 2) the formation and release of the oxytocic hormone, oxytocin; and 3) the formation and release of hormonal substances which regulate certain secretory functions of the anterior pituitary (1–3).

The antidiuretic activity of posterior pituitary extract was established clinically when the extract was found to decrease urine volume in patients with diabetes insipidus. Vasopressin and oxytocin are synthesized in the hypothalamic nuclei in the form of secretory vesicles enclosed by membranes. These secretory vesicles are transported down the neurohypophysial tract to the posterior pituitary.

Neurophysiological and chemical studies have established the existence of an area of the hypothalamus, the hypophysiotrophic area, which is involved in the control of anterior pituitary hormone release. Current data on mapping of this area locate the site of control of adrenocorticotropin (ACTH) secretion in the posterior hypothalamus. The release of thyroid-stimulating hormone by the pituitary is under control of thyro-

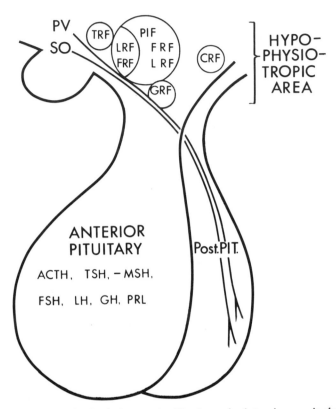

Figure 12.1. Hypothalamic-pituitary axis. The hypophysiotropic area is depicted with the loci of release of the various releasing and inhibitory neurohormones. The details are described in the text. The anterior part of the medial aspect is site of release of spurts of the gonadotropin-releasing factors.

tropin-releasing factor (TRF) area in the anterior hypothalamus. Control of basal gonadotropin release resides in the middle regions of the hypothalamus while spurts of release are controlled by an area just anterior. The ventral aspect of the hypothalamus is concerned with control of growth hormone (GH) release (Figure 12.1).

Chemical and Physical Characteristics of Neurohypophysial Hormones

Vasopressin The hormone is made up of 8 amino acid residues containing 5 amino acids linked by an S–S bond and a tail composed of 3 amino acids. The structure of human vasopressin was discovered by du Vigneaud (3) who also showed that species differences between vasopressins resided in the replacement of arginine in the "tail" (human vasopressin contains arginine) by lysine which is unique to pig vasopressin. These molecules are small enough to be dialyzable; the active hormone is bound electrostatically to a carrier protein of approximate molecular weight 30,000.

Oxytocin Oxytocin is a peptide hormone of octapeptide structure sequence

$$Cys-Tyr-Ile-Glu(NH_2)-Asp(NH_2)-Cys-Pro-Leu-Gly(NH_2)$$

and molecular weight around 1,200. Like vasopressin, this peptide is produced in the hypothalamus and incorporated into neurosecretory granules. The major synthesis occurs in the paraventricular nuclei. The hormone is then transported along the axons into the posterior pituitary for storage. Release of oxytocin from the posterior pituitary is stimulated by many factors, such as pain or anesthesis. These stimuli release vasopressin and oxytocin simultaneously. Suckling causes a release of oxytocin and, to a small extent, vasopressin.

Hyperosmolality and carotid occlusion or hemorrhage stimulate vasopressin release, but some oxytocin may also be released. Independent release has been shown to occur also. The afferent reflex pathway for oxytocin release consists of sensitive receptors in the nipple areas from which fibers enter the spinal and dorsal roots in the lateral funiculus to the brain stem. Fibers reach from there to the hypothalamus, transmitting the impulses for release of oxytocin. The released oxytocin enters the circulation and is carried to the appropriate target organs, viz., the myoepithelial cells in the mammary gland. Contraction of these cells surrounding the alveoli of the mammary gland leads to milk ejection. Absence of the pituitary (as after hypophysectomy) or blockage of oxytocin action on the cells (as by catecholamines) results in failure of lactation. This hormone also causes uterine contraction, but its physiological role in the precipitation and progress of labor is not known. Oxytocin causes contraction of the postpartum uterus by inducing a removal of Ca^{++} from the myometrial cell membrane, entrance of sodium, and membrane depolarization. Contracture of the endometrium is caused by larger doses of this hormone.

Oxytocin is degraded by the kidney and, to some extent, by the liver. Significant amounts of the hormone are trapped and degraded in the target cells, breast, and uterus. The degradation involves reduction of the S—S bonds and possibly enzymatic destruction of the amide groups which are necessary for biological activity.

Hypothalamic Neurohormones Regulating Anterior Pituitary Functions Hypothalamic regulation of the anterior pituitary is mediated by several neurohormones which are transported by a portal system to the anterior pituitary (4–6). The stimulatory neurohormones include somatotropin-releasing hormone (SRF) or growth hormone-releasing hormone, thyrotropin-releasing hormone (TRH), corticotropin-releasing factor

(CRF), and gonadotropin-releasing hormone (GnRH), which is now considered to be the stimulus to release of both FSH and LH and is, therefore, also called FSH/LH-RH. The inhibitory neurohormones whose functions have been clearly identified are prolactin inhibitory factor (PIF), melanocyte-stimulating hormone inhibitory factor (MIF), and somatotropin release inhibitory factor (SRIF or somatostatin). There are suggestions that additional inhibitory hormones corresponding to the stimulatory ones may exist, but their presence is not definitively proved.

SRF is a peptide of known sequence containing 11 amino acid residues. Its biological activity in stimulating growth hormone release has been confirmed in vivo and in vitro. TRH is a tripeptide with the sequence pyro-Glu-His-Pro(NH$_2$) which is active in stimulating the release of pituitary TSH and prolactin. Both actions are now employed in assessment of pituitary activity. Absence of a TSH increase after TRH challenge is indicative of pituitary hypothyroidism, but there are proved cases of hypothalamic hypothyroidism in which TRH is lacking. There are two CRF peptides (α and β) which possess biological activity in stimulating the release of ACTH from the anterior pituitary. α-CHF is thought to be quite similar to α-MSH in chemical structure, and β-CRF may be similar to vasopressin. PIF represents the biological activity which suppresses the release of prolactin by the anterior pituitary. Some aspects of dynamics of prolactin release are presented in Chapter 13. The chemical structure of PIF is not clear, but it is probably a peptide of similar small size as the other neurohormones. A peptide structure of MIF has been suggested, but this is not definite. This hormone increases release of MSH by the anterior pituitary. SIF, SRIF, or somatostatin has been identified as a tetradecapeptide from the hypothalamus. This hormone inhibits the release of GH by the anterior pituitary. Its participation in the sleep-associated rhythmicity in GH secretion, and its usefulness in disorders resulting from excess GH, are now being actively investigated. Inhibition of insulin and glucagon release by somatostatin was described (Chapter 1).

The gonadotropin-releasing hormone is a small basic peptide of estimated molecular weight between 1,200 and 2,000 which lacks disulfide bridges. The amino acids in the peptide are known to be aspartic acid, glutamic acid, glycine, alanine, lysine, histidine, threonine, serine, proline, and leucine. Its biological activity in releasing FSH and LH by the pituitary is well known, and it is now used in standard tests to determine integrity of the hypothalamic-pituitary-gonadal axis. Some studies have suggested that the FSH- and LH-releasing activities may be dissociated as may be required in regulation of the menstrual cycle. It is probable, however, that the sequential release of FSH and LH under hypothalamic control depends on time-related changes in responsiveness of the appropriate gonadotrope cells.

Effects of Pharmacological Agents on Activity of Hypophysiotropic Area

Transducer neurons, the neurons which stimulate releasing factors, are located in the hypophysiotropic area in the ventral hypothalamus. Their axons extend into the median eminence where the releasing factors are secreted into the capillary plexus which eventually discharges into the portal system supplying the anterior pituitary. Factors which influence the activity of these transducer neurons affect the function of the hypophysiotropic nuclei. It has been suggested that neurotransmitters within the neurons may also affect function of this hypophysiotropic area. Undoubtedly, neurons located higher than the transducer neurons alter the activity of this system (7).

Catecholamines and serotonin, derivatives of tyrosine and tryptophan respectively, are known to affect neurotransmitter function. Drugs such as the phenothiazines block the receptor site to norepinephrine, dopamine, and serotonin. This blockage leads to increased synthesis of these monoamines by a negative feedback control. Uptake of these neurotransmitter agents by their respective nerve terminals is blocked by tricyclic antidepressant drugs, such as imipramine and desipramine. Amphetamines release newly formed norepinephrine and dopamine. Reserpine depletes norepinephrine, serotonin, and dopamine and interferes with their storage. The effects of various pharmacological agents on secretion of the hypophysiotropic releasing factors are presented in Table 12.1.

VASOPRESSIN: PHYSIOLOGICAL CONSIDERATIONS

The major physiological role of vasopressin or antidiuretic hormone (ADH) is in the regulation of water balance by the renal tubule. Increasing the osmotic pressure of plasma in the distribution of the internal carotid leads to a release of antidiuretic hormone, and the resultant formation of a concentrated urine. The receptors responding to the osmotic challenge are located in the anterior hypothalamus. Conversely, dilution of body fluid suppresses the release of ADH, with the resultant excretion of urine hypotonic in relation to the body fluids. A feedback between the renal tubule and the anterior hypothalamus serves to maintain the normal tonicity in body fluids. A close anatomical and physiological interrelation between the anterior hypothalamic ADH mechanism and a thirst center serves to maintain normal fluid balance in the body. It has been shown that there are stimuli of a nonosomotic nature which apparently influence the release of ADH; these include pain, emotional states, nerve stimulation of certain nerves, as well as pharmacological agents, such as alcohol (which inhibits the release), nicotine, morphine, acetylcholine, barbiturates, bradykinin, ferritin, and cinchoninic acid.

Table 12.1. Pharmacological Effects on Releasing Factors Secretion

Factor	Increased by	Decreased by
CRF	Reserpine (transient), amphetamines, endotoxin	Phenothiazines, cortisol
TRH		T_4, T_3
GnRH (FSH/LH-RH)	Dopamine, L-dopa, estrogens (at certain levels)	Serotonin, melatonin (?), estrogens
PIF	L-dopa, dopamine	Reserpine, phenothiazines, tricyclic antidepressants, α-methyldopa
GRF	Amphetamines, dopamine, L-dopa	Reserpine, phenothiazines, imipramine, progesterone

Various studies have revealed that second to the osmotic factors in the regulation of vasopressin activity is a reduction in effective plasma volume. The mechanism involves the participation of right atrial stretch (volume) receptors which sense decreased plasma volumes and stimulate a release of vasopressin in an attempt to conserve fluid volume. This physiological pathway has been shown to be operative even in the presence of hypotonicity, suggesting that osmolality as a stimulus may well be secondary under certain conditions.

Physiological studies reveal that the pool of neurohypophysial vasopressin is heterogeneous with a readily releasable pool of 10–20% of the total pituitary content. After discharge of this pool by appropriate stimuli, the neurohypophysis may continue to release the hormone, but at an attenuated rate.

The antidiuretic hormone exerts its action water balance by increasing the permeability of the distal tubular luminal cells to water so that hypotonic luminal fluid becomes equilibrated with interstitial fluid. This action is independent of sodium or other solute reabsorption. There are some data which suggest that, because of its ability to induce water retention, ADH may secondarily induce sodium excretion via a suppressed aldosterone secretion caused by increased glomerular filtration rate.

Under certain conditions, vasopressin, as the name implies, may exhibit a significant vasopressor activity. Antidiuretic levels of vasopressin cause widespread vasoconstriction affecting peripheral and visceral vessels. A decrease in cardiac output may occur. This action, coupled with coronary artery vasoconstriction, may be dangerous in patients with decreased coronary reserve.

Vasopressin is distributed in the blood stream attached to a protein, but it is not certain what proportion is actually protein bound. The hormone is metabolized by the liver and the kidneys, but measurable amounts are also recoverable in the urine. The metabolism of ADH by the kidney exceeds that of the liver by a factor of 2.

Clinical Disorders Associated with Changes of Vasopressin Secretion

Vasopressin Deficiency (Diabetes Insipidus) The most significant and important result of a deficiency of vasopressin is the secretion of dilute urine with resultant increase in serum osmolality. This may be compensated for by activation of the thirst center and the induction of a secondary polydipsia. In the absence of sufficient fluid intake, the rise in serum osmolality will lead to serious clinical symptoms eventually culminating in death. However, in the presence of an active thirst center, such dire consequences are rare, but may occasionally occur in patients with unconsciousness caused by trauma, coma, or anesthesia.

Causes of Vasopressin Deficiency These causes are classified as primary and secondary. Primary diabetes insipidus includes idiopathic, which constitutes approximately 45% of all cases, and familial, which is responsible for 1% of all cases of diabetes insipidus. The familial type often will start in infancy, and the idiopathic type in childhood or later life. The secondary causes of diabetes insipidus include head trauma, accidents, head surgery, primary neoplasms, metastatic neoplasms (especially breast carcinoma), sarcoid disease, birth injuries, eosinophilic granuloma, and certain metabolic disorders.

The major manifestations of diabetes insipidus are secondary to the loss of fluid volume, patients being described as excreting 5–10 liters daily, with associated polydipsia. The urine specific gravity ranges from 1.001–1.005, with corresponding low urine osmolality. With fluid restriction, the specific gravity may increase somewhat. There are no other major clinical manifestations ascribable to the diabetes insipidus per se, but if there is an associated defect in the thirst center or in the ability to consume the required fluids, then death may ensue.

Differential Diagnosis Diabetes insipidus, a deficiency of antidiuretic hormone, has to be distinguished from two other conditions which are associated with polyuria and hyposthenuria. They are inability of the kidney to elaborate a concentrated urine despite adequate vasopressin secretion, and persistent excessive water intake, such as in psychogenic polydipsia which may itself result in a relative insensitivity of renal tubule responsiveness to antidiuretic hormone.

Any interference of the normal renal concentrating mechanism to render it unresponsive to the action of vasopressin may result in a syndrome clinically indistinguishable from diabetes insipidus, although, in some disorders, the manifestations are less severe. Hypercalcemia, such as in primary hyperparathyroidism, and hypokalemia caused by various factors, may impair the maximum concentrating ability of the renal tubules. In most such patients, the urine specific gravity is lower than normal, but only in a few is it sufficiently decreased and the osmolality sufficiently low to suggest diabetes insipidus. Renal concentrating ability may also be significantly decreased in chronic renal disease of several etiologies; such defects are usually accompanied by other evidence of the basic renal disorders. The natural history of acute tubular necrosis, caused by infection, trauma, or renal transplantation, will include a polyuric phase following the oliguric phase. Clinical stigmata of the respective underlying disorder aid in differentiating them from diabetes insipidus.

Clinical States Associated with Increased Secretion of ADH Bartter and Schwartz (8) described a syndrome of hyponatremia and decreased concentration of blood urea nitrogen, unassociated with cardiovascular decompensation, in patients with bronchogenic carcinoma. An interesting feature was the presence of significant amounts of sodium in the urine.

This latter finding distinguishes this syndrome from the hyponatremia caused by congestive heart failure or hepatic cirrhosis. These findings essentially duplicated those observed in normal human subjects who were given injections of a long acting vasopressin and allowed access to a normal fluid intake. The syndrome has been reported in several unrelated clinical states, the common feature in each being a secretion of ADH inappropriate to the extant water balance status. The clinical states include bronchogenic carcinoma, pancreatic carcinoma, lymphosarcoma, duodenal adenocarcinoma, subdural hematoma, brain tumors, subarachnoid hemorrhage, cerebrovascular thrombosis, skull fractures, cerebral atrophy, seizure disorders, Guillain-Barre syndrome, tuberculous meningitis, acute intermittent porphyria, and myxedema. Similar clinical findings have also been noted after administration of morphine, barbiturates, and anesthesia. Measurable amounts of ADH have been found in some of the tumors associated with the syndrome of inappropriate ADH.

In the clinical evolution of this syndrome, there is an apparently paradoxical natriuresis ascribed to an escape from the maximal renal effect of ADH caused by intra- and extrarenal response to the progressive expansion of total body water. The essential clinical laboratory features of this syndrome include hyponatremia, decreased serum osmolality, decreased blood urea nitrogen, natriuresis inappropriate to the hyponatremia, urine and increased urine osmolality, normal adrenal function, and normal renal function (8).

Procedures for Establishing Diagnosis of Diabetes Insipidus

Methods of Increasing Serum Osmolality

Water Restriction The principle of this method is to determine the changes in urine volume, specific gravity, and osmolality after a measured period of fluid restriction. Normal subjects on fluid restriction may reduce their urine flow to 0.5 ml/min or less, increase the urine specific gravity to 1.020 or greater, and increase the urine osmolality to 300 mOsm/kg or greater. The test should be carefully supervised, especially in patients in whom there is a strong possibility of diabetes insipidus. Water or other fluid intake should be restricted completely for up to 24 hr, depending on the tolerance of the patient. The body weight should be determined at the inception of the water restriction, and should be checked frequently. A body weight loss of less than 5% is safe, but any excessive weight loss may lead to circulatory collapse. Patients with diabetes insipidus, or with nonresponsiveness to ADH, will excrete urine with specific gravity of 1.001 to 1.005 persistently unless severe dehydration supervenes. The urine volume will not decrease to the 0.5 ml/min or less as occurs in normal subjects, nor will the urine osmolality increase significantly. It is possible, however, if dehydration supervenes, that the urine osmolality may rise to 300–400 mOsm/kg; these occurrences of dehydration will be avoided if the test is discontinued before the patient has lost 5% body weight.

The patient who fails to increase urine specific gravity and osmolality significantly, or to reduce the urine volume in a like manner, should then be studied further. The screening test does not provide conclusive evidence between the alternative possibilities of inadequate vasopressin secretion versus tubule nonresponsiveness.

Intravenous Infusion of Hypertonic Saline (Hickey-Hare Test) This procedure is an alternative method of increasing serum osmolality in order to determine the release of antidiuretic hormone. The principle of the method is that the increased serum osmolality should induce the release of ADH which should then act on the renal tubules to decrease urine output and increase urine concentration.

As recommended by Hickey and Hare, the patient is hydrated initially with glucose in water (8–10 ml/min) sufficient to induce a diuresis of 5 ml/min. The glucose-water infusion is then replaced with a 2.5% sodium chloride solution and infused at the rate of 0.25 ml/min/kg body weight; this is continued for 45 min. Voided urine flow is determined every 15 min. Normal subjects should exhibit a sharp decrease in urine volume with the hypertonic saline infusion. (This test is hazardous in patients with decompensated cardiovascular disease.) Failure to respond in this test with decreased urine volume still does not distinguish between inadequate ADH release or a nonresponsiveness of the kidneys.

Nicotine Infusion Test A third variant of inducing ADH release is accomplished by pharmacological means. The principle of this test is based on the fact that intravenously administered nicotine (0.5–1 mg in non-smokers and up to 3 mg in smokers) stimulates the release of ADH by the neurohypophysial system. Normal subjects will exhibit a significant decrease in urine volume and increase in specific gravity and osmolality following the injection of nicotine. Failure to respond suggests either inadequate ADH release or inadequate renal response to ADH, or both.

Test to Determine Responsiveness to Exogenous Vasopressin The principle of this method is that an adequate amount of exogenous vasopressin is administered, and the urine volume, specific gravity, and osmolality are monitored. In the presence of responsive renal tubules, normal subjects and patients with diabetes insipidus should exhibit maximal urine concentration (i.e., specific gravity of > 1.025 and urine osmolality of around 700 mOsm/liter).

The patient is instructed to empty his bladder at the start of the study. Vasopressin in normal saline, 5 milliunits/min, is infused over a 1-hour period (total of 0.3 unit). Voided urine volumes every 15 min should be obtained, and measurements made of the specific gravity (and osmolality). An alternative procedure is to use pitressin tannate in oil. This more convenient procedure is performed as follows: the patient is given an intramuscular injection of 5 units of pitressin tannate in oil at 7 p.m. He is instructed to empty his bladder at bedtime. On arising, a urine specimen is collected, as are voided specimens at three hourly intervals thereafter, during which time he is restricted from fluid intake. Significant concentrating ability indicates tubular responsiveness. The above procedures readily distinguish between diabetes insipidus and nephrogenic diabetes insipidus, the latter failing to respond to the vasopressin challenge. Failure to concentrate urine after exogenous vasopressin is a reflection of tubular nonresponsiveness to the hormone. This could result from a tubular insensitivity associated with long standing compulsive water drinking-psychogenic polydipsia. Hence, it is occasionally difficult on the basis of the above tests to distinguish between diabetes insipidus and psychogenic polydipsia. It has been suggested that if, after water restriction, the urine concentrating ability exceeds that found after vasopressin, then the ability to secrete ADH is normal, regardless of how low the urinary concentration may be. If vasopressin infusion is followed by higher urine concentration ability than after water restriction, then it should be concluded that ADH secretion is abnormal, regardless of how high the urine concentration is.

Management of Diabetes Insipidus (DI)

Replacement therapy of DI is indicated mainly for the discomfort associated with the disorder, and for patients whose ability to replace water loss is impaired. Aqueous pitressin in a nasal spray (20 units/ml) or posterior pituitary snuff are administered every 2–6 hr as indicated. In event of upper respiratory tract irritation the aqueous hormone is applied on a cotton pledget to the oral or vaginal mucosa. Injection of a suspension of pitressin tannate in oil (0.5–1.0 ml) may provide relief for 24–72 hr, and may be repeated on recurrence of symptoms. The diuretic drug chlorthiazide paradoxically reduces the polyuria in DI by two-thirds in many patients. Its mechanism of action is related to induction of a sodium deficit. A limiting factor in its use is induction of hypokalemia. Chlorpropamide induces antidiuresis by suppression of cAMP degradation in the renal tubule cell, by some stimulation of ADH release, and by inhibiting prostaglandins which suppress tubule cell adenylate cyclase. Hypoglycemia is a limiting factor in prolonged use. Phenformin and carbamazepine (Tegretol) are also useful in management of DI presumably by similar mechanisms.

Management of Syndrome of Inappropriate Antidiuretic Hormone (SIADH)

In the absence of severe dilutional hyponatremia the treatment of SIADH is fluid restriction (basal intake only) until restitution of normal serum osmolality. Cerebral complications associated with serum sodium below

115 mEq/liter respond dramatically to infusion of hypertonic saline. Fluid restriction should be continued, as the improvement is only temporary as natriuresis continues due to volume expansion. Severe hyponatremia is correctable by inducing diuresis with furosemide and replacement of urinary electrolyte losses (monitored hourly). Desired fluid loss is calculated on the basis of plasma osmolar deficit (normal P_{osm}/L − patient's P_{osm}/L), and total body water (0.65 × body weight (kg), as follows:

Desired fluid loss (L) =

$$\frac{(\text{Normal } P_{osm}/L - \text{patient's } P_{osm}/L)}{\text{Normal } P_{osm}/L} \times \text{body water (liters)}$$

LITERATURE CITED

1. Guillemin, R. 1967. The adenohypophysis and its hypothalamic control. Am. Rev. Physiol. 29:313–348.
2. Guillemin, R. 1964. Hypothalamic factors releasing pituitary hormone. Recent Prog. Horm. Res. 20:89–130.
3. du Vigneaud, V. 1956. Hormones of the posterior pituitary gland: Oxytocin and vasopressin. Harvey Lect.
4. Schally, A. V., A. Arimura, C. Y. Bowers. 1968. Hypothalamic neurohormones regulating anterior pituitary function. Recent Prog. Horm. Res. 24:497–588.
5. McCann, S. M., and J. C. Porter. 1969. Hypothalamic pituitary stimulating and inhibiting hormones. Physiol. Rev. 49:240–284.
6. Martini, L., and J. Meites. 1970. Neurochemical Aspects of Hypothalamic Function. Academic Press, New York.
7. Frohman, L. A. 1973. Clinical neuropharmacology of hypothalamic releasing factors. N. Engl. J. Med. 286:1391–1397.
8. Bartter, F. C., and W. B. Schwartz. 1969. The syndrome of inappropriate secretion of antidiuretic hormone. Am. J. Med. 42:790–806.

13 _____ Anterior
_____ Pituitary

The anterior pituitary gland (adenohypophysis) influences a variety of biological processes through the production of polypeptide and glycoprotein hormones. Body growth is regulated through the synthesis and release of growth hormone (somatotropic hormone, STH) and the structure and activity of several other endocrine glands are regulated by the secretion of various tropic hormones by the anterior pituitary. The gland is derived from ectodermal cells (Rathke's pouch) in the roof of the primitive oral cavity. After migration of these cells upward, and separation from the oral cavity by mesoderm, the cells eventually assume a position anterior to the neurohypophysis. The pituitary gland (adenohypophysis and neurohypophysis) weighs approximately 500 mg in the normal adult male, and may increase to 1 g in the pregnant female. The adenohypophysis accounts for approximately 75% of the entire pituitary size. The pituitary gland rests in the sella turcica which is a bony structure in which the gland is surrounded on all sides except the superior surface. The anterior pituitary is supplied by a system of portal veins from a capillary network around the median eminence and the neural stalk (1). In the gland, the portal system divides into sinusoids so that the cells are separated from blood by the endothelium and perisinusoidal space (1).

CONTROL OF ANTERIOR PITUITARY GLAND

There are several stimulatory and inhibitory factors (correctly termed hypothalamic neurohormones) which are transported by the portal blood supply to the pituitary. The stimulatory hormones include somatotropin-releasing factor (SRF), luteinizing hormone-releasing factor (LRF), follicle-stimulating hormone-releasing factor (FRF), thyrotropin-releasing factor (TRF), and corticotropin-releasing factor (CRF). There are some data showing close similarities between FRF and LRF. The inhibitory neurohormones prolactin inhibitory factor (PIF) and melanocyte-stimulating hormone inhibitory factor (MIF) inhibit release of prolactin and melanocyte-stimulating hormone (MSH), respectively. The existence of a growth hormone inhibitory hormone (GHIF, SRIF, somatostatin) is now proved. There are suggestions that inhibitory factors corresponding to all stimulatory neurohormones may exist, but this has not been definitively proved. The various specific secretory cells of the anterior pituitary are under immediate control by the hypothalamic neurohormones. These neurohormones are formed at axonal terminals of tracts which ultimately respond to circulating levels of hormones produced by the target glands, to various metabolic stimuli, e.g., amino acids, and to higher neural control. These higher neural stimuli may supercede the usual negative feedback circuit (see Chapter 12).

HORMONES PRODUCED BY ANTERIOR PITUITARY

The anterior pituitary gland is composed of several types of cells which have been characterized by staining and immunofluorescent techniques. Different cell types presumably secrete specific hormones. The general groups of cells include the acidophilic cells which secrete growth hormone and prolactin; the basophilic cells which secrete thyroid-stimulating hormone, follicle-stimulating hormone, luteinizing hormone, and adreno-corticotropic hormone. Chromophobe cells may also participate in the secretion of the pituitary hormones.

The anterior pituitary hormones ACTH, the melanocyte-stimulating hormones (α-MSH, β-MSH), GH, and prolactin, possess protein or polypeptide structures whereas TSH, LH, and FSH are glycoproteins. The tropic hormones TSH, ACTH, LH, and FSH maintain the structure and biological activities of specific target endocrine glands. GH affects several organ systems and is involved in several biochemical reactions. ACTH, TSH, and LH increase the activity of adenylate cyclase in the cell membranes of the adrenal cortex, thyroid, and ovary, respectively, accelerating the formation of cyclic adenosine $3':5'$-monophosphate (cAMP) from ATP. cAMP serves as the intracellular mediator of the action of these hormones. Growth hormone is a single chain polypeptide composed of 188 amino acids with a molecular weight of 21,500. There is an intrachain disulfide bond which forms a ring structure (2). Recent studies reveal the existence of "big" and "little" components of GH, the latter presumably the active hormone. The "big" fraction possesses a molecular weight of 40,000–45,000 (3). There are species differences in immunological activity as well as in biological activity; only primate GH has significant biological activity in man. GH influences several biochemical mechanisms, such as stimulation of protein synthesis, intracellular transport of amino acids, increased ribosomal protein synthesis, and intracellular lipolysis, a process leading to increased plasma free fatty acids and enhancement of fatty acid oxidation and ketogenesis. Carbohydrate metabolism is affected by GH in decreasing the responsiveness to insulin, decreasing conversion of glucose to fat in adipose tissue; the hormone is also diabetogenic in certain species. GH stimulates collagen synthesis, increases intestinal absorption of calcium, induces hypercalcemia, stimulates the retention of sodium and phosphate, and increases serum alkaline phosphatase. GH probably requires further transformation before it is biologically effective in growth stimulation. This activation may require renal uptake of the hormone. The ability of somatomedin (sulfation factor) to stimulate growth in the absence of GH has been proved. It is likely that GH is either a precursor to, or stimulates production of, somatomedin (4).

It is estimated that the pituitary contains 5–10 mg of GH/gland. In normal individuals in the fasting and resting state, the plasma GH concentration is less than 5 ng/ml and the half-life of the circulating hormone is 20 min. GH levels in the plasma are increased by exercise, hypoglycemia, and infusion or ingestion of certain amino acids, e.g., arginine. The hormone levels decrease in the presence of hyperglycemia. Assessment of pituitary GH secretion is best done after challenging with one of the above stimuli. These are discussed later.

Prolactin is a polypeptide hormone of molecular weight of 23,000; the molecule contains an intrachain disulfide bond. Secretion of this hormone is stimulated by hypothalamic TRH and suppressed by PIF. Prolactin plays an important role in growth and development of the breasts and in lactation, but these actions of the hormone are dependent on the presence of GH, corticosteroids, estrogens, and progesterone. The mammotropic and lactogenic actions of this hormone have been utilized in a biological assay. This hormone is now measured by a radioimmunoassay method and by a method based on its biological potency.

Follicle-stimulating hormone has a glycoprotein structure and has an estimated molecular weight of 29,000. Its biological activity is confined to the gonads, stimulating maturation of the ovarian follicle in the female and increasing the growth of the seminiferous tubules and the process of spermatogenesis in the male. FSH administration in women is followed by increased levels of urinary estrogens and pregnanediol. FSH extracted from human postmenopausal urine has been employed for induction of ovulation and pregnancy in patients with ovulatory failure, with a high incidence of multiple births. A radioimmunoassay method for FSH quantitation is now available. The secretion of FSH by the pituitary is inhibited by estrogens; conversely, in estrogen deficiency, e.g., hypogonadism, there are increased levels of FSH in the urine. In the male, testosterone is relatively ineffective in inhibiting FSH release.

Luteinizing hormone is a glycoprotein hormone with an approximate molecular weight of 30,000. This hormone stimulates the secretion of progesterone by the corpus luteum, and the released cAMP functions as the intracellular mediator of the steroidogenic action of LH. In the male, LH (called interstitial cell-stimulating hormone, ICSH) stimulates the production of testosterone by the interstitial cells of the testis. The ability of LH to increase the weight of the ventral prostate in the rat has been the basis of a biological assay method for LH. Radioimmunoassay has been employed in the measurement of LH in the plasma. In prepubertal children, the level of LH was estimated to be 0.5 ng/ml. At puberty in males, the levels reach 0.7 mg/ml, increasing up to 1.7 ng/ml in the 4th decade. In females, the postpubertal level is 1.2 ng/ml in the follicular phase, and 1.0 ng/ml in the luteal phase of the menstrual cycle. Detailed patterns of plasma LH during the menstrual cycle have been described (5).

The regulation of LH secretion is dependent on the activity of the central nervous system (6). Estrogens inhibit LH release, and, conversely, low levels of estrogens, as in ovarian insufficiency, result in increased LH release. However, a positive feedback between estrogens and LH is necessary for the LH spurt before ovulation. In the male, testosterone has been shown to decrease LH levels (7).

Thyroid-stimulating hormone is a glycoprotein hormone which contains glucosamine and galactosamine. The estimated molecular weight of this hormone is 28,000. TSH increases adenylate cyclase in thyroid tissue and, thus, stimulates the release of cAMP which serves as the intracellular mediator of TSH action. TSH is also suggested to have an extrathyroidal action in accelerating lipolysis in rat adipose tissue, but the significance of this finding is not clear.

TSH increases the thyroidal uptake of ^{131}I, as well as the discharge of thyroid hormone. The release of TSH is determined in large part by the circulating level of thyroid hormone by a negative feedback circuit in which hypothalamic TRH plays a role. This role is superseded by the thyroid-pituitary feedback system, however. By radioimmunoassay procedures (8), it has been estimated that TSH levels in human plasma range from 0–10 microunits/ml, with marked elevations in patients with hypothyroidism and low to undetectable levels in primary hyperthyroid states.

Adrenocorticotropic hormone is a single-chained polypeptide made up of 39 amino acids; species differences reside in amino acids at positions 25 and 33. Amino acids 1 to 24 of the peptide possess biological activity of the full ACTH molecule. The major function of ACTH is to maintain the structure and secretory activity of the adrenal cortex. ACTH stimulates the production of cortisol, corticosterone, and 17-ketosteroids (17-KS) by the adrenals by activation of adrenal cell membrane adenylate cyclase, which leads to release of cAMP which serves as the intracellular mediator of ACTH action (9). ACTH possesses a melanocyte-stimulating activity, but increased pigmentation observed in patients with high levels of ACTH is probably caused by associated increased MSH levels. There is a circadian variation in ACTH release, with peak levels occurring at the time of awakening, followed by a steady decline at the time of sleep. The level of ACTH is also dependent on the circulatory levels of cortisol by a negative feedback system mediated by hypothalamic CRF. ACTH depletes the adrenal stores of cholesterol and ascorbic acid, and the latter finding is basis for a biological assay for ACTH. The steroidogenic action of ACTH in the hypophysectomized rat's adrenal is another method of biological assay of ACTH. Employing bioassay methods, it was shown that plasma ACTH ranges between 0.1 and 0.5 milliunit/100 ml at 6:00 a.m., with undetectable levels at 6:00 p.m. Yalow et al. (10), employing radioimmunoassay, demonstrated somewhat higher levels of plasma ACTH.

α-MSH is a polypeptide composed of 13 amino acids, and β-MSH is made up of 22 amino acids. There are certain features in these structures which are similar to the amino acid sequence in ACTH. MSH produces dispersion of melanin granules in the skin; this activity has been separated from similar action by ACTH.

Laboratory Diagnosis of Anterior Pituitary Disorders

These have been outlined in detail (11) and are summarized here.

Assessment of Growth Hormone Functions Clinical disorders may involve decreased and excessive GH secretion. These clinical states may be suspected on the basis of the target organ effects of GH.

The clinical features of various pituitary disorders are presented in Tables 13.1 and 13.2. In the unihormonal deficiency state involving GH, dwarfism is the resultant clinical condition. In the adult, the major clinical laboratory finding is of a hypoglycemia which may be symptomatic occasionally. In the child with decreased GH, the most important manifestation is decreased bone age; the epiphyses do not develop at a normal rate; hence, "bone age" on an x-ray of the wrists, for example, is retarded. Serum phosphate and alkaline phosphatase are often decreased.

Direct Assessment of Decreased Growth Hormone The following studies are useful:

1. Basal Fasting Serum Immunoreactive GH Levels Basal fasting serum immunoreactive GH levels of less than 1 ng/ml are found in hyposomatotropinism associated with panhypopituitarism and with unihormonal deficiency.

Table 13.1. Clinical Features and Laboratory Diagnostic Studies in Hypopituitary States

Disorder	Etiology and mechanism	Clinical effects	Diagnostic studies
Hypopituitarism	Surgery or radiation	Decreased water diuresis	Water loading test: HGH and cortisol after hypoglycemia, cosyntropin challenge
		Nausea, vomiting, hypotension, death (early changes 4–14 days)[a]	
		Cold intolerance, dry skin, myxedema, (4–8 weeks postoperative)[b]	T_4, TSH levels, TSH stimulation
		In males, testes smaller and softer; decreased libido and potency aspermia[c]	Sperm count; plasma FSH and LH
		In females, amenorrhea; vaginal and uterine atrophy[c]	Cytology; FSH, LH after LRH or clomiphene
		Loss of axillary and pubic hair in both	
Spontaneous panhypopituitarism	Postpartum necrosis of pituitary; granulomas; infarction from vessel disease; infection; Hand-Schuller-Christian disease; craniopharyngioma	Same as above in altered sequence	Same as above; skull x-ray may show evidence of tumor erosion of dorsum sella, posterior clinoids intrasellarcalcification and separation of sutures may be found in craniopharyngioma
		As late manifestations[a]	
		May occur 5–10 years later; hair loss and coarse voice[b]	
		Gonadal manifestations are earliest in postpartum pituitary necrosis[c]	

	Etiology	Manifestations	Diagnostic tests
	Pituitary apoplexy in tumor	Shock from adrenal insufficiency is earliest manifestation	
Unihormonal (dwarfism)	Often unknown etiology: hereditary in few; possible hypothalamic defects	Body growth and facial features; immature eruption of secondary teeth late; subclinical hypoglycemia[d]	Bone age; height; plasma GH after insulin or arginine infusion
Nonresponse to GH-ACTH deficiency	African Pygmies; possible defect in GRF from hypothalamus	Decreased growth, hypoglycemia; Nausea, vomiting, weakness, hypotension decreased axillary and pubic hair[a]	Plasma cortisol or urine 17-OHCS pre- and postvasopressin, hypoglycemia or metyrapone ACTH levels
TSH Deficiency	Possible defect in hypothalamus	Cold intolerance, dry skin, myxedema, anemia[b]	RAI uptake pre- and post-TSH; TSH levels;
Gonadotropin deficiency	X-linked trait; others	Anosmia, eunuchoidism in males, complete and incomplete forms—in latter, there is delayed puberty; aspermia; decreased Leydig cells[c] In females, amenorrhea, decreased pubic and axillary hair	sperm count; testicular biopsy; urine or plasma gonadotropins; Vaginal cytology; endometrial biopsy

[a] Caused by secondary defect in adrenal.
[b] Caused by secondary defect in thyroid.
[c] Caused by secondary defect in gonads.
[d] Caused by defect in growth hormone.

Table 13.2. Clinical Features and Laboratory Diagnostic Studies in Hyperpituitary States

Disorder	Etiology	Clinical effects	Diagnostic studies[a]
Hyperpituitarism: Hypersomatotropinism	Acidophilic and chromophobe tumors of pituitary; chromophobe tumors most frequent in 3rd–5th decades; may spread; acidophilic tumors, not metastatic	Prepubertal onset: gigantism, excessive proportional growth, later acral changes; postpubertal onset: acromegaly, periosteal growth, widening of bones, broad hands, widened fingers with blunted ends; prognathism, teeth widely separated, macroglossia, deepened voice, osteoarthritis, cardiomegaly, cardiomyopathy, congestive heart failure, and diabetes mellitus; hypogonadism is frequent; osteoporosis, hirsutism, and persistent lactation in some patients; visceromegaly—liver and kidney may have increased GFR; perhaps an increased incidence of parathyroid and islet cell hyperplasia	Diabetic type GTT; bone changes by x-ray; Plasma GH—baseline and failure to suppress after hyperglycemia; skull x-ray: erosion of posterior clinoids, dorsum sella; thickening of calvarum and enlargement of frontal sinuses

Hypersecretion of prolactin	Hypothalamic defect	Chiari-Frommel syndrome: postpuerperal persistent lactation and secondary amenorrhea	Serum prolactin by RIA
	Pituitary tumors—mainly chromophobe adenoma	Forbes-Albright: nonpuerpertal lactation and amenorrhea; in both types: vaginal and uterine atrophy	
Hypersecretion of ACTH and MSH	Basophilic adenomas mainly	Hypercortisolism, Cushing's syndrome: hypertension, phlethora, moonfacies, striae centripetal fat distribution, obesity, and polycythemia; hyperpigmentation, occasional hirsutism, and clitoromegaly	Plasma and urine cortisol and 17-OHCS before and after dexamethasone suppression; ACTH radio-immunoassay, MSH radio-immunoassay
Ectopic ACTH production	Bronchogenic small cell, or undifferentiated, carcinoma; pancreatic and thymic carcinoma	As above, except for absence of obesity, weight loss may be caused by tumor growth	As above ACTH radioimmunoassay (?)

^{a}Specific laboratory tests are underlined.

2. Serum GH Levels after Insulin Hypoglycemia A baseline blood sample is obtained for glucose and GH determinations. The patient is given crystalline insulin by intravenous injection (0.05 unit/kg body weight in children, and 0.1–0.15 unit/kg in adults). Blood samples are obtained at 20, 60, and 90 min after the injection of insulin. An adequate stimulus is a drop of blood sugar to less than 50% of basal value, or below 50 mg/100 ml. Baseline plasma and at least two in the hypoglycemic range are used for GH radioimmunoassay. Normal subjects show levels of GH 2–3 times the basal level of GH, or at least exhibit GH levels of > 10 ng/ml at the hypoglycemic peak. Patients with pituitary insufficiency causing decreased GH, as well as obese individuals, fail to show increased levels of GH. It is suggested that nonresponsiveness of HGH to hypoglycemia should be confirmed by the arginine challenge.

3. GH Levels after Arginine Infusion A baseline blood sample is obtained for glucose and GH determinations. The patient is given an arginine solution 0.5 mg/kg body weight by intravenous infusion over a period of 30 min. Blood samples for GH levels are taken at the end of the infusion (30 min) at 60, 90, and 120 min after start of the infusion. Normal subjects show increases in the GH levels to 2–3 times the basal value. Patients with defective GH secretion fail to show values above 10 ng/ml.

4. GH Levels after Glucagon In this test, a similar protocol as in Section 3 is employed. The baseline GH level is compared with those taken 20, 60, and 90 min after the subcutaneous injection of 1.0 mg of glucagon. The criteria for diagnosis are those in Section 3 above. This procedure is safer than that in Section 2 above.

5. GH Response to Vasopressin Challenge Baseline plasma and plasma obtained 30 and 60 min after intramuscular injection of 10 units of vasopressin is followed by a significant rise of GH in normal subjects. Failure to show GH above 10 ng/ml is consistent with hyposomatotropinism.

6. GH Levels after Exercise and during Sleep GH levels after vigorous physical exercise or during sleep are methods employed, especially in pediatric practice, for assessment of hyposomatotropinism.

7. GH Levels in Plasma after Challenge with L-dopa Several studies show that normal individuals exhibit a prompt and significant increase in plasma LGH after oral ingestion of 0.5 g of L-dopa (dihydroxyphenylalanine). This test is readily performed on an outpatient basis.

It should be pointed out that the above procedures should not be performed unless the patient is euthyroid, as hypothyroidism will attenuate or obliterate the expected rises in GH after the various challenges.

Hypersomatotropinism (excessive GH) in the prepubertal child will cause gigantism. After puberty, the excess GH will lead to acromegaly. Indirect clinical tests consistent with hypersomatotropinism include an abnormal diabetic type glucose tolerance test and often an elevated serum inorganic phosphorus level, without the normal circadian variation, as well as hypercalciuria and hydroxyprolinemia. Virilization ascribable to increased 17-KS levels is often found in these patients.

Direct Assessment of Growth Hormone Excess These methods involve the determination of GH levels by radioimmunoassay.

Basal GH levels in the fasting male subject are 5 ng/ml or less, and a level greater than 5 ng/ml is, therefore, consistent with hypersomatotropinism. In female patients, the basal fasting levels may fluctuate widely. It is necessary to conduct a hyperglycemic challenge before assessing the GH levels.

GH levels during the oral or intravenous glucose tolerance test (GTT)— In male and female patients with acromegaly, there is less than 50% decrease in plasma immunoreactive GH after infusion of glucose intravenously. Normal subjects exhibit an almost complete suppression of GH production during the hyperglycemia. Patients with hypersomatotropinism show plasma HGH levels of >10–300 ng/ml, regardless of the level of blood sugar elevation.

Assessment of Pituitary ACTH Function Diseases of the pituitary may cause hyperadrenocorticotropinism and hypoadrenocorticotropinism. Both are manifested clinically by their effects on adrenocortical functions.

Hyperadrenocorticotropinism results in bilateral adrenocortical hyperplasia (Cushing's disease), hypercortisolemia, as well as increased levels of adrenal 17-KS androgens. Clinical manifestations of hypercortisolemia are caused by the effects of the hormone on protein, fat, and carbohydrate metabolism, as well as on blood pressure, connective tissues, and bone structure. The androgenic effects include virilization and hirsutism in the female. These clinical effects are described in Chapter 15.

Indirect clinical laboratory effects of hypercortisolemia include an increased blood sugar and impaired GTT, decreased total eosinophil count in peripheral blood, and an increase in serum Na:K ratio. These parameters are not diagnostic of hypercortisolemia, however.

Assessment of Pituitary Hyperadrenocorticotropinism These methods involve quantitation of adrenocortical steroids or their metabolites after appropriate physiological manipulations. These tests are described more fully in Chapter 15.

1. In the overnight dexamethasone suppression test, the patient is given 1 mg of dexamethasone orally at 12 midnight, and a plasma cortisol level is determined on blood drawn at 8:00 a.m. Normal individuals show a plasma cortisol level <5 μg/100 ml, whereas non-Cushing obese patients show values <10 μg/100 ml. Levels of cortisol >10 μg/100 ml are found in

patients with hypercortisolemia caused by hyperadrenocorticotropinism (as well as adrenal adenoma, carcinoma, or ectopic ACTH).

2. With circadian variation of plasma cortisol, plasma samples drawn at 8:00 a.m. and at 5:00 p.m. contain levels of 5–25 μg/100 ml and 2.5–12.5 μg/100 ml respectively in normal subjects. Patients with increased ACTH exhibit values of 25 μg/100 ml or greater at both times, demonstrating a lack of circadian variation.

3. Basal urinary excretion of 17-hydroxycorticosteroids (17-OHCS) and 17-ketogenic steroids (17-KGS) will be increased in patients with hyper-corticotropinism, adrenal adenoma, adrenal carcinoma, and ectopic ACTH excess. Urinary 17-KS is also increased in the above conditions excepting adrenal adenoma. Methods for urinary steroid determinations are described in Chapter 15.

4. Dexamethasone suppression tests utilizing urinary 17-OHCS (total or after sequential extraction) or 17-KGS reveal no suppression of urinary steroids after the low dexamethasone dosage (0.5 mg every 6 hours for 3 days) in patients with hypercorticotropinism. Suppression occurs after higher doses of dexamethasone (2 mg four times daily for 3 days).

5. Urinary 17-OHCS (total or fractionated), 17-KGS, or plasma 11-deoxycortisol after metyrapone (oral or intravenous)—Patients with hypercorticotropinism exhibit significant increases in the high baseline levels of urinary steroids after metyrapone challenge (see Chapter 15).

6. Plasma ACTH levels—The biological assay methods of measuring ACTH levels are not readily applicable to clinical practice. The radio-immunoassay of ACTH promises to be quite helpful in diagnosis of pituitary-adrenal disorders. In hypercorticotropinism, the levels of ACTH are significantly higher than the normal 0.1–0.5 milliunit/100 ml.

Hypoadrenocorticotropinism (decreased ACTH secretion) is manifested clinically by evidence of adrenal insufficiency as described in Chapter 15. Patients with hypoadrenocorticotropinism lack the pigmentary and marked electrolyte disturbances seen in primary adrenal disease.

The best tests to evaluate a defect in ACTH production involve methods of stimulating the release of ACTH. The effects of ACTH release are measured by study of plasma cortisol or urinary corticosteroids. After establishing that the adrenal cortex is responsible (see intravenous cosyntropin test and 8-hour ACTH test described in Chapter 15), these tests may be done:

1. In our experience, the vasopressin stimulation test is very reliable and considerably less cumbersome than any of the other procedures employed. Plasma cortisol increase of 100% or greater after injection of vasopressin

(10 units intramuscularly) is reliable evidence of intact pituitary ACTH secretion.

2. Repeated 8-hour intravenous ACTH tests show incremental increases in urinary 17-KS, 17-KGS, or 17-OHCS in patients with hypoadrenocorticotropinism. A simpler procedure is repetitive (0.25 mg every hour for 3 doses) cosyntropin stimulation. Incremental increases are seen in hypoadrenocorticotropin disorders (11).

3. The various procedures employing metyrapone challenge are quite reliable for assessment of pituitary ACTH function and are especially helpful in differentiating primary from secondary adrenal insufficiency. The lack of increased levels of plasma 11-deoxycortisol, or of urinary 17-KGS, 17-OHCS, or THS after metyrapone, would be consistent with decreased pituitary ACTH production (provided the adrenal is ascertained to be intact).

Assessment of Pituitary Gonadotropic Functions   These activities of the pituitary are reflected by the functions of the targets of the gonadotropic hormones, viz., testes in the male and ovaries in the female. Indirect methods are vaginal cytology and endometrial development in the female and sperm counts and testicular biopsy in the male. These are discussed in sections on ovaries and testes. The differential diagnosis of hypopituitarism from primary gonadal insufficiency requires the determination of plasma or urinary pituitary FSH and LH. In primary gonadal failure, the pituitary gonadotropin levels are markedly elevated, whereas, in pituitary insufficiency, these levels are lower than normal. These tests are especially useful in the diagnosis of hypopituitarism in the postmenopausal women; in these patients, the increase in urinary gonadotropins associated with the postmenopausal state is absent. In younger patients, normal plasma values for FSH range from 6–30 mIU/ml and, for LH, essentially the same. Low values are difficult to interpret, and it is necessary to perform stimulation tests to assess pituitary gonadotropic responsiveness. These tests include the clomiphene stimulation test in which 50 mg of clomiphene is given orally two or three times daily for 7 days. Plasma is obtained before and after the clomiphene ingestion for FSH and LH determinations. A significant increase in LH after clomiphene is a normal response. FSH does not show as marked a rise. Patients with gonadotropin deficiency fail to show a significant increase in LH. In the FSH/LH-RH stimulation test, the hypothalamic neurohormone LRH (100 µg are injected intravenously) and plasma LH and FSH are determined before and after the injection. The integrity of pituitary gonadotropic activity is reflected by significant increases in these gonadotropins at 60–90 min. The reliability of this test is now being questioned as there are factors which may attenuate this response.

Assessment of Pituitary Thyrotropic Function The target organ effects of TSH on the thyroid are employed in testing for pituitary TSH activity. In the TSH stimulation test, a basal epithyroid ^{131}I uptake is increased to normal or supranormal levels in patients with decreased thyrotropic function. But in some patients with very long standing hypopituitarism with marked thyroid involution, no increase is seen after TSH stimulation.

Direct Assessment of Pituitary TSH Function In primary thyroid insufficiency, the TSH levels are higher than normal ($>$ 10 microunits/ml); in pituitary insufficiency the levels are between 0–10 microunits/ml which is the normal range. It is, therefore, necessary to perform the TRH stimulation test. In this test, the hypothalamic neurohormone TRH is given by intramuscular injection 50–100 μg, and plasma TSH levels are measured before and after the TRH administration. A significant increase within 20–30 min in TSH reflects integrity of pituitary thyrotropic activity.

Assessment of Pituitary Prolactin Release The TRH stimulation test is employed to assess pituitary release of prolactin. Normal individuals show a marked increase in plasma prolactin after TRH injection. (It is well to note (Chapter 12) the close proximity of the site of TRH production in the hypophysiotropic area and that for gonadotropin release.) There is a direct correlation between plasma osmolality and PRL release, and alterations in this parameter are being used in testing.

Combined Pituitary Challenge Test The studies are detailed above to present the methods, rationale, and interpretations of the individual tests. It is now recommended that most of the information derived from those tests may be obtained by the combined pituitary challenge test (12). In this procedure, the patients are studied in the fasting state with the test commencing between 9:00 and 10:00 a.m. Regular insulin is administered intravenously (0.05–0.03 unit/kg body weight) and followed immediately by a mixture of 200–500 μg of TRH and 100 μg of FSH/LH-RH in 5 ml of sterile water. Blood samples are obtained at 0, 30, 60, 90, and 120 min after the infusion for quantitation of glucose, growth hormone, and cortisol. TSH, FSH, and LH are determined only at 0-, 20-, and 60-min intervals. The results obtained in this manner are essentially comparable to those obtained with the separate test procedures. Normal subjects exhibit significant elevations in GH (values reaching in excess of 10 ng/ml by 60 min, with mean values around 120 ng/ml), cortisol (values at least 7 μg/100 ml greater than baseline or a 3- to 4-fold increase by the 20- to 60-min sampling times). Patients with panhypopituitarism fail to show significant increases in these hormones after the combined challenge.

Clinical Disorders of Anterior Pituitary Function Clinical patterns in disorders of the anterior pituitary depend on the hormones affected and on the time of onset of the disorder. Because of the multiplicity of anterior pituitary hormones, either hyperfunctional or hypofunction states may be manifest by combination of disturbances in the target effects of various or isolated (single) pituitary hormones. Etiologies and clinical manifestations of the various clinical disorders are summarized in Tables 13.1 and 13.2. Disturbances in the production of the tropic hormones are manifested mainly by clinical and laboratory parameters relative to the target organs of the specific tropic hormones. Disturbances in GH secretion are reflected by disturbances in the various tissues effects of GH.

Hypopituitary States Clinical manifestations depend on both age of onset, as well as on the hormones affected. In panhypopituitarism in childhood, there are several clinical manifestations; namely, a major manifestation secondary to GH deficiency is marked growth retardation detected by serial height-weight measurements noted during the 1st year of life. Certain landmarks will not appear at correct times; for example, on x-ray examination of the wrists, bone age is retarded and epiphyseal development is slowed. The ratio of upper (crown to pubis) to the lower (pubis to floor) body segments will approach 1:1 in contrast to the infantile 1.7:1. Gonadotropin deficiency is reflected by retarded pubertal development. In the male, the penis and testes are small, and secondary sexual characteristics, axillary, facial, and pubic hair, and deepening of the voice do not take place; there is also lack of spermatogenesis. In the female patient, there is lack of female sexual characteristics such as pubarche and thelarche, and there is no evidence of estrogen effect on the vagina. In both sexes, linear growth may continue into 3rd or 4th decade because of lack of epiphyseal closure. Manifestations caused by lack of ACTH may not be overt and may occur only during stress characterized by occasional episodes of hypoglycemia and weakness. Hypothyroidism caused by lack of TSH may be mild compared to the clinical manifestations in primary hypothyroidism.

The manifestations of panhypopituitarism in the adult are referable mainly to deficiencies of the tropic hormones, since there are no overt clinical manifestations of GH deficiency in the adult. Hypoglycemia may occur under certain stress situations and in the presence of infections. The clinical patterns of this disorder, as well as of unihormonal deficiencies, are presented in Table 13.1.

Treatment of Pituitary Diseases Most of the hyperpituitary states presented in Table 13.2 are caused by tumors. The available methods for therapy of these tumors are surgical hypophysectomy, conventional radiation, radiation with proton beam, yttrium, radioactive gold implants, and cryosurgery. These methods have been evaluated in several centers, and final data are not available. Conventional radiation has been employed for patients without extrasellar spread, but is probably not satisfactory.

Proton beam therapy is moderately effective, especially in patients without extrasellar extension. Surgery has been performed in patients with local tumor extension with some degree of success. Cryosurgery has been quite successful and has been followed by early decreases of HGH in acromegalic patients treated. The transsphenoidal implantation with yttrium-90 is also worthwhile but may be complicated by infection and cerebrospinal fluid rhinorrhea. Medical management of acromegaly with progesterone and phenothiazines has been attempted with some evidence of improvement. In the hypothalamic disorder associated with suppression of prolactin inhibitory factor resulting in inappropriate prolactin release, newer information on pharmacological agents, e.g., L-dopa, bromoergocryptine, and others may provide a rationale for therapy (see Chapter 11).

Clinical disorders secondary to deficiencies in the tropic hormones are not treated by the pituitary hormones since all of the hormones of the target glands are available and have been extensively employed. Replacement therapy includes the use of thyroid hormone, corticosteroids, and gonadal hormones appropriate to the sex of the patient. Gradual restitution of replacement doses of thyroxin, 0.05 mg daily (or 15 mg of thyroid extract), is started. The dosage should be increased gradually until a full replacement dose of 0.15–0.20 mg of thyroxin (or 60, 90 mg of desiccated thyroid) is achieved. The presence of arteriosclerotic heart disease and angina may necessitate slower progression, to lower final dose. In myxedema coma, the faster acting preparation triiodothyromine is recommended. The usual replacement dose of glucocorticoids is between 12.5 and 37.5 mg of cortisone acetate daily, but larger doses may be required in stressful situations. Replacement with a mineralocorticoid is rarely needed in pituitary ACTH deficiency. Male patients are treated with methyl testosterone sublingually 20–30 mg daily. Fluoxymesterone 10–15 mg daily is more convenient since it is swallowed. Injections of testosterone cypionate 300 mg every 3–4 weeks have been employed in several patients. These therapies restore libido and potency as well as general vigor in hypopituitary males. Young female patients are treated with estrogens to prevent osteoporosis and atrophy of the genital organs and vaginal mucosa. The rare occurrence of unihormonal deficiency of pituitary tropic hormones is treated by appropriate target gland product as above.

In the treatment of pituitary dwarfism, human growth hormone in doses of 1 mg/day is followed by markedly accelerated growth, up to 3–5 inches/year within the 1st year. Thereafter, the growth rate is somewhat slower. Occasionally antibody formation precludes further therapy, but reinstitution after several months may again cause growth. The supply of human growth hormone is limited, as it is harvested from cadaver pituitaries, but synthetic growth hormone will probably be available soon.

Androgenic therapy should be used only in patients over age 15 years for whom GH is unavailable. Nonvirilizing doses of androgens may cause a limited growth spurt. The treatment potential of sulfation factor (somatomedin) is not yet known.

LITERATURE CITED

1. Harris, G. W. 1955. Neural Control of the Pituitary Gland. London.
2. Li, C. H., W. Liu, and J. S. Dixon. 1966. Human pituitary growth hormone. XII. The amino acid sequence of the hormone. J. Am. Chem. Soc. 88:2050–2051.
3. Gorden, P., C. M. Hendricks, and J. Roth. 1973. Evidence for "big" and "little" components of human plasma and pituitary growth hormone. J. Clin. Endocrinol. Metab. 36:178–184.
4. Daughaday, W. H. 1971. Regulation of skeletal growth by sulfation factor. Adv. Intern. Med. 17:237–263.
5. Odell, W. D. 1968. Gonadotropins: Present Concepts in the Human. Calif. Med. 109:467–485.
6. Everett, J. W. 1964. Central neural control of reproductive functions of the adenohypophysis. Physiol. Rev. 44:373–431.
7. Odell, W. D., G. T. Ross, and P. L. Rayford. 1966. Radioimmunoassay for human luteinizing hormone. Metabolism 15:287–289.
8. Utiger, R. D. 1965. Radioimmunoassay of human plasma thyrotropin. J. Clin. Invest. 44:1277–1286.
9. Gill, G. N. 1972. Mechanism of ACTH action. Metabolism 21:571–589.
10. Yalow, R. S., S. M. Glick, J. Roth, and S. Berson. 1964. Radioimmunoassay of human plasma ACTH. J. Clin. Endocrinol. Metab. 24:1219–1225.
11. Bacchus, H. 1972. Endocrine profiles in the clinical laboratory. In M. Stefanini (ed.), Progress in Clinical Pathology. Vol. 4, pp. 1–101. Grune & Stratton, Inc., New York.
12. Harsoulis, P. J. C., S. F. Marshall, C. W. Kuku, D. K. Burke, D. K. London, and T. R. Fraser. 1974. Combined test for assessment of anterior pituitary function. Brit. Med. J. 4:326–329.

14

Thyroid
Gland

The human thyroid gland consists of two lobes joined by an isthmus and attached to the anterior aspect of the trachea. In the adult, the entire gland weighs between 15 and 20 g. The gland is derived from the alimentary tract and arises in the fetus at about the 17th gestation day. The anlage for the medial part of the gland is the floor of the pharynx at the level of the first and second pharyngeal pouches. The anlage for the lateral areas is thought to be from the area of the fourth pouches. In the evolutionary scale, this gland probably functioned as an exocrine gland. Compared with other endocrine glands, the thyroid is unique in storing its products in colloid-containing vesicles enclosed by epithelium. The thyroglobulin present in the vesicles contains iodinated iodotyrosines, monoiodotyrosine (MIT) and diiodotyrosine (DIT), and iodothyronines, thyroxin (tetraiodothyronine, T_4) and triiodothyronine (T_3). MIT and DIT are precursors which are coupled to form T_3 and T_4. The parathyroid glands are anatomically closely related to the thyroid and are derived from the third and fourth branchial arches. The parathyroid glands produce parathyroid hormone. It is of interest that the ultimobranchial body of the sixth arch is incorporated into the human thyroid gland and is the origin of the parafollicular or "C" cell which is the source of calcitonin.

Early thyroid gland development is not dependent on TSH from the anterior pituitary, but by the 13th week of gestation, at which time the gland forms colloid, development and regulation of the gland become dependent on the tropic hormone. There is a general correlation between the height of the follicular epithelial cells and the levels of TSH; indeed this correlation has been previously employed in a biological assay procedure for TSH activity. Removal of TSH activity by pituitary surgery or disease is followed by atrophy of the thyroid gland. Enlargement of the thyroid by excess pituitary TSH is extremely rare. Ectopic TSH, such as from hydatidiform mole, has been reported to be a cause of hyperthyroidism.

SYNTHESIS OF THYROID HORMONES

The synthesis of T_4 and T_3, the active hormones of the thyroid, requires as substrates the amino acid, tyrosine, and iodine. Tyrosine is present in thyroglobulin molecule which is stored in the follicles as thyroid colloid. Each thyroglobulin molecule contains 115 tyrosyl residues. Iodination of tyrosine takes place at certain strategically located tyrosyl residues of thyroglobulin. The various steps in T_3 and T_4 synthesis are considered below (1–2).

Iodine in food and water is the eventual source of iodine in thyroid hormone synthesis. It is reduced to iodide in the gastrointestinal tract where it is rapidly absorbed. Iodide is taken up by the salivary glands, the stomach mucosa, and mammary tissue, but the iodide-trapping mechanism in the thyroid is several times more efficient than the others so that 90% of total body iodine is found in the thyroid gland. The thyroid iodine pool, mainly organic iodide in thyroglobulin, is 5,000–7,000 μg, and there is a turnover of approximately 1% daily.

BIOSYNTHETIC PROCESSES IN THYROID HORMONE PRODUCTION

Formation of Thyroid Hormone

Several steps are involved in the formation of T_3 and T_4 by the thyroid gland. These are conveniently considered under the following processes: 1) iodide trapping by thyroid cells; 2) organification of thyroid iodine; 3) coupling of iodotyrosines; 4) release of T_3 and T_4 from thyroglobulin; 5) deiodination of iodotyrosines (Figure 14.1); and 6) other metabolic processes in thyroid cells.

Iodide Trapping by Thyroid Cells Iodide is trapped by the thyroid cells by the "iodide pump" or "iodide trap." The development of this process antedates the development of the follicular structure. Iodide is concentrated against strong electrical as well as concentration gradients. The iodide diffuses rapidly into the follicular lumen. Considerably less antigradient accumulation of iodide occurs in gastric mucosa, salivary gland, mammary tissue, small intestine mucosa, and placenta. This process is inhibited by agents such as thiocyanate, perchlorate, nitrites, dinitrophenol, and cardiac glycosides. The trapping process requires energy, integrity of the cell membranes and cellular organelles, and the ability to transport Na^+ and K^+, probably involving the Na^+-K^+-dependent ATPase. The process is increased by TSH and increased iodide ingestion. The oxidation of iodides to iodine is essential to further participation in hormone synthesis. Iodide is converted to iodine by a thyroid peroxidase system; possibly other oxidizing systems may be involved to some extent.

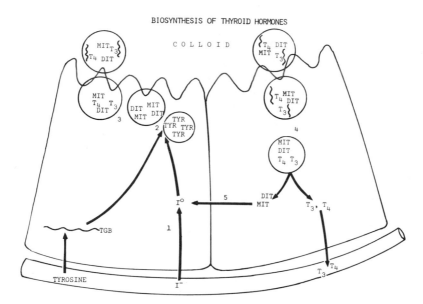

BIOSYNTHESIS OF THYROID HORMONES

Figure 14.1. Biosynthesis of thyroid hormones. Steps in the synthesis of thyroxin (T_4) and triiodothyronine (T_3) by thyroid cells are depicted. Enzymatic steps are as follows: (1) peroxidase; (2) iodination of tyrosyl moieties (organification of $I°$ may be nonenzymatic or may be mediated by an iodinase system); (3) the coupling reaction, which is probably enzymatic; iodothyronines are synthesized as constituents of thyroglobulin produced on ribosomes and transferred to soluble droplets and carried to the cell-colloid interface where steps (1) and (2) take place; (4) proteolysis, whereby T_4, T_3, diiodotyrosine (DIT) and monoiodotyrosine (MIT) are released from thyroglobulin; and (5) deiodination.

Organification of Thyroid Iodine   In the follicular lumen, there is spontaneous iodination of accessible tyrosyl molecules in thyroglobulin. This proceeds at or near the surface of the thyroid follicle cells. There are some data suggesting an enzymatic (iodinase) process also in organification of iodine. Under normal conditions, approximately equal amounts of MIT and DIT are formed. Iodide deficiency is accompanied by a relative decrease in the amount of DIT, with preferential synthesis of T_3, the biologically more powerful thyroid hormone, presumably to maintain euthyroidism in the face of iodide deficiency. Organification is blocked by thionamide drugs, such as propylthiouracil and methimazole, agents which have found application in medical management of hyperthyroidism.

Coupling of Iodotyrosines   Molecules of MIT and DIT suitably located along thyroglobulin at the cell:colloid interface undergo a coupling reaction (probably enzymatic) to form T_3, triiodothyronine (MIT + DIT) or T_4, thyroxin, tetraiodothyronine (DIT + DIT). The former reaction is relatively increased in iodide deficiency states.

Release of T_4 and T_3 from Thyroglobulin   Epithelial follicular cells take up droplets of thyroglobulin colloid by pinocytosis. This process is stimulated by TSH. Lysosomes coalesce with these droplets and release hydrolases which degrade thyroglobulin with the release of T_4, T_3, MIT, and DIT. The active hormones T_4 and T_3 are secreted into the parafollicular capillaries with small amounts of thyroglobulin and perhaps minute amounts of iodotyrosines. TSH stimulation of pinocytosis by the thyroid epithelial cell is caused by activation of membrane adenylate cyclase with release of cyclic adenosine monophosphate (cAMP).

Deiodination of Iodotyrosines   Deiodinase in the follicle cells removes iodine from the iodotyrosines but not from iodothyronines. The released iodine is utilized for iodination of thyroglobulin tyrosyl molecules. A defect in deiodinase in thyroid and in peripheral tissues is associated with clinical sequelae. It is estimated that two-thirds of the intrathyroidal iodide pool is derived from this step.

Other Metabolic Processes in Thyroid Cells   The biosynthetic processes in the thyroid cells require energy and cofactors. TSH stimulates glucose metabolism and oxygen consumption in thyroid cells. Phospholipid and RNA synthesis are also increased by TSH. These effects are all ascribed to TSH activation of membrane adenylate cyclase which is noted within a few minutes after TSH administration.

Transport of Thyroid Hormones

Thyroxin (T_4) and triiodothyronine (T_3) are reversibly, but firmly, bound to circulating serum proteins. The major binding globulin (TBG) is a glycoprotein that migrates between the α_1 and α_2 regions. The second binding protein is a thyroid-binding prealbumin (TBPA) that probably is identical with prealbumin 1. Albumin itself possesses the ability to transport thyroid hormones. The binding ability of TBG and TBPA is saturable, but that of albumin is not. It is estimated that TBG levels in the serum probably do not exceed 1 mg/100 ml; this amount has the ability to bind 20 μg of T_4. TBPA may amount to 30 mg/100 ml of serum, and 1 mole of T_4 is bound/mole of TBPA. The binding affinity of T_3 and T_4 to TBG and TBPA depends on the structures of the thyroid hormones; T_3 is not appreciably bound to TBPA. T_3 is weakly bound to TBG and is readily displaced by T_4. The affinity of the TBG for T_4 is much greater than that for T_3. The protein-binding phenomenon undoubtedly affects both the biological activities, as well as the metabolism, of thyroid hormones.

It is estimated that approximately 0.04% of serum T_4 is free, whereas the remaining 99.96% is distributed among TBG (60%), TBPA (30%), and albumin (10%). The proportion of free T_3 is 10 times greater than that of

T_4, i.e., 0.4% is free and the remaining 99.6% is bound. The decreased affinity of T_3 for protein binding underlies its rapid onset of action compared with that of T_4. The intrinsically greater potency of T_3 in biological activity is probably not related to differences in binding affinity.

The protein-bound iodine (PBI) in the absence of contamination (see later) is largely a measure of T_4, but this value is influenced by alterations in binding proteins, e.g., an increased TBG in pregnancy or after estrogen treatment or decreased TBG in TBG deficiency. Serum levels of free T_4 amount to about 3 ng/100 ml and of free T_3 approximately 1.0–1.5 ng/100 ml.

Metabolism of Thyroid Hormones

The binding proteins influence the degradation of T_4 and T_3 considerably. By limiting the amount of free T_4 in the circulation, TBG plays a very important role in degradation of the hormone. The exchangeable cellular T_4 influences thyroid hormone flux. Approximately 10% of T_4 secreted daily is excreted in the bile, mainly as free T_4 and partly as the glucuronide conjugate. The remainder of thyroid hormone degradation takes place in various tissues, especially liver, muscle, and kidney. The cellular degradation mechanism involves the process of deiodination, which occurs in essentially all tissues affected by thyroid hormones. There are species differences in the steps and rates of deiodination of thyroid hormones. After deiodination, the conversion of the hormones to their pyruvic and acetic acid analogues is accomplished by deamination, transamination, or decarboxylation reactions. These degradative steps in the liver take place in the endoplasmic reticulum. After secretion of T_4 into the circulation, it undergoes conversion to T_3 to an extent estimated to be 50% of the daily production of T_3. It is now known that T_4 is both an active hormone as well as a prohormone.

Regulation of Thyroid Activity

Pituitary-Thyroid Axis and Hypothalamus   Activity of the thyroid gland is controlled by TSH. TSH influences many aspects of thyroid structure and function, including the size and vascularity, the height of the epithelial cells, and the amount of stored colloid. In addition, several metabolic parameters are stimulated by TSH, viz., glucose oxidation, phospholipid synthesis, and RNA synthesis. Release of TSH is dependent on the levels of free thyroid hormones. The pituitary thyroid axis is unique in that there is greater intrinsic pituitary control in this system than in the other pituitary-target organ control mechanisms. TSH secretion is inversely related to the metabolic effects of T_4 and T_3 in the pituitary. (It is of some interest that salicylates and dinitrophenol may also influence pituitary TSH release.) The hypothalamus exerts a modulating influence on TSH excretion, but is not the final regulator of feedback control of the pituitary thyroid axis.

Autoregulation of Thyroid There are intrathyroidal mechanisms designed to maintain a relative constancy of hormonal stores within the gland which operates essentially independent of the levels of TSH. Large doses of iodide acutely depress organic binding and coupling reaction within the thyroid. This response, called the Wolf-Chaikoff effect, is apparently designed to prevent massive increases in hormone synthesis. An acute depletion of iodide in the extracel induces an increased iodide clearance and uptake of iodide by the thyroid. Under chronic conditions, the glandular content of organic iodine is inversely related to the activity of iodide transport system. This transport mechanism of the thyroid is more responsive to TSH in a gland depleted of iodine compared with the responses in the gland rich in iodide.

Decreased levels of thyroid hormone stores reflecting decreased synthesis initiate changes in intrinsic function and in TSH response designed to increase thyroid hormone biosynthesis. When hormone stores are increased secondary to increased synthesis, TSH release by the pituitary is inhibited and the biosynthetic pathways are suppressed.

METABOLIC EFFECTS OF THYROID HORMONES

Thyroid hormones (T_4 and T_3) affect several metabolic parameters. The presence of alanine in the side chain confers significant biological activity to the molecule. Replacement of iodine by other halogens is associated with biological activity, but at a decreased level. The iodines on the T_4 and T_3 structures provide molecular stability and prevent free rotation around the ether oxygen of these iodothyronines, hence maintaining the configuration necessary for attachment to the target receptors.

A single regulatory reaction has not been found to explain the multiple effects of thyroid hormones, but there are some data which suggest that the primary action may well be to increase synthesis of mitochondrial RNA. Thyroid hormones are known to increase the incorporation of amino acids into mitochondrial proteins.

The following are also known effects of the thyroid hormones:

1. They increase oxygen consumption and calorigenesis in heart, liver, kidney, and skeletal muscle, considered the target organs for the calorigenic effect of thyroid hormones. Oxygen consumption and calorigenesis in brain, testis, and lymph nodes are not similarly stimulated. The effects on cellular respiration were ascribed to uncoupling of oxidative phosphorylation, but this phenomenon is now considered a pharmacological effect.

2. They increase the activities of several mitochondrial enzymes, including L-glycerophosphate dehydrogenase which is important in the metabolism of fats and carbohydrates, and glutamic dehydrogenase.

3. They increase the incorporation of amino acids into ribosomes.

4. Thyroid hormones decrease glycogen synthesis, but the oral glucose tolerance test is often of a diabetic type in patients with hyperthyroidism. This is ascribed to increased glucose absorption from the gastrointestinal tract. In addition, excessive thyroid hormones increase the caloric needs and induce a type of resistance to insulin effects (e.g., metathyroid diabetes).

5. Thyroid hormones affect cholesterol and fatty acid metabolism. Hepatic cholesterol biosynthesis is increased by large amounts of T_4 and T_3. This phenomenon is related to availability of glycogen and ATP.

6. The biliary excretion of cholesterol is decreased in hypothyroidism and increased in the presence of excess thyroid hormones. Cholic acid excretion is decreased in hypothyroid states.

7. Thyroid hormones increase lipolysis and also support the action of catecholamines in this activity as well as affecting utilization of carbohydrate and synthesis of fats. The calorigenic action of catecholamines is dependent on the presence of thyroid hormones.

8. Thyroid hormones increase the renal plasma flow and glomerular filtration rate and decrease the sensitivity of the renal tubules to antidiuretic hormone (ADH). In hypothyroid states, impaired diuresis and hyponatremia, perhaps with the syndrome of inappropriate ADH, are often found.

9. Excessive thyroid hormones increase bone turnover and hypercalciuria is often found in hyperthyroidism.

10. Thyroid hormones are required for the conversion of carotene to vitamin A. Vitamin A deficiency may occur in hypothyroid subjects as a result.

11. The requirements for B vitamins and vitamin C are probably increased in hyperthyroid states.

PHYSIOLOGICAL EFFECTS OF THYROID HORMONES

Thyroid hormones exert the following effects:

1. They increase basal metabolism and oxygen consumption. T_3 is 3–4 times more powerful than T_4 in increasing oxygen consumption. Administration of a single intravenous dose of T_4 requires 10 days for its peak effect on the BMR, the effect having a half-time of 15 days after the peak. The peak effect of T_3 administered similarly is noted within 24–36 hours with a decay half-time of 8 days.

2. They stimulate and support growth processes in various tissues and organs, e.g., mammary glands and the reproductive system.

3. Thyroid hormones support oxygen consumption by myocardium; an excess of T_4 or T_3 increases heart rate and may eventually lead to myocardial hypertrophy and subsequent necrosis. Systolic blood pressure is elevated by excess thyroid hormones. The heart seems to be the first organ to respond to T_4 and T_3, and this effect is not necessarily correlated with the increased rate of metabolism. T_4 and T_3 localize in the bundle of His and are thought to inhibit cardiac monoamine oxidase, epinephrine dehydrogenase, and catechol O-methyltransferase, with the result that higher levels of biogenic amines may remain in the cardiac muscle.

4. They enhance maturation of the central nervous system.

5. They increase the motility of the gastrointestinal tract and decrease the production of mucoid substance by the mucosal cells.

6. They increase blood flow to the skin.

Assessment of Thyroid Function

The various useful tests will be considered under the headings: tests of thyroid gland activity; tests of thyroid hormone levels; and tests of thyroid hormone effects.

Tests of Thyroid Gland Activity Several measurements have been derived to determine the uptake, clearance, and discharge rates of labeled iodine by the thyroid gland. Variations in time of observation may aid in determining certain specific steps in thyroid function, e.g., measurements of ^{131}I uptake within a short period (up to 3 hr) may aid in determining the iodide trapping potential of the gland.

Thyroid Radioiodine Uptake The most practical and widely employed procedure in this category is the ^{131}I uptake by the thyroid. The patient is given 2–15 μCi of ^{131}I by mouth, and the concentration of the isotope in the gland is determined by epithyroid counts. The uptake is usually determined after approximately 24 hr, but there are occasions when earlier uptake measurements are helpful, e.g., in extremely thyrotoxic patients in whom the uptake and discharge of ^{131}I are relatively rapid. This measurement is standardized in each laboratory, but, in general, the normal 24-hr uptake is between 10–35%. Values below 10% are considered abnormally low and would suggest hypothyroidism. Other disorders characterized by decreased ^{131}I uptake include chronic thyroiditis, subacute (de Quervain's) thyroiditis, biosynthetic defects in the thyroid, acute therapy with antithyroid drugs, and pituitary hypofunction. Other causes, not necessarily associated with thyroid hypofunction, include exogenous iodide (by dilutional effects on iodide pool and by affecting the intrathyroidal regulatory mechanisms), renal and cardiac failure rarely, extreme hyperthyroidism with rapid (before 24-hr) discharge of the labeled iodine.

Epithyroid ^{131}I uptake values greater than 35% are consistent with hyperthyroidism. Other states which may be associated with elevated ^{131}I uptakes include rebound from thyroid suppression, recovery from subacute thyroiditis, and recent withdrawal from an antithyroid drug. In the presence of excess loss of T_4 and T_3, the thyroid ^{131}I uptake may be high as in nephrosis, chronic diarrhea, and spontaneous or induced malabsorption states. It is also possible that in a biosynthetic defect (as in some forms of Hashimoto's thyroiditis) the ^{131}I uptake may be high because of synthesis and discharge of abnormal iodoproteins. Representative values for epithyroid ^{131}I uptake are presented in Table 14.1.

Triiodothyronine Suppression of Increased Thyroid Radioiodide Uptake Euthyroid individuals given 50–75 μg of T_3 daily will exhibit a significant suppression of their normal thyroid radioiodide uptake. Patients with diffuse toxic goiter fail to show a suppression of their elevated radioiodide uptake after similar T_3 therapy. This test has been especially useful in the diagnosis of T_3 toxicosis patients in whom the baseline radioiodine uptake is often normal.

Perchlorate or Thiocyanate Washout Test This procedure is useful in detecting defects in the biosynthetic pathways, induced or congenital, in the thyroid. If the iodide-trapping mechanism is intact, then the thyroid radioiodide uptake appears normal. If a significant falloff of radioactivity in the gland follows administration of either perchlorate or thiocyanate,

Table 14.1. Radioiodide Uptake by Thyroid in Clinical States

Diagnosis	Thyroid uptake (%)		
	1 hr	6 hr	24 hr
Euthyroid	5–10	8–16	10–35
Hypothyroid	<7	2–7	<10–12
Hyperthyroid	>15	>35	40–90
De Quervain's thyroiditis			
Acute	?,<7	?,<7	0–20
Subsiding	N^a or ↑	N; ↑	N, or ↑
Hashimoto's thyroiditis	N	N	N
Nontoxic nodular goiter	5–15	5–25	10–50
Endemic goiter (euthyroid)	↑	10–35	50–70
Reidel's disease	N?	N,?	N

[a] N, normal.

then an error in organification of iodine is likely. Normal individuals show less than 5% loss of radioactivity after this challenge.

The test is performed as follows: a tracer dose of ^{131}I or ^{125}I is given orally and the iodide uptake by the thyroid is measured at 60 min. Potassium perchlorate or sodium thiocyanate is given by mouth, and uptake readings are made at 90 and 100 min. A decrease of 10% or more of the uptake at 60 min is considered as diagnostic of an error in organic binding of iodine. This finding is noted in patients with congenital hypothyroidism caused by peroxidase defect, in iodide goiter, in thionamide-induced organification defect, in Hashimoto's thyroiditis, in radioiodine-treated thyrotoxicosis, and occasionally in severe thyrotoxicosis.

TSH Stimulation Test This test is most useful in evaluating findings of a low radioiodine (RAI) uptake. After the baseline RAI uptake study, the patient is given 5–10 units of TSH intramuscularly for 3 days (or 1 day occasionally). If, on repeat RAI uptake, there is no increase, then primary hypothyroidism is likely. Normal individuals exhibit an increment in RAI uptake of at least 15%. Patients with pituitary hypothyroidism will often show a greater increment than 15%. (Serum T_4 or PBI determinations may also be performed before and after TSH stimulation.)

Thyroid Uptake of Pertechnate $99^m TC$ The pertechnate ion is trapped by the thyroid, but it does not undergo organic binding. The nucleide is given intravenously, and epithyroid counts are made up to 30 min after administration. Maximal epithyroid counts are noted in about 20 min. Normal individuals show values less than 2% at this interval. Thyrotoxic patients exhibit an uptake of 5–25% in 20 min. Values in this range may also be found in iodine deficiency and biosynthetic defects in the thyroid (dyshormonogenesis and autoimmune thyroiditis).

Tests of Thyroid Hormone Levels Several methods are available for estimating the levels of thyroid hormones in the plasma. Some methods involve quantitation of iodine attached to proteins on the assumption that most circulating thyroxin is protein bound. Other newer methods include the quantitation of T_4 and T_3 by radioimmunoassay.

Protein-bound Iodine (PBI) The principle of this measurement involves precipitating serum proteins, digestion or ashing of the precipitate, and determination of the iodine in the precipitate. Normal values of PBI range from 4–8 μg/100 ml. Patients with myxedema usually have PBI values below 2 μg/100 ml. Hyperthyroid patients have PBI values of greater than 10 μg/100 ml. Newborn babies show PBI values up to 12 μg/100 ml between 5 and 7 days of life and between 4 and 8 μg/100 ml later. The method does not eliminate inorganic or organic iodides ingested in medications, foods, or employed in tests. For this reason, values of PBI greater than 25 μg/100 ml should be viewed with suspicion for the probability of contamination. Iodotyrosines are also quantitated in this method, so that increased levels of these substances, either in disease or after drugs, contaminate the application of the PBI method.

Butanol-extractable Iodine (BEI) Butanol extraction eliminates inorganic iodides as contaminants. Ingested and absorbed iodides are excluded by this method, but iodoproteins are not. Discrepancies between the PBI and BEI levels are useful in estimating levels of iodoproteins in the presence of biosynthetic defects in the thyroid. Development of methods for T_3 and T_4 measurements render the PBI and BEI methods relatively obsolete, except in the situations cited above.

Total Thyroxine Iodine Thyroid hormone is separated by column chromatography, and quantitation of the iodine content gives a value for T_4 iodine by column. This method provides more reliable data than the previously described procedures for thyroid iodine.

Serum Thyroxine Radioimmunoassay or competitive protein binding (CPB) methods for total thyroxin are not dependent on quantitation of iodine levels in the hormones and are free of contamination by exogenous iodinated materials. Normal values range from 5–13 μg/100 ml.

Serum "Free" Thyroxin This is determined after a dialysis procedure after which the CPB method is applied. This is the most sensitive and accurate method of quantitating the active levels of T_4 in the serum.

Method of Calculating Free Thyroxine Index This method employs the total T_4 level or PBI and the assessment of the amount of binding proteins after this formula:

$$\text{Adjusted } T_4 = \text{total } T_4 \times \frac{\text{resin } T_3 \text{ uptake (patient)}}{\text{resin } T_3 \text{ uptake (normal)}}$$

Normal values range from 5–13 μg/100 ml.
If the PBI is employed:

$$\text{Thyroid index} = \text{PBI} \times \frac{\text{resin } T_3 \text{ uptake (patient)}}{\text{resin } T_3 \text{ uptake (normal)}}$$

Normal values range from 4.2–7.8 μg/100 ml.

Serum Triiodothyronine Levels (T_3) by Radioimmunoassay This was devised by Hollander et al. (4). Circulating levels in normal subjects range from 60–220 ng/100 ml. Hyperthyroidism is associated with values considerably in excess of 220 ng/100 ml, and such high values may antedate elevations in the other parameters of estimating thyroid gland function.

Thyroid Hormone Binding by Serum Proteins as Index of Thyroid Function

Resin T_3 Uptake When a tracer amount of ^{131}I-labeled T_3 is added to serum containing an insoluble anion exchange resin or charcoal, the amount of labeled T_3 retained in the insoluble phase represents the resin T_3 uptake. This value is a measure of the reserve binding capacity in the serum. Increased thyroid hormone in the serum leads to a greater saturation of the binding capacity, so that the insoluble resin takes up more of the labeled T_3, i.e., an increased resin T_3 uptake is found in hyperthyroidism. In hypothyroidism, decreased levels of thyroid hormones leave a larger amount of unsaturated binding sites, hence the labeled T_3 is picked up by these sites instead of onto the insoluble resin, hence there is a decreased resin T_3 uptake in hypothyroidism.

It should be emphasized that there are several factors which may alter the binding thyroid capacity of the serum proteins. Pregnancy or estrogen administration induces increased levels of TBG. It is not unexpected, therefore, that the resin T_3 uptake is low in these states despite the absence of thyroid disease. This information used in combination with the T_4 or PBI can be employed in the calculation and provides a reliable index of thyroid function as free T_4 is proportional to total T_4 concentration and inversely proportional to the unsaturated binding capacity (Figure 14.2).

Tests of Thyroid Hormone Effects   Clinical procedures to measure biological activity of its hormones include basal metabolic rate (BMR), Achilles tendon reflex time, and miscellaneous tests.

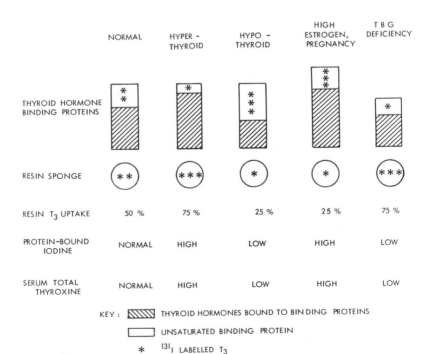

Figure 14.2. Principles in the resin uptake of ^{131}I-labeled T_3 (RUT$_3$).

Basal Metabolic Rate This rate varies directly with the level of thyroid function. In euthyroidism, the BMR ranges between −10 and +10% of normal. Myxedematous patients exhibit a value of below 30%, while hyperthyroid subjects may show values of +25 to +75%. This procedure, despite its usefulness, is not widely employed now. Several technical problems, including leaks in the metabolometer, lack of patient cooperation, the emotional state of the patient, as well as non-thyroidal illnesses, may alter the basal metabolism rate.

Achilles Tendon Reflex Measurement This test is based on the observation that there is a significant delay in the relaxation phase of the deep tendon reflexes. The procedure is recommended only to provide secondary confirmation of hypothyroidism.

Miscellaneous Tests These include the measurement of serum cholesterol which is inversely related to the level of primary function. Elevated serum cholesterol levels are found in patients with primary hypothyroidism, and decreased levels in hyperthyroidism. Secondary (pituitary) hypothyroidism is not followed by hypercholesterolemia.

LONG-ACTING THYROID STIMULATOR

Long-acting thyroid stimulator (LATS) is an immunoglobulin of the IgG class produced by lymphocytes. It is found in patients with Graves' disease and occasionally with Hashimoto's thyroiditis. Several studies suggest that this substance is pathogenetically related to the onset of Graves' disease. The circulating titer of LATS correlates well with the pervasiveness of the disorder as well as with improvement. This is especially true in patients with Graves' disease who improved with the use of thionamide drugs. LATS levels correlate well with the occurrence of thyrotoxic dermopathy (pretibial myxedema).

Experimental studies reveal an effect of LATS on the release of membrane adenylate cyclase in the thyroid, in several respects quite similar to the effect of TSH. Strong evidence implicates LATS in the onset of neonatal thyrotoxicosis in babies of mothers with Graves' disease, but a recent report (3) casts some doubt on this observation. It seems likely now that, while LATS cannot be considered the sole cause of Graves' disease, it may nevertheless play a contributory role in its pathogenesis.

HYPERTHYROIDISM

Hyperthyroidism refers to the multisystem disorders arising from increased circulating levels of thyroid hormones, thyroxine (T_4) and triiodothyronine (T_3), the iodothyronines. Etiology of the various types of

Table 14.2. Hyperthyroidism

I. Goitrous
  A. Diffuse
    1. Graves' disease
      a) With ophthalmopathy
      b) With dermopathy
      c) With acropachy
      d) Neonatal
      e) Ectopic TSH
  B. Nodular
    1. Multinodular
      a) Toxic multinodular
      b) Iod-Basedow, if induced by iodides
    2. Uninodular
      a) Plummer's
      b) Follicular adenoma
      c) Follicular carcinoma
      d) Subacute granulomatous thyroiditis
      e) Ectopic TSH secretion (hydatidiform mole)
II. Nongoitrous
  A. Struma ovarii
  B. Factitious
  C. Medicamentosa

hyperthyroidism is presented in Table 14.2. The clinical manifestations may be present in patients with hyperthyroidism regardless of type or etiology. Many of these features are caused by the interaction of thyroid hormones and catecholamines as there is synergism in many of the actions of both types of hormones. The symptoms and signs of hyperthyroidism are summarized in Table 14.3. Special manifestations in variant patterns of hyperthyroidism are now recognized (Table 14.4).

Hypertriodothyroninemia or T_3 toxicosis has been described by Hollander et al. (4) and others, and is undoubtedly more prevalent than previously recognized. In the past, the diagnosis was suspected in patients who exhibited all of the features of hyperthyroidism, lacking laboratory confirmation by standard methods, but demonstrating nonsuppressibility of thyroid RAI uptake by exogenous T_3. With new methodology, the diagnosis is made more readily with the following criteria: 1) clinical picture of hyperthyroidism and hypermetabolism; 2) normal levels of PBI and of total T_4; 3) normal levels of free T_4; 4) normal or slight to moderate increase in epithyroid RAI uptake which is not suppressible by the T_3 suppression test (triiodothyronine (T_3) 25 μg three times daily for 7–10 days); 5) an increased total T_3 level (normal level = 80–220 ng/100 ml); and 6) demonstration of pituitary thyrotropic suppression by absent TSH levels or by lack of pituitary response to TRF. In addition to the full-fledged T_3 toxicosis pattern, certain variants have been described.

Table 14.3. Clinical Manifestations of Patients with Hyperthyroidism

I. Symptoms of hyperthyroidism
  A. Referrable to enhanced catecholamine effects (nervousness; tremors; palpitations; rapid heart rate; increased perspiration; heat intolerance)
  B. Referrable to hypermetabolism (mild hyperpyrexia; increased appetite and hyperphagia; weight loss usually, but weight gain may occur as in early manifestations)
  C. Increased autonomic activity (diarrhea caused by decreased transit time)
  D. Miscellaneous (myopathy with muscle weakness; periodic paralysis; dyspnea caused by weakness of respiratory muscles; personality changes; psychosis; criminal behavior; hypermentation; restlessness; hair loss; symptoms of high output failure; lid retraction with staring; ophthalmopathy)
II. Clinical signs in hyperthyroidism
  A. Skin and appendages (smooth pink elbows; soft, smooth velvety skin texture; fine hair structure; palmar erythema; onycholysis; increased sweating; vitiligo or hyperpigmentation)
  B. Cardiovascular and respiratory systems (increased pulse pressure caused by increased systolic blood pressure; increased pulse rate; increased cardiac stroke volume; dilated peripheral vascular bed; high output cardiac failure, depending on severity, atrial fibrillation (10–15%); decreased pulmonary compliance; weakness in respiratory muscles leading to dyspnea)
  C. Gastrointestinal system (diarrhea and/or hyperdefecation; hypochlorhydria (30% have antibodies to parietal cells); hepatocellular dysfunction; lipid infiltration; increased clearance of various substrates; hypoalbuminemia may be caused by hepatocellular disease or hypercatabolism)
  D. Nervous system (hyperkinesis; tremors; increased energy followed by fatigability; hyperreflexia followed by hypo- or areflexia if myopathy becomes severe)
  E. Ocular system (ophthalmopathy in Graves' disease, variable and including unilateral or bilateral exophthalmos; proptosis; edema of the eyelids; conjunctival injection; chemosis; ophthalmoplegia caused by edema of extraocular muscles, lid retraction (Dalrymple's sign); lid lag (von Graefe's sign); globe lag; loss of sight from optic nerve involvement)
  F. Locomotor system (proximal muscle weakness, may be unable to climb stairs because of thigh muscle weakness; periodic paralysis may be associated with hypokalemia (seen especially in Orientals)
  G. Reproductive system (delayed sexual maturation if hyperthyroidism starts early in life; accelerated skeletal growth; increased libido in both sexes; an ovulatory menstrual cycle, oligomenorrhea, or amenorrhea)
  H. Renal system (increased renal blood flow and glomerular filtration rate (GFR); increased tubular reabsorption and secretion)
  I. Hematopoietic system (occasionally erythrocytosis, but anemia may also occur; relative lymphocytosis and granulocytopenia)
  J. Pituitary and adrenocortical function (exaggeration of circadian variation of plasma cortisol; accelerated disappearance of cortisol from blood stream; increased conversion of cortisol to cortisone, the latter being biologically less active; increased reduction of the Δ^4,3-ketone structure of ring A, thus inactivating the biological activity; attenuated growth hormone response to insulin)

Table 14.4. Special Manifestations of Different Forms of Hyperthyroidism

	Graves'	Plummer's	Subacute thyroiditis	Exogenous thyroid	Follicular carcinoma	Struma ovarii	TSH ectopic (or pituitary)
Thyroid structure	Diffuse goiter	Goitrous: uni- or multinodular	Tender ± goitrous	Normal	Normal or nodular	Normal	Normal
Ophthalmopathy: exophthalmos, chemosis, swelling, conjunctivitis, paresis	Prominent						
Pretibial myxedema	Present						
Acropachy	Present						
Lymphoid hyperplasia	Present						
T_4 and or T_3 levels	Increased	Increased	Increased	Increased	Increased	Increased	Increased
Resin T_3 uptake	Increased	Increased	Increased	Increased	Increased	Increased	Increased
RAI uptake (epithyroid)	Increased	Increased	N[a] or ↑	Decreased	N or ↑	N over thyroid; ovarian	N, ↑
TSH levels (serum)	Decreased	Decreased	Decreased	Decreased	Decreased	Decreased	Increased
Mechanism	Unknown: autoimmune; LATS (?)	Autonomous nodule(s); LATS not involved	Destruction of many follicles	Exogenous thyroid substance	Neoplastic radiation exposure (?)	Teratoma ectopic thyroid(?)	Trophoblastic tumor production of TSH-like substance
Incidence	Highest between age 30–40 years; more in females	Multinodular; in over 50 years of age; uninodular among 30–40-year-olds	Young adults; more females	Variable	Usually after age 40 years; more females		women of childbearing age

[a] N, normal.

These include hyperthyroninemia as a premonitory manifestation of thyrotoxicosis (4), T_3 elevation during antithyroid drug therapy for hyperthyroidism, T_3 toxicosis as an early manifestation of recurrent hyperthyroidism (e.g., following inadequate thionamide drug therapy or after inadequate ^{131}I therapy), and T_3 elevation in iodine deficiency. There are data suggesting that the T_3 levels in T_3 toxicosis may vary according to the type of gland involvement so that, in diffuse toxic goiter, the T_3 levels are higher than in uninodular and multinodular toxic goiter. Hyperthyroidism without evident goiter has been described in 1–3% of hyperthyroid patients (1). Hyperthyroidism without overt hypermetabolism has also been described by Werner and Hamilton (5). The absence of hypermetabolism was established by BMR values which were within normal ranges, but PBI and RAI uptake were elevated. Both these parameters reverted to normal after therapy. Ophthalmopathy has been described in overtly euthyroid patients who nevertheless had some evidence of autonomous thyroid activity (euthyroid Graves' disease with ocular changes). Apathetic hyperthyroidism describes the clinical state of elderly patients with laboratory evidence of hyperthyroidism but with many of the other clinical manifestations of hyperthyroidism overtly lacking except for the cardiovascular components. These patients are prone to progress rapidly into thyroid storm and die suddenly if the diagnosis is not made and the disorder treated.

Natural Course of Hyperthyroidism

This discussion refers more specifically to diffuse toxic goiter, but may, in some considerations, apply also to nodular toxic goiter. Etiology of these disorders is not known despite the preferred relationship between LATS and Graves' disease. Many predisposing factors have been described, including genetic susceptibility, familial tendency, and previous nutritional history. Precipitating factors include physical or emotional trauma, stress, illness, accident, pregnancy, puberty, and labor among others.

There are old data which indicate that significant numbers of patients may undergo spontaneous remission (6). The reason for these remissions is not clear either. It is not possible now to design a study to determine the natural course of this disorder. Older statistics indicate that about 15–20% of patients died during the active phase of thyrotoxicosis (presumably of the disorder) if not treated (7). Spontaneous remission in 26–50% of untreated patients and 15–30% rate of improvement have been described (8). It is now becoming apparent that, in a large number of patients, Graves' disease evolves first into euthyroidism followed by hypothyroidism. Follow-up of patients treated with high dose ^{131}I revealed 20% become hypothyroid within 1 year of therapy, with an additional 3%/year thereafter. When a low dose of ^{131}I was employed, it became apparent

346   Habeeb Bacchus

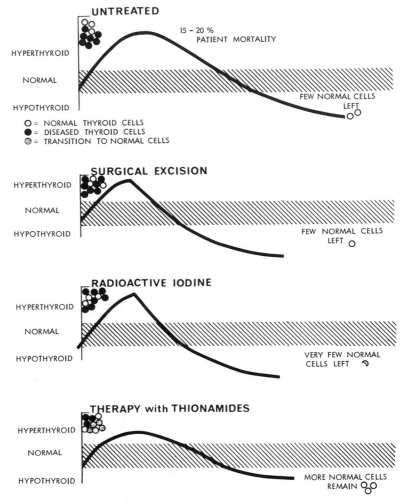

Figure 14.3. Natural history of diffuse toxic goiter and effects of different methods of management. It is shown that radioiodine therapy and surgical excision remove a number of euthyroid cells from the total thyroidal cell pool. It is suggested that the thionamide drugs may alter some hyperthyroid cells to the euthyroid state, hence potentially altering the natural progression toward hypothyroidism.

that the rate of development of hypothyroidism was slowed for the first 1–3 years, but the subsequent course was similar to those treated with the higher doses of radiation. Careful follow-up of patients treated by surgery revealed a similar evolution into hypothyroidism. The above data suggest that the natural course of hyperthyroidism in the patient who survives the acute phase evolves through a period of remission followed by hypothyroidism (Figure 14.3).

Treatment of Hyperthyroidism

Management will depend on the type of hyperthyroidism. Major consideration will be given to the management of diffuse toxic goiter, but
multinodular and uninodular toxic goiters will also be considered.

Three therapeutic measures are available: surgery, antithyroid drugs,
and radioiodine therapy. Surgery has been extensively employed in the
management of all types of hyperthyroidism. In the properly prepared
patient, removal of part of the thyroid was followed by remission in a high
percentage of patients, but later follow-up revealed an increasing incidence
of permanent hypothyroidism in a large number of patients. In addition,
even though there was a low postoperative mortality rate (0–3%), the
morbidity rate was significant. When parameters such as recurrence,
hypoparathyroidism, tetany, vocal cord paresis, wound problems, and
thyrotoxic storm were assessed, the morbidity ranged from 4% to over
30%, the higher percentages with more meticulous follow-up (9). The
surgical approach is now de-emphasized in the management of diffuse
toxic goiter. Uninodular toxic goiter, when treated by surgical excision, is
not associated with significant postoperative hypothyroidism and is
reasonably highly recommended. Multinodular toxic goiter may be treated
by surgery depending on the size and the presence of tracheal obstruction.

Three classes of antithyroid drugs have been employed: thionamides,
perchlorate, and iodine. Thionamide drugs decrease the organification of
iodine and the coupling of iodotyrosines in the thyroid. One member of
this group, propylthiouracil, also decreases the peripheral conversion of T_4
to T_3. The more widely used preparations are propylthiouracil (PTU) and
methimazole in the U.S.A. and carbamizole in Europe. The duration of
action of these drugs is relatively short, so that they are usually
administered every 6–8 hr. In some situations, single doses per day have
been successful. The degree of thyrotoxicosis influences the duration and
efficacy of the preparations, so that higher dosages are required in the
most toxic patients. Accordingly, the starting dose range is from
200–1200 mg/day for PTU and 20–120 mg/day for methimazole. These
drugs rapidly block hormone synthesis, but clinical effects may not be
immediately apparent since it may take 1–2 weeks for colloid-stored T_4
and T_3 to be dissipated. Within 2–3 weeks, clinical improvement is noted
in most patients, first a decrease in nervousness and diaphoresis, then a
slowing of the pulse rate, and a change in the weight curve. A good
prognosis is revealed by a decrease in the size of the gland. In many cases,
useful alternative prognostic indices are the suppressibility of ^{131}I uptake
by T_3 and the perchlorate washout test. Depending on the response, it is
recommended that the patient be committed to 6–12 months of the first
course of therapy. Dosage of drugs is decreased soon after there is evidence
of improvement or may be increased if there is no improvement within

2–3 weeks. An enlargement of the gland, after initial decrease in size, indicates over-treatment and induction of hypothyroidism. This may be confirmed by a plasma TSH level. This is not a frequent problem with reasonably careful follow-up. Cutaneous allergies and agranulocytosis may occur in a few patients on these drugs. The incidence of such problems is from 0.7–3.0%. Occasional leukocyte counts may be made, but they are not necessarily of predictive value. The patient should be cautioned to stop the drug if an unexplained sore throat or rash should appear after institution of the medication. In that event, an alternative drug is tried. Worldwide statistics indicate a 40–60% permanent remission rate with one course (6–18 months) of therapy. A secondary course of therapy is followed by a similar remission rate. Most authorities recommend an alternative method of management after failure with two courses. Tertiary courses have occasionally been successful, however. The low incidence of permanent hypothyroidism following medical therapy suggests that the natural history may well be altered by this method.

Short-term medical therapy is often used for preoperative preparation. Iodine is added for several days before surgery.

Perchlorate prevents iodide uptake by the thyroid, and this method has been used therapeutically. Because of the occurrence of aplastic anemia following its use, the drug is now restricted.

^{131}I is quite useful in the management of diffuse toxic goiter and in many cases of multinodular toxic goiter. Extensive use permits statistical evaluation of its efficacy. The heavy dose therapy 14,000 rads is followed by reasonably prompt remission of the disorder (3–4 months), but a 20% occurrence of permanent hypothyroidism is noted within 1 year, increasing roughly 5–6%/year thereafter. Conventional dose (7,000 rads) therapy also produces reasonably rapid remission, but a 10–15% incidence of hyperthyroidism within 1 year and 3% each succeeding year has been observed. One-half of the conventional dose (3,500 rads) is followed by a measurable rate of hypothyroidism also. The use of β-adrenergic blocking agents (e.g., propranolol) has recently been advocated in long-term treatment, as well as for preoperative management of Graves' disease.

Treatment of Eye Changes in Graves' Disease

Management of the more severe ocular changes of Graves' disease is extremely difficult. Because local edema contributes to the fulness, lacrimation, and ophthalmoplegia, a useful procedure is to have the patient sleep with the head elevated. Corneal injury may be prevented by the use of glasses as well as of lubricant drops or ophthalmic ointments. Local therapy with guanethidine drops to produce Horner's syndrome has occasionally been helpful. In severe proptosis, decompression measures may become necessary.

Because of the possibility that surgical ^{131}I therapy for hyperthyroidism may be associated with exacerbation of the eye changes, many physicians prefer therapy with antithyroid drugs. Despite this method of therapy, however, exophthalmos may progress. Systemic drug therapy has been attempted with some degree of success. Prednisone therapy (100–125 mg daily) has been used to suppress the muscle and visual impairment. In severe cases, therapy may be continued for 6–8 months, during which time many of the untoward effects of steroids become apparent. Milder degrees of eye involvement have been treated with smaller doses of steroids. It is essential that patients receiving heavy doses of prednisone should receive potassium supplements and other protective measures. Diuretic therapy for exophthalmos of Graves' disease has met with only a mild degree of success. X-ray therapy to the pituitary is not particularly helpful, but radiation to the retobulbar areas has aided several patients. Surgical decompression measures are required when the lids are tense and edematous precluding surgical procedures to produce lid adhesions.

Thyrotoxic storm (thyroid storm) represents an exaggerated phase of thyrotoxicosis in which the etiology of the acute complication is unknown. It has frequently been precipitated by surgery and by several medical stresses, e.g., diabetic ketoacidosis, fright, toxemia of pregnancy, and parturition. Withdrawal from iodine therapy has also been suggested as a precipitating cause. The mechanism is ascribed to suppressed hormone release while the patient is on iodine, with rapid release of hormone from an iodine-enriched gland upon sudden withdrawal of the drug. Radioiodine therapy, by causing postradiation thyroiditis, may also precipitate this clinical emergency. Ether anesthesia is associated with increased dissociation of T_4 from tissue stores and may precipitate this disorder. Other factors include alterations in differential protein binding of T_3 and T_4.

Thyrotoxic storm is seen mainly in diffuse toxic goiter, but has occasionally arisen in multinodular toxic goiter. It is usually of abrupt onset, and hyperpyrexia is a sine qua non of the diagnosis. The fever may reach lethal levels within 1–2 days. The patient usually has most of the stigmata of thyrotoxicosis. Atrial fibrillation or other tachyarrhythmias may be present, and acute pulmonary edema or congestive heart failure may supervene. Systolic hypertension, as in uncomplicated hyperthyroidism, may later change to hypotension and shock. The usual CNS manifestations of hyperthyroidism may be replaced by stupor or coma. Diarrhea may be a major manifestation.

Differential diagnosis to rule out intercurrent problems superimposed or hyperthyroidism is important as therapy for the storm and for hyperthyroidism are similar but an intercurrent problem will require definitive therapy.

Laboratory data are not of any additional help over and above the diagnosis of hyperthyroidism. Specific therapeutic goals in management of thyrotoxic storm are designed to halt the increased synthesis and secretion of T_4 and T_3, to suppress the iodothyronine-catecholamine target effects, to treat the precipitating illness, and to support body defense mechanisms by treating congestive failure, atrial fibrillation, and shock when present. Antithyroid drugs should be instituted first to achieve the first goal above. Propylthiouracil (PTU 1,200–1,500 mg/day, or tapazol 120–150 mg) is given by mouth, or crushed and given by nasogastric tube if necessary. PTU is probably better, as it depresses conversion of T_4 to T_3 in the periphery. Iodine therapy is instituted to decrease the release of T_4 and T_3 from the gland. (Lugol's iodine, 30 drops/day orally, or NaI, 1–2 g by slow intravenous drip, is recommended.) Antithyroid drugs should precede the use of iodine, as they will block the organification and coupling of iodine in the gland. Blockage of the iodothyronine-catecholamine interaction requires the use of drugs which deplete catecholamines or prevent their action. These drugs include reserpine, guanethidine, and propranolol. Reserpine up to 2.5 mg intravenously four to six times a day is recommended because of its depressant effect, but should be avoided in shock.

Guanethidine (50–150 g/day) is also quite effective in this function, but should be avoided in shock. Propranolol, a β-adrenergic blocker, may be administered parenterally 1–2 mg intravenously under EKG control, and the dose is repeatable in 2 min. A vigorous search for coexistent or precipitating disorders such as febrile, inflammatory, or infectious disease should be undertaken, and the appropriate therapy instituted. Supportive management of the associated physiological or biochemical aberrations may require the use of cardiac glycosides and diuretics for congestive heart failure. Measures for alleviation of hyperpyrexia, including replenishment of fluids if dehydration is a factor or glucose infusion for caloric replacement, are employed when required. Some may elect to use glucocorticoids 100–300 mg of solucortef daily. The rationale may be that the effective cortisol levels are lower because of the activation of 11-dehydrogenation of cortisol (with formation of cortisone, biologically less active) by excess thyroid hormones. With employment of the above therapeutic procedures, most patients should show improvement within 24–36 hr, with complete recovery from this complication within 5 days. Further therapy of hyperthyroidism is discussed in another section.

Thyrotoxicosis in Pregnancy

Hyperthyroidism complicates pregnancy in 0.047–0.1% of patients. Despite alterations in menstrual cycle by hyperthyroidism, such patients may become pregnant. It has been suggested and discounted that pregnancy may be a precipitating factor in the pathogenesis of hyperthyroidism. Many features of pregnancy imitate hyperthyroidism, for example, skin texture, slight systolic hypertension, a slight temperature rise, and often an enlargement in the thyroid gland. However, if true hyperthyroidism is present, there are usually several additional features.

Laboratory diagnosis is relatively simple if the alterations in TBG induced by pregnancy (via estrogens) are kept in mind. Accordingly, even in the non-pregnant state, the PBI and total T_4 are elevated, while the resin uptake of T_3 is depressed. Calculation of the thyroid index from these data will confirm euthyroidism. Hyperthyroidism superimposed in pregnancy will be associated with higher levels of PBI and total T_4, and the RU T_3 will be increased, so that the calculated thyroid index will be unquestionably in the hyperthyroid range (see section on laboratory methods). (Determination of a free T_4 by dialysis will confirm the diagnosis, but this is unnecessary under most conditions.) It should be emphasized that diagnostic thyroid ^{131}I uptake is not recommended in pregnancy, because of potential hazard to the fetal thyroid.

Treatment of Hyperthyroidism in Pregnancy

Therapeutic abortions are not needed for conventional hyperthyroidism as medical management is reasonably effective. The goals of management are to achieve euthyroidism before time of delivery, to avoid thyroid storm, and to achieve euthyroidism by measures which are not harmful to mother or baby. There are two available safe methods applicable in pregnancy, either antithyroid drugs or surgery. The use of iodine is absolutely contraindicated because the ingested iodine, on reaching the fetal thyroid, suppresses thyroid hormone release. Negative feedback regulation precipitates an increased release of TSH with consequent induction of a goiter. Radioiodine therapy is contraindicated as stated above. Surgery is not recommended in the first or third trimester, and is considered only in the second trimester. By this time the patient should be essentially euthyroid if the precipitation of thyroid storm and all its hazards are to be avoided. It is, therefore, essential that the patient be given a course of antithyroid drugs to achieve euthyroidism by the second trimester. Since the natural outcome of a given hyperthyroid gland is not predictable, as indeed there may well be spontaneous remissions, some thought should be given to continuing antithyroid drugs and avoiding ablative surgery.

Of the antithyroid drugs, the thionamides commonly employed block the organic binding of iodine and the coupling of iodotyrosines in the thyroid. In addition, one of these, propylthiouracil, blocks the conversion of T_4 to the more active T_3. Management of the pregnant patient with antithyroid drugs requires awareness that these drugs cross the placental barrier and will affect the fetal thyroid and thyroid-pituitary axis. This effect is directly correlated with the dosage of the drugs used. The required dosage is also related to the degree of thyrotoxicosis in the mother, as the biological decay of the drugs will be enhanced by increased hypermetabolism. It is, therefore, necessary to employ dosages sufficient to suppress maternal thyroid overactivity, while not sufficient to significantly affect fetal hormonogenesis and TSH release.

Propylthiouracil (600 mg/day) or tapazol (60 mg/day) may be employed in early pregnancy. These doses are given as ¼ every 6 hr or ⅓ every 8 hr. With this dosage, it is possible in most patients to achieve euthyroidism before the start of the third trimester, at which time a considerably lower dose may be used. Some authorities have used thyroid extract or thyroxin concurrently in order to suppress fetal TSH overproduction in the event of significant antithyroid drug effect on the fetal thyroid. This concept may in part be fallacious, as the high TBG levels in the maternal circulation may effectively deter much transfer of T_4 to the fetal compartment. It might be more useful to use T_3 supplements because of their weaker affinity for TBG. We have rarely added thyroid hormone supplements in the management of our thyrotoxic pregnant patients, although data from previous surveys have occasionally shown the occurrence of fetal goiters following the maternal use of antithyroid drugs, but these occurred when larger doses were employed and occasionally when iodides were added to the regimen.

Pediatric Aspects of Hyperthyroidism

Special features of fetal and neonatal thyroid activity should be considered in order to understand some of the dynamics in thyroid disease in the pediatric population.

Intrauterine Thyroid Function Iodide concentration activity is evident by 11–12 weeks of gestation. Thereafter, all processes in thyroid biosynthesis, viz., trapping, organification, coupling, and secretion, increase progressively until term. The fetal thyroid radioiodine uptake is 3–4 times that of the adult gland and is adjusted for size. Fetal PBI and T_4 are low in midgestation and increase progressively toward term, representing increases in TSH and TBG as well as in free T_4. Placental permeability to maternal iodothyronines may be variable, but progressively increases with duration of pregnancy. Circulating levels of TBG in the maternal compartment undoubtedly retard exchange of iodothyronines. TSH does not cross the placenta, so that the pituitary thyroid axis in the fetus is relatively independent of maternal control. TSH has been detected in fetal blood at 8–10 weeks of gestation.

Thyroid Function at Birth and Infancy Serum T_4 level in the newborn increases progressively and is only 10–20% less than that in the maternal circulation. PBI and BEI increase progressively over the first few hours of extrauterine life. By 24–48 hr of age, the PBI is normally 8–16 μg/100 ml, without increased levels of TBG or TBPA; an increased free T_4

level is also found. This is ascribed to increased TSH in the neonatal period. Within 1 hr after delivery, the TSH levels may reach 80–90 microunits/ml; this gradually falls off 10–15 microunits/ml by 48–72 hr. It is assumed that this increased thyroid activity mediated by TSH stimulation is precipitated by the decreased body temperature which occurs at the time of exposure to extrauterine life.

Thyroid Function in Childhood During the first 2 years of life, the mean PBI is higher than in the adult, children having mean PBI levels of 6.4 μg/100 ml. By 13–15 years, the mean value decreases to 4.8 μg/100 ml, and by age 19–22 years the values are comparable to the adult range of 4–8 μg/100 ml. These changes are in part undoubtedly related to gonadal maturation and its influence on the binding proteins.

Hyperthyroidism in Infancy Neonatal Graves' disease is extremely rare; only about 40 patients with proved neonatal Graves' have been reported. About 0.07% of total population of Graves' disease is found in infancy, and these are usually infants of hyperthyroid mothers. It is essential that infants of mothers with thyrotoxicosis should be carefully checked at intervals for the possibility of neonatal Graves' disease.

The clinical manifestations include: irritability, flushing, tachycardia, increased appetite, weight loss or slow weight gain, exophthalmus, and thyroid enlargement. An occasional patient may have thrombocytopenia with hepatosplenomegaly, and rarely jaundice. The birth weight is usually slightly below normal. The clinical features may not become evident for 8–9 days and, if untreated, may subside in a few weeks, but the mortality rate, if not treated, approaches 25%. Serum T_4, PBI, and resin T_3 uptake are all diagnostic, but an ^{131}I uptake is not helpful in neonatal Graves' as it is normally up to 90% at this age. Treatment of neonatal Graves' disease requires the use of sedatives and digitalis preparations. Propylthiouracil, preferably, or methimazole, in doses of 5–10 mg/kg/day or 0.5–1 mg/kg/day, respectively, in divided doses at 8-hr intervals should result in a clinical response within 24–36 hr. Lugol's iodine, 1 drop three times a day, is also recommended. Surgery is employed only if there is evidence of obstruction from the enlarged thyroid.

Juvenile Hyperthyroidism Hyperthyroidism in childhood and adolescence accounts for 1–5% of all hyperthyroid patients, the female to male preponderance being 4:1 to 6:1. The important clinical features include, in order of incidence: goiter, prominent eyes, tachycardia, nervousness, exophthalmos, increased perspiration, increased appetitie, weight loss, deterioration of school work, emotional disturbances, heat intolerance, breathlessness, and diarrhea. Diagnosis is made by standard laboratory studies, including T_3 levels, T_4 levels, resin T_3 uptake, and epithyroid ^{131}I uptake.

Most pediatricians prefer the use of antithyroid drugs in the treatment of diffuse toxic goiter in children. Medical therapy should be tried in most cases unless there are contraindications, such as drug reactions, lack of patient cooperation or physician interest, or unreliability of patient. An adequate trial requires sufficient drug and a treatment period of 6–18 months at least. Radioiodine treatment is a second choice provided the patient is informed of the probability of subsequent permanent hypothyroidism.

For uninodular hyperthyroidism, surgical management is recommended, and, for multinodular hyperthyroidism, a combination of antithyroid drugs and radioiodine therapy has been employed successfully.

HYPOTHYROIDISM

Hypothyroidism is caused by a deficiency of thyroid hormones with a resulting decrease in or absence of the peripheral effects of the hormones. Hypothyroid states are conveniently classified according to Table 14.5. Regardless of the basis of the deficiency of iodothyronine hormones, there are several features common to all hypothyroid states. Special features relative to either age of onset or to specific types of disorders are discussed later in the chapter. A major cluster of complaints in the hypothyroid patient includes apathy, lethargy, somnolence, and cold intolerance. De-

Table 14.5. Hypothyroid State

I. Goitrous
   A. Congenital goitrous cretinism caused by biosynthetic defects
      1. Iodide-trapping defect
      2. Organification defect
      3. Coupling defect
      4. Deiodinase defect
      5. Secretion of abnormal iodoproteins caused by abnormal synthesis or defective proteolysis
      6. Congenital calcified goiter
      7. Congenital deaf mutism, goiter, and elevated T_4; possible refractoriness to T_4
   B. Endemic cretinism
   C. Caused by goitrogens: drugs, foods
II. Nongoitrous
   A. Idiopathic myxedema
   B. Congenital athyreosis
   C. Thyroid destruction: surgical, x-ray, radionucleides
   D. Congenital hypothyroidism with impaired response to TSH
   E. Caused by TSH deficiency
      1. Isolated TSH deficiency
      2. Panhypopituitarism
      3. Hypothalamic hypothyroidism

creased metabolic rate and oxygen consumption are associated with brady-cardia, slight to moderate weight gain, and constipation. The patient may have dyspnea caused by alveolar hypoventilation. Hair loss, loss of lateral third of the eyebrows, and coarse skin structure are seen. Female patients complain of hypermenorrhea, male patients of impotence, and both sexes of decreased libido. The clinical signs of hypothyroidism are presented in Table 14.6. The laboratory tests for diagnosis of hypothyroidism and their rationale are presented in Table 14.7.

Treatment of Hypothyroidsm

The goal of therapy of hypothyroidism is to achieve euthyroid levels by replacement with thyroid hormone. The clinical end points are the well-being of the patient, skin structure, pulse rate, as well as improvement in several of the parameters affected by the disorder. Three thyroid prepara-tions, desiccated thyroid extract, thyroxin, and triiodothyronine, are avail-able for therapeutic use. In all cases of hypothyroidism, full replace-ment doses of one of these preparations is recommended. Conditions which contraindicate full replacement dosages are arteriosclerotic heart disease with angina pectoris and myxedema-induced heart disease.

Table 14.6. Clinical Signs of Hypothyroidism

I. Skin and appendages
  A. Dermal glycoprotein deposition (myxedema) with non-pitting puffi-ness especially around eyes and hands
  B. Decreased sweating
  C. Coarse, brittle hair (especially on back and extremities in children)
  D. Follicular hyperkeratosis
  E. Malar flush and yellowish discoloration in other areas
II. Cardiovascular system
  A. Bradycardia, decreased stroke volume, and decreased cardiac output
  B. Increased vascular resistance, dilated heart with pale flabby myo-cardium
  C. Electrocardiogram may be normal or may show low P, ORS, and T, occasional rightward T vector
  D. Increased susceptibility to cardiac glycosides
  E. Cerebral blood flow decreased
  F. Some evidence of increased atherogenesis
III. Respiratory system
  A. Decreased maximum breathing capacity
  B. Alveolar hypoventilation
IV. Gastrointestinal system
  A. Delayed dentition seen in children
  B. Broad, thick tongue
  C. Hypochlorhydria
  D. Enlargement of intestinal tract in some patients

continued

Table 14.6. *continued*

    E. Delayed absorption of carbohydrates, fats, proteins, vitamins, and minerals

    F. Distention, abdominal pain, and vomiting leading to paralytic ileus

    G. Decreased hepatic clearance of several substrates

V. Nervous system

    A. Slowing of intellectual function

    B. Slow and clumsy movements

    C. Occasional cerebellar ataxia

    D. Diminished deep tendon reflexes

    E. Dysarthria

    F. Carpal tunnel syndrome

    G. Myxedematous dementia

    H. Cretinous deafness and deaf mutism in Pendred's syndrome

VI. Locomotor system

    A. Decreased growth and bone maturation

    B. Decreased bone turnover

VII. Reproductive system

    A. Menorrhagia, metrorrhagia, and, occasionally, amenorrhea may occur

    B. Male patients on rare occasions may have oligospermia or normal sperm counts with low inability percentage

VIII. Renal system

    A. Decreased glomerular filtration rate

    B. Decreased renal blood flow

    C. Tubular dysfunction manifested by decreased resorptive and secretory maximal capacities

    D. Decreased water diuresis

IX. Hematopoietic system

    A. Decreased red cell mass with normocytic normochromic anemia; presumably decreased O_2 dissociation prevents erythropoietic release

    B. Occasionally pernicious anemia may be secondary to achlorhydria and lack of intrinsic factor production in the gastric mucosa in hypothyroidism

    C. A malabsorption of B_{12} intrinsic factor complex caused by ileal mucosal defect has been noted occasionally

    D. Clotting factors VIII and IX are decreased

X. Pituitary-adrenocortical axis function

    A. Peripheral metabolism of cortisol is altered in primary hypothyroidism

    B. Because of the influence of the 11-dehydrogenation reaction on thyroid hormone, there is a decreased conversion of cortisol to cortisone

    C. Because of its greater effect on feedback suppression of ACTH release by cortisol, a decreased ACTH production is quite likely

    D. Urinary 17-OHCS and 17-KS are decreased in hypothyroidism

    E. Plasma cortisol levels are lower than normal, and an attenuated circadian cortisol rhythmicity correlates well with the severity of hypothyroidism

    F. ACTH or cosyntropin tests reveal no evidence of adrenocortical failure, especially in the repetitive stimulation test

Table 14.7. Differential Diagnostic Procedures in Hypothyroidism

Disorder[a]	RAI uptake	RAI after TSH	Perchlorate washout[b]	TSH levels	TRH stimulation	Special tests
Goitrous defects in						
Iodide trapping	↓	↓	Discharged	↑		
Organification	↑	↑	Discharged	↑		
Coupling	↑	↑	N	↑		Low MIT and DIT
Deiodinase				↑		Measure iodotyrosines
Abnormal iodoprotein				↑		Measure iodotyrosines
Deaf mutism with end-organ resistance		↑		↑		Separation of iodoproteins
Endemic cretinism	↓	↓		↑		
Goitrogens Rx[c]	↑ N[d] ↓	N	N or Discharged	↑		
Nongoitrous						
Idiopathic myxedema	↓	↓		↑		
Congenital athyreosis	↓	↓		↑		
Thyroid destruction	↓	↓		↑		
TSH deficiency	↓	↑		↓ N	↕	
Panhypopituitarism	↓	↑		↓ N	↕	
Hypothalamic hypothyroidism	↓	↑		↓ N	↑	

[a] In the disorders listed, T_4, T_3, PBI, and resin uptake of T_3 are decreased, except in deaf mutism with end-organ resistance, where their values are normal. A disorder of deaf mutism and goitrous hypothyroidism is Pendred's syndrome in which there is a biosynthetic defect. Biosynthetic defects may also occur in Hashimoto's (lymphocytic) thyroiditis.

[b] Blank spaces, tests not required.

[c] Depends on the type of antithyroid drug, e.g., perchlorate will decrease trapping and thionamide drugs cause organification and coupling defects.

[d] N, normal.

The average daily full replacement dose of thyroid extract is 90–120 mg of thyroxine 0.15–0.25 mg, and of triiodothyronine, 25–50 μg, with the dose chosen given once daily. T_3 has a faster onset of action and its effect is more rapidly dissipated. T_3 is especially useful in elderly patients with the cardiovascular disorders listed above because of the relatively short half-life in comparison to the other preparations. Such patients are given suboptimal doses 5–10 μg of T_3, 0.05 mg of T_4, or 15 mg of desiccated thyroid daily for 2 weeks or more, and observed for any manifestations of worsened heart disease. The dosage is gradually increased to the closest to full replacement dose tolerable. The replacement program in myxedema coma is described separately. The best current method of gauging adequacy of replacement therapy in primary hypothyroidism is the measurement of plasma TSH levels. Euthyroidism is reflected by TSH values of 0–10 microunits/ml.

Secondary hypothyroidism may be caused by panhypopituitarism or isolated TSH deficiency. If panhypopituitarism is also present, then the manifestations include those of deficiencies of the various tropic hormones and of growth hormone (see Chapter 13). Isolated TSH deficiency as a cause of hypothyroidism exhibits some clinical features different from primary hypothyroidism, viz., the skin changes are less noticeable, plasma TSH is not elevated, a TSH stimulation test shows good response, and TSH levels do not increase after TRH injection.

Myxedema coma describes an emergency clinical state caused by severe deficiency of thyroid hormones. Clinical features include cachexia in most patients, lethargy progressing to stupor and coma, hypothermia, hypoventilation and respiratory acidosis, hyponatremia, elevated plasma lactate, hypoglycemia, inappropriate antidiuretic hormone, disturbed cerebral metabolism, and rapid progression to death if not treated. There is no spontaneous remission. It is most often seen in the elderly poor, often in patients treated with ^{131}I in the past, and in patients with unknown cause of hypothyroidism. The acute state may be precipitated by drugs which depress respiration.

If this diagnosis is suspected, it is essential that blood be obtained immediately for T_4, T_3, and TSH levels. Without awaiting the results, treatment is instituted to replace the body pool of thyroid hormones and to manage secondary problems. Thyroid hormone replacement is rapidly achieved by the intravenous infusion of sodium L-thyroxine (100–200 μg). Alternatively, 75–100 μg of T_3 may be administered orally. It is essential that a clear airway is established and adequate ventilation is maintained employing assisted breathing if necessary. Sedative drugs are contraindicated during the management of this emergency, and, if pressor agents are needed for shock, only small amounts are recommended lest the synergism with thyroid hormones precipitates arrhythmias. A blanket is used, but active warming is contraindicated since vascular collapse and increased O_2 consumption may ensue. In rare cases, the use of glucocorticoids may be indicated.

THYROID CANCER

Malignant tumors of the thyroid are relatively rare, and deaths from this cause constitute about 0.35% of all cancer deaths in the U. S. The three major types of thyroid cancer are the papillary, follicular, and medullary forms. Papillary carcinoma constitutes 50% of thyroid cancers and is most prevalent between the 2nd and 5th decades with a 4:1 female to male preponderance. This tumor may spread by lymphatic channels to regional lymph nodes. The prognosis is reasonably good after surgical removal.

Follicular carcinoma constitutes 25% of thyroid cancer and occurs in young adults, with a higher incidence in women. The tumor is spread by local extension; distant metastases considerably alter the prognosis. This type of tumor is responsive to TSH and is capable of iodide uptake. Therapy includes surgical excision and radioiodide therapy for metastases.

The lesions of medullary carcinoma are large and hard and may be present in both thyroid lobes. This form of malignancy constitutes about 10% of all thyroid cancers. The hormone calcitonin is produced in significant amounts by this tumor, and the detection of this hormone by radioimmunoassay will serve both for diagnosis and follow-up of disease progression. Medullary carcinoma often occurs concurrently with pheochromocytoma (Sipple syndrome) and with pancreatic tumors.

LITERATURE CITED

1. Werner, S. C., and S. H. Ingbar (eds.). 1971. The Thyroid. 3rd Ed., pp. 1–876. Harper & Row, Publishers, New York.
2. Rawson, R. W., W. L. Money, and R. L. Grief. 1969. Diseases of the thyroid. In P. K. Bondy (ed.), Diseases of Metabolism, pp. 753–826. W. B. Saunders Co., Philadelphia.
3. Solomon, D. H., and I. J. Chopra. 1970. LATS and Graves' disease. Calif Med. 113:50–55.
4. Hollander, C. S., T. Mitsuma, and A. J. Kastin, L. Shenkman, M. Blum, and D. G. Anderson. 1971. Hypertriiodothyroninemia as a premonitory manifestation of thyroxicosis. Lancet 2:731–733.
5. Werner, C. S., and H. Hamilton. 1961. Hyperthyroidism without hypermetabolism. JAMA 146:450–455.
6. Means, J. H. 1948. The Thyroid and Its Diseases. J. B. Lippincott Co., Philadelphia. 292 pp.
7. Hagen, C. A. 1968. Treatment of thyrotoxicosis with ^{131}I and posttherapy hypothyroidism. Med. Clin. North Am. 52:417–445.
8. Stattler, H. 1952. Basedow's Disease. Grune & Stratton, Inc., New York.
9. Swerdloff, R. S. 1970. Treatment of thyrotoxicosis. Calif. Med. 113:55–65.

15
The Adrenal
Cortex

Adrenal cortical cells are derived from mesodermal elements in close connection with the renal and gonadal anlagen. The morphological zonation into the zona glomerulosa, zona fasciculata, and the zona reticularis has been shown to be of significance in terms of biosynthetic activity (1–3). The zona glomerulosa secretes the mineralocorticoid hormone aldosterone, and the inner zones produce the glucocorticoid hormone cortisol, as well as the androgens and estrogens. In the human (and other mammalian) adrenal glands, the cortical cells are supplied by arterial branches which enter sinusoidal circulation in the cortex; the blood then drains into a single vein from each gland.

REGULATION OF GLUCOCORTICOID SECRETION

Pituitary ACTH stimulates the secretion of the glucocorticoid hormones, cortisol and corticosterone, by the zona fasciculata. Secretion and release of the mineralocorticoid principal aldosterone depend on the renin-angiotensin mechanism. Biosynthetic activities in this zone are dependent on the availability of steroid substrates which are provided from cholesterol through ACTH action on the inner zones. (ACTH supports growth of adrenal cells by increasing RNA replication.)

ACTH release is under the control of the hypothalamus; it is probable that higher central nervous system centers also influence the hypothalamic corticotropin-releasing factor (CRF). Circulating levels of cortisol regulate ACTH release by a negative feedback mechanism, whereby high levels of cortisol depress release of hypothalamic CRF and subsequently of pituitary ACTH. Low levels stimulate increased ACTH release by the intact pituitary. In primary adrenocortical insufficiency, for example, there are high circulating levels of ACTH. Cortisone and aldosterone possess some of the ACTH suppression activity. The mineralocorticoid, deoxycorticosterone, which may accumulate in certain biosynthetic defects in the adrenal, possesses $1/50$ of this ACTH suppression activity, while androgens and estrogens lack this ability.

REGULATION OF MINERALOCORTICOID SECRETION

Regulation of secretion and release of aldosterone by the adrenal cortex is mediated mainly by the renin-angiotensin system, and secondarily by plasma sodium and potassium concentrations. Availability of the biosynthetic precursors of the aldosterone is under control of ACTH.

RENIN-ANGIOTENSIN MECHANISM

The source of renin is known to be the juxtaglomerular cells situated next to the macula densa located at the first segment of the distal convoluted tubule. These highly specialized juxtaglomerular cells line the terminal part of the different arteriole just before the glomerulus. The juxtaglomerular cells and the macula densa constitute the juxtaglomerular apparatus. Increase in stretch of the renal arteriolar wall results in an increase in granulation in the juxtaglomerular cells, and decreased stretch is followed by degranulation of the cells and release of renin. The renal afferent arteriole functions as a stretch receptor which signals release of renin. The macula densa may serve as a volume sensor or as a chemoreceptor responsive to sodium concentration. Reduction of intravascular volume, induced by low sodium intake, blood loss, or change from recumbent to upright posture, induces a degranulation in the juxtaglomerular cells and release of renin into the blood stream and lymph. In the blood stream, renin, a proteolytic enzyme, catalyzes the transformation of a circulating globulin angiotensinogen (produced in the liver) to angiotensin I. This decapeptide is acted on by "plasma angiotensin converting enzyme" with the cleavage of 2 amino acid residues leaving an octapeptide angiotensin II.

Angiotensin II, the most potent vasopressor agent known, also functions as the main physiological stimulant for aldosterone release. Angiotensin II is destroyed by "angiotensinases" in the plasma; these enzymes may be produced in the adrenal gland. The longevity of angiotensin II in the blood stream is estimated to be 4–20 min. In addition to causing a release of aldosterone, angiotensin II may also stimulate the release of corticosterone, deoxycorticosterone, and, to a small extent, cortisol. There are data which indicate that catecholamines may also be released by angiotensin II. When the perfusion pressure in the renal arteriole is sufficiently low, increased aldosterone is released and sodium reabsorption is induced. Increased water reabsorption associated with this process enhances the perfusion pressure in the region of the afferent arteriole. If tubular luminal sodium concentration is sufficiently low, the macula densa chemoreceptors signal renin release with eventual release of aldosterone by the adrenal cortex, designed ultimately to correct the hyponatremia. Reduction in intravascular volume may induce a decrease in the inactivation of aldosterone in the liver, resulting in increased circulating levels of aldosterone. The synthesis of aldosterone is ultimately dependent on the presence of appropriate steroid precursors. Since the formation of these precursors in the adrenal is ACTH dependent, certain aspects of aldosterone kinetics are undoubtedly responsive to anterior pituitary function.

BIOSYNTHESIS OF ADRENAL CORTICAL HORMONES

All physical signs and symptoms of adrenal disorders are ultimately related to increased or decreased levels of certain biologically active hormones. The bulk of the abnormal metabolites is biologically inactive. Discernible effects in adrenal diseases are caused by either increased or decreased glucocorticoids, mineralocorticoids, androgens, estrogens, or combinations thereof.

The immediate precursor for corticosteroidogenesis is cholesterol. This substrate is provided from dietary intake as well as from synthesis from acetyl-CoA. This synthetic reaction involves the participation of several cofactors, including pantothenic acid (for coenzyme A), NADH, and NADPH as well as energy from high energy phosphate bonds. The availability of cholesterol for corticosteroidogenesis is enhanced by ACTH. At low levels of ACTH activity, plasma cholesterol enters the synthetic pool; this action is mediated by adenosine $3':5'$-monophosphate (cAMP) which is released from ATP by an ACTH-activated membrane adenylate cyclase. Higher levels of ACTH through the cAMP mechanism make cholesterol from liposomes available for corticosteroidogenesis (4).

The first reaction in the corticosteroid synthetic chain is the desmolase reaction, a multistep process which results in the cleavage of the cholesterol side chain with the release of Δ^5-pregnenolone and isocaproic acid. Pregnenolone has two alternative fates in the biosynthetic sequence (Figure 15.1). The $\Delta^5,3\beta$-ol structure is converted to the $\Delta^4,3$-ketone group by a two-step microsomal reaction described at the $\Delta^5,3\beta$-ol dehydrogenase system, resulting in the formation of progesterone. The alternative fate of pregnenolone is the hydroxylation at C-17 by a cytoplasmic 17α-hydroxylase to form 17α-hydroxypregnenolone. The major purpose of this pathway is synthesis of androgens and estrogens. To this end, the side chain is cleaved off leaving a ketone group at C-17, i.e., formation of Δ^5-androsten, 3β-ol-17-one, or dehydroepiandrosterone (DHEA). As shown in Figure 15.1, a microsomal $\Delta^5,3\beta$-ol dehydrogenase then converts DHEA to Δ^4-androsten-3,17-dione. Reduction of the 17-ketone group of androstenedione results in the formation of testosterone. Hydroxylation of androstenedione at C-19 permits subsequent aromatization

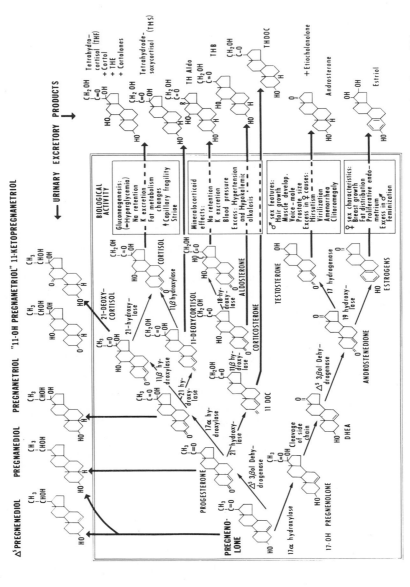

Figure 15.1. Biosynthesis of adrenocortical hormones. The compound Δ⁵-pregnenolone, which is the substrate for all steroid hormone synthesis, is derived from cholesterol. ACTH activates the "desmolase reaction" which results in the release of pregnenolone and isocaproic acid. The small rectangular areas list the clinical effects of the various hormones. The compounds outside the double-lined borders are urinary end products of the various adrenocortical hormones. (Reprinted from Bacchus (3) with permission of the publisher.)

of ring A of the steroid nucleus, with the resulting formation of estrone, an estrogen. An alternative fate of 17-hydroxypregnenolone is 17-hydroxy-progesterone as shown in Figure 15.1. This 17-hydroxyprogesterone is an intermediate in the formation of cortisol.

Progesterone formed from pregnenolone is the precursor to all biologically active C-21 adrenal cortical hormones. The Δ^4,3-ketone structure is essential to the biological activity of these hormones. Progesterone has two alternative fates in the adrenal, viz., it can be converted to 17-hydroxy-progesterone by a 17α-hydroxylase in the cytosol, or it can be converted to 11-deoxycorticosterone (DOC) by a soluble 21-hydroxylase enzyme. The intermediate 17α-hydroxyprogesterone is converted to the biologically inactive intermediate 11-deoxycortisol (S) by 21-hydroxylase. A mitochondrial 11β-hydroxylase converts 11-deoxycortisol to cortisol, the definitive glucocorticoid in the human adrenal. The intermediate 11-de-oxycorticosterone is converted to corticosterone by 11β-hydroxylase. The normal human adrenal produces cortisol and corticosterone in a ratio between 10:1 and 4:1. Corticosterone is converted to aldosterone by the enzyme 18-hydroxylase; this transformation confers powerful mineralo-corticoid activity to the hormone. It is probable that in some situations 11β hydroxylation may precede 21-hydroxylation.

The normal secretory rate of cortisol in the adult man is estimated to be from 20–30 mg/24 hr, and of corticosterone, 4–6 mg/24 hr. Aldosterone secretion rate on a normal 5 to 10-g sodium chloride intake ranges from 60–170 μg/24 hr.

TRANSPORT OF ADRENOCORTICAL HORMONES

It is estimated that 60–70% of cortisol is secreted during the period from midnight to 8:00 a.m., and the remaining 30–40% during the rest of the day. This circadian variation in cortisol secretion, which is evident when plasma cortisol determinations are done at 8:00 a.m. and 5:00 p.m., is obliterated in certain disease states. There is also a semblance of circadian variation of corticosterone secretion. Under maximal stimulation, the adrenal cortex can produce up to 300 mg of cortisol/24 hr, the circadian variation being obliterated under such conditions.

Cortisol is transported in the circulation in a form bound to an α-globulin, cortisol-binding globulin (CBG). There are specific chemical characteristics in the steroid molecule which determine affinity to CBG. Approximately 50–60% of cortisol is bound to CBG; and 10% circulates as free cortisol. The remainder of secreted cortisol is rapidly inactivated by the liver. The protein binding renders the hormone soluble in plasma and prevents its inactivation by the liver. Certain clinical states are associated with changes in CBG, thereby affecting cortisol kinetics. Plasma cortisol levels in the adult man range from 5–25 μg/100 ml at 8:00 a.m. and 2.5–12.5 μg/100 ml at 5:00–6:00 p.m. Plasma corticosterone levels are normally in the range of 0.5–2.5 μg/100 ml. Mean plasma concentration of aldosterone in the adult is reported to be 0.008 μg/100 ml.

FURTHER CONSIDERATIONS ON SYNTHESIS OF ANDROGENS BY ADRENAL CORTEX

As presented in Figure 15.1, the precursor to the series is 17α-hydroxy-pregnenolone which, after cleavage of the side chain, becomes dehydro-epiandrosterone. This compound is biologically a very weak androgen. It is a source of androstenedione which may be hydroxylated to 11β-hydroxy-androstenedione. DHEA may be hydroxylated to C-11 to form Δ^5-andro-stenediol. In the adrenal cells there is a sulfatase which transfers sulfate to the OH group at carbon 3, hence the formation of DHEA sulfate. A similar conjugation of testosterone, DOC, and corticosterone is possible. Cortisol, cortisone, and aldosterone are not sulfated to any significant degree.

STEROID HORMONE PRODUCTION IN FETAL ADRENALS

The fetal adrenal responds to fetal ACTH as maternal ACTH fails to traverse the placental barrier. For this reason, in an anencephalic fetus with atrophic pituitary, adrenal development does not progress beyond the 20th week of gestation. From the 10th week of gestation on, normal fetal adrenals possess all the enzymes necessary for synthesis of cortisol, as well as of 17-ketosteroids. There may be a partial deficiency in Δ^5,3β-ol dehydrogenase system, and this could be the basis of the preponderance of C-19 compounds produced by fetal adrenals. Recent data reveal a unique relationship between placental HCG (chorionic gonadotropin) and the fetal zone. It is suggested that stimulation of this zone is a major function of HCG from the placenta.

BIOLOGICAL ACTIONS OF ADRENOCORTICAL HORMONES

These activities are discussed under the categories of their potencies as glucocorticoids, mineralocorticoids, and androgens (5). The secretory rate of adrenal estrogens is small under normal conditions and does not warrant a discussion of biological actions. For certain pathological states, estrogen levels may be significant.

Glucocorticoid Actions

The definitive glucocorticoid in man is cortisol, although measurable amounts of a weaker glucocorticoid, corticosterone, are also produced;

corticosterone also possesses mineralocortical activity. The prime effect of cortisol is on the process of gluconeogenesis. Cortisol increases the synthesis of the enzymes essential to gluconeogenesis, e.g., PEPCK among others. Because of the gluconeogenic and anti-insulin actions of glucocorticoids, hyperglycemia and a metacorticoid diabetes may be induced. Such a diabetic state is not usually accompanied by ketoacidosis.

Glucocorticoids also affect fat metabolism, excessive cortisol activity causing centripetal redistribution of fat. Cortisol also induces fat synthesis partly as a result of the induced hyperglycemia which then stimulates insulin release and eventually lipogenesis. Chronic cortisol excess may lead to hyperlipidemia and hypercholesterolemia. Many deamination and transamination enzymes are activated by glucocorticoids.

Glucocorticoids enhance water diuresis so that, in adrenocortical insufficiency, a water load is not readily excreted. Cortisol prevents the shift of water intracellularly, hence maintaining a higher extracel water volume. This causes a higher glomerular filtration rate and water diuresis. It has been suggested that cortisol has a direct antagonistic effect on ADH action on the renal tubule, increases ADH inactivation by the liver, and suppresses the production of ADH by the neurohypophysial system.

Glucocorticoids produce a lymphopenia by lysis of circulating and fixed lymphocytes. In this process, antibody proteins are released initially, but the continued production of antibodies is depressed by the continued thymicolymphocytolysis. Cortisol, cortisone, and aldosterone induce a depression of circulating eosinophils (and basophils) by sequestration of these cells in the lungs and spleen and by lysis to some extent. Total neutrophils are increased by glucocorticoids, resulting in a leukocytosis with neutrophilia. Glucocorticoids also influence the numbers of erythrocytes culminating in a pattern of steroid-induced or stress-induced erythrocytosis. Occasionally, cortisol-induced thrombocytosis may precipitate thromboembolic phenomena. Cortisol increases muscle performance to the extent that much activity was used in the past as an assay for glucocorticoid activity.

Glucocorticoids lower the threshold for excitation of the central nervous system; this is the basis of certain psychiatric disorders precipitated by pharmacological doses of cortisol and similar steroids. Many patients with Cushing's syndrome exhibit psychiatric abnormalities. Pharmacological doses of glucocorticoids cause an increase in gastric acidity, a probable decrease in protective mucopolysaccharides, and an increase in uropepsin excretion. These factors may underlie the high occurrence of peptic ulcer disease in patients treated with cortisol or in patients under stress.

Glucocorticoids also affect bone turnover by decreasing osteoblast activity and bone matrix formation (antiprotein-anabolic action), by decreasing calcium deposition, by decreasing the hepatic conversion of vitamin D to a more active biological form, and by increasing the clearance and urinary loss of calcium. These effects of cortisol are demonstrated by the severe osteoporosis following long-term use of pharmacological doses of cortisol, or in patients with endogenous cortisol excess such as in Cushing's syndrome.

Glucocorticoids also exert effects on the cardiovascular system through different mechanisms which include an effect on sodium retention, a mineralocorticoid effect of large amounts of cortisol. Cortisol is also known to enhance the production of angiotensinogen which would eventually lead to increased levels of angiotensin. A well known effect of cortisol is to sensitize the vasculature to the pressor effects of catecholamines. Perhaps this "sensitization" action is the basis of the occasional benefits of glucocorticoid therapy in patients with shock. It is well known that decompensated cardiovascular disease is a major cause of death in Cushing's syndrome.

Glucocorticoids have been shown to possess marked anti-inflammatory effect, altering the response of connective tissues to injury. Fibroblast activity is decreased by these hormones; fibroblast activity is increased by desoxycorticosterone, a mineralocorticoid, as is the inflammatory reaction. It is suggested that the ability of cortisol to stabilize lysosomal membranes underlies the anti-inflammatory effects of these compounds.

Biological Actions of Mineralocorticoid Hormones

The prototype mineralocorticoid aldosterone is secreted by the zona glomerulosa of the adrenal cortex; at least two other natural steroids possess significant mineralocorticoid activity, deoxycorticosterone and corticosterone, which are produced in the human adrenal to a small extent normally and in excessive amounts in certain pathological states. Deoxycorticosterone possesses approximately $1/30$ of the sodium-retaining potential of aldosterone, and corticosterone possesses even less of this activity.

The major effect of aldosterone is on the reabsorption of sodium in the distal renal tubule. This permits the intracellular sodium to increase in the tubule cell and potassium and hydrogenions to escape into the tubular lumen. The studies of Feldman, Fundar, and Edelman (6) revealed that aldosterone induces DNA formation and thereby increases extranuclear RNA production. These RNAs direct an increased synthesis of enzymes which increase oxidative phosphorylation from carbohydrate breakdown, thereby producing sufficient intracellular high energy phosphate bonds to supply the energy for the sodium pump. Deoxycorticosterone, a less powerful mineralocorticoid, also induces a sodium retention, but it is thought to possess a somewhat higher potassium-excreting activity. The sodium retention caused by aldosterone is not associated with edema, presumably because of the ability to increase glomerular filtration pressure and, thereby, water excretion. Deoxycorticosterone does not have this ability; hence, edema is often an accompaniment of excess deoxycorticosterone action.

Aldosterone has been shown to decrease carbohydrate metabolism ascribable to the associated hypokalemia. Replenishment of potassium effectively corrects this abnormal carbohydrate tolerance. It is assumed that deficiency of K^+ ions impairs the secretion and release of insulin by the β cells of the pancreas.

Biological Actions of Adrenal Androgens

The androgenic substances in adrenal hormone synthesis are dehydroepiandrosterone, androstenedione, and, in minimal amounts, testosterone. All except testosterone are 17-ketosteroids. The 17-KS compounds enhance amino acid incorporation into protein synthesis and oppose the deamination and transamination catabolic reactions of glucocorticoids. Testosterone is more powerful in this regard, but the amounts produced normally in the adrenals are minimal. The effect of these adrenal 17-KS and testosterone is more important in females since they lack any major other source of androgen production. Excessive amounts of these androgens induce hirsutism, a male habitus and clitoromegaly in females. In the male, large amounts of these androgens enhance the male habitus, cause deepening of the voice, and increase acne. If there is an excess of these compounds in the female fetus before birth, development of a male urogenital tract occurs.

CATABOLISM OF ADRENOCORTICAL SECRETIONS

As described previously, cortisol, the definitive glucocorticoid, circulates largely in a form bound to CBG, and small amounts in free form. It has been shown in some studies that, in the presence of large amounts of cortisol production, a small fraction may be loosely bound to albumin. Conditions which alter the levels of CBG may alter the ratio of bound cortisol to free cortisol. For example, patients receiving estrogens and birth control pills have an increase in CBG. Progesterone also has a strong affinity for CBG so that, in pregnancy and in the progesterone phase of the menstrual cycle, there is sufficient displacement of cortisol from CBG to result in somewhat higher levels of free cortisol. However, during later stages of pregnancy, the estrogen-induced CBG levels may be so high that the circulating total cortisol levels are elevated. In the presence of hepatocellular disease, nephrosis, amyloid disease, multiple myeloma, and congenital CBG deficiency, the levels of CBG are quite low. The protein binding permits the solubility of the steroids as well as protects the steroids from inactivation by the liver. Free cortisol is readily metabolized by the liver by certain enzymatic reactions which render the steroid biologically inactive. The biological half-life of cortisol is estimated to be 90 min; this is prolonged in liver disease and hypothyroidism and shortened in thyrotoxicosis. The major catabolism of cortisol takes place in the liver, but under certain conditions the extrahepatic catabolism may be considerable.

Steps in Cortisol Metabolism in Liver

The steps involved in the hepatic degradation of cortisol are similar to those involving aldosterone, cortisone, and corticosterone as well as many of the biosynthetic intermediates. For this reason, the steps in cortisol degradation will be considered as prototype for most of the other C-21 compounds from the adrenals. There are four pathways for cortisol degradation in the liver (and perhaps in extrahepatic tissues) (Figure 15.2).

1. The first pathway involves reduction of the Δ^4,3-ketone structure in ring A by a two-step reaction, first involving Δ^4-hydrogenase and requiring NADPH whereby cortisol is converted to dihydrocortisol. This compound is biologically inactive. This reductive step is impaired in hepatocellular disease. The second step is the reduction of the ketone group at C-3 by an α-hydroxysteroid dehydrogenase in the presence of NADH or NADPH. The resultant compound is tetrahydrocortisol. This compound is then conjugated to glucuronic acid at the hydroxyl group at C-3. The reaction involves the participation of uridine disphosphoglucuronic acid in the presence of glucuronyltransferase, with the resulting formation of a tetrahydrocortisol glucuronoside (glucuronide) (THF glucuronide). This transformation renders the compound water soluble, permitting excretion by the kidneys without any significant tubular reabsorption. This pathway of cortisol reduction amounts to approximately 45–50%.

2. In the second pathway, a small fraction of cortisol (5–10%) is degraded to 17-ketosteroid derivatives by cleavage of the side chain. The end products include 11β-hydroxyandrosterone and 11-ketoetiocholanolone. This pathway is also decreased in the presence of hepatocellular disease.

3. In the third pathway, there is reduction of the ketone group at C-20 to form the glycol side chain. This reaction may precede the reduction of the Δ^4,3-ketone group in some conditions.

4. In the fourth pathway, there is hydroxylation of the ring structure of cortisol by certain inducible hydroxylase enzymes, e.g., 6β hydroxylation which occurs in liver disease, pregnancy (7), following estrogen therapy, and after phenobarbital. This pathway is not a major one normally, but may assume some significance in the clinical states described above. Under such conditions also, other hydroxylations have been known to occur. For example, the newborn infant who has significant 6β hydroxylation path-

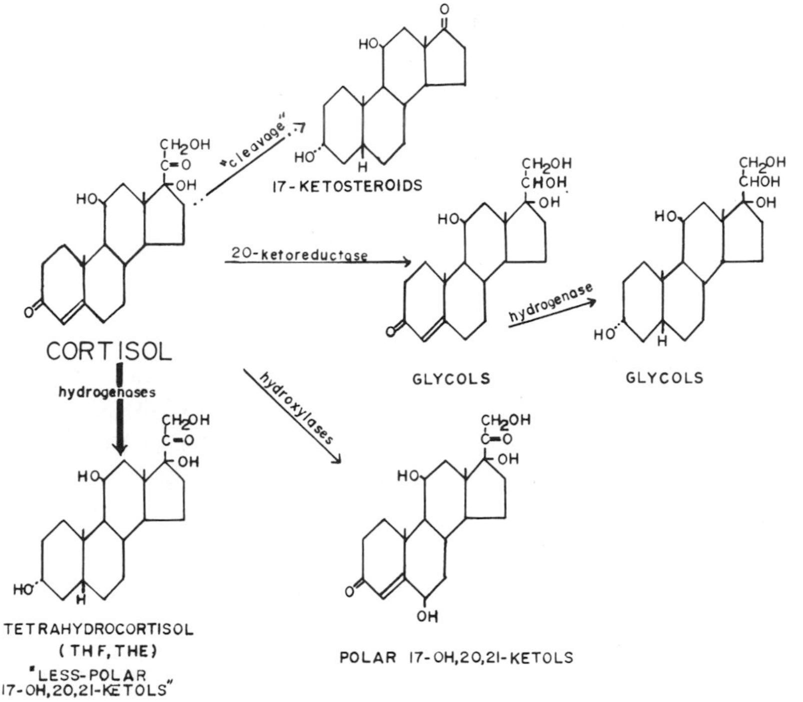

Figure 15.2. Pathways of cortisol degradation. The "cleavage" process involves the "desmolase" reaction. A portion of secreted cortisol is converted to glycine. The reduction of these two compounds to tetrahydrocortisol (THF) and tetrahydrocortisone (THE) involves two steps. The glycol derivatives may be formed directly from cortisol without prior reduction of ring A, as well as following ring A reduction. The process of 6β hydroxylation may represent an alternative excretory pathway when the THF-THE and 17-KS pathways are decreased, e.g., in hepatic cirrhosis and in the newborn. Enzymes involved are indicated in the figure. (Reprinted from Bacchus (3) with permission of the publisher.)

way may also produce 2α-hydroxyl derivatives of cortisol (8). These products are relatively water soluble and are excreted without prior glucuronosidation.

Catabolism of Aldosterone

The major pathway of aldosterone catabolism reported is via Step 1 listed above, i.e., by the formation of tetrahydroaldosterone and conjugation through glucuronyltransferase.

Catabolism of 17-Ketosteroids

Dehydroepiandrosterone is converted to the sulfate in the liver and kidneys, and most of circulating DHEA is present as the sulfate. Normal values range from 60–260 μg/100 ml, decreasing with age. DHEA, androstenedione, and testosterone, may all be reduced in ring A to form androsterone and etiocholanolone which are then excreted after glucuronide formation.

Catabolism of Certain Biosynthetic Intermediates

Progesterone This intermediate in adrenal hormone synthesis may accumulate whenever there is a synthetic block just distal to it, e.g., 17α-hydroxylase deficiency or C-21 hydroxylase deficiency. This compound is inactivated mainly through step 1 listed above, i.e., reduction of ring A with formation of pregnanediol (Figure 15.2). This end product is biologically inactive.

17-Hydroxyprogesterone This intermediate may also accumulate in the presence of certain biosynthetic defects. The pathway of degradation is mainly via step 1 listed above, i.e., with the formation of 17-hydroxy-pregnenolone (Figure 15.2). Further reduction at C-20 via step 3 listed above would result in the formation of pregnanetriol (Figure 15.1).

21-Deoxycortisol This compound accumulates when there is a defect in 21-hydroxylation. The reduction end product via step 1 above is 5β-pregnane-3α,11β,17α-triol,20-one. This on further reduction at C-20 will result in the formation of pregnane 3α,11β,17β,20-tetrol. It is well to note that the liver may dehydrogenate the 11-hydroxy group with the resultant formation of 11-ketopregnanetriol (Figure 15.1).

11-Deoxycortisol This compound accumulates when there is a defect in 11-hydroxylase, spontaneous or induced by metyrapone. The degradation product via step 1 above is tetrahydrocortisol (THS) (Figure 15.3) which is excreted as the glucuronide. In the presence of very large amounts of this compound, additional step 3 results in the formation of pregnan-3,17,20,21-tetrol.

Corticosterone (B) This compound may occur in the presence of 17α-hydroxylase deficiency in man. The degradation pathway is mainly via step 1 above to tetrahydrocorticosterone THB which is then excreted as the glucuronide or sulfate.

Deoxycorticosterone (DOC), similar to corticosterone, is excreted as tetrahydrodeoxycorticosterone (THDOC) glucuronide or as the sulfate.

CLINICAL DISORDERS OF ADRENOCORTICAL FUNCTION

Adrenocortical Insufficiency

The clinical manifestations of adrenal insufficiency are caused by a deficiency or absence either of cortisol or of aldosterone, or of both hormones. For this reason, it is occasionally possible to distinguish the glucocorticoid or the mineralocorticoid deficiency effects. The insufficiency patterns may be of a chronic nature or of acute onset; they may be caused by primary adrenal disease or be secondary to pituitary disease.

Acute Adrenocortical Insufficiency Acute adrenocortical insufficiency is a medical emergency in which the clinical manifestations are caused by a relative or absolute deficiency of cortisol and aldosterone. Acute clinical symptoms include lassitude, headache, confusion, restlessness, abdominal pain, nausea, and vomiting. Circulatory collapse which may lead to unconsciousness and shock. This constellation of symptoms caused by decrease in both glucocorticoids and mineralocorticoids is usually found in acute adrenal destruction. Such destruction may be caused by cellular necrosis and lipid depletion of cortical cells, with widened adrenal sinusoids filled with blood; this type of adrenal damage often follows meningococcemia, but other infections may be responsible; these include pneumococci, streptococci, and H. influenzae. Several features of the adrenal destruction suggest intravascular coagulopathy. Other etiologies include trauma of prolonged labor (found in newborns), pemphigus, leukemias, hemorrhagic disorders, anticoagulant therapy, and adrenal thrombosis. A fairly common form of acute adrenocortical insufficiency is now seen in patients maintained on pharmacological doses of glucocorticoids who subsequently develop latent adrenal insufficiency.

Clinical Diagnosis of Acute Adrenocortical Insufficiency Adrenal hemorrhage should be suspected in the presence of fulminating sepsis especially if complicated by cutaneous hemorrhages, petechiae, and purpura. Postoperative vascular collapse should also suggest this diagnosis.

Laboratory Diagnosis of Acute Adrenocortical Insufficiency In this medical emergency, there is almost invariably insufficient time for laboratory confirmation. Occasionally, a high total eosinophil count ($>50/\text{mm}^3$) may be strongly suggestive, since, in shock of other cause, there is usually an eosinopenia. A serum sodium to potassium ratio is occasionally helpful if it drops from the usual 30 toward 20. It is occasionally possible to measure serum cortisol by the fluorimetric method as an emergency procedure. In adrenocortical insufficiency, the values are low or normal, whereas, in shock of other cause, the adrenals are capable of increasing cortisol release by severalfold. It is suggested that suspected cases should be treated with glucocorticoids after a plasma sample is obtained for cortisol determination to be done later.

Chronic Adrenocortical Insufficiency Chronic adrenocortical insufficiency may be caused by primary adrenal disease or secondary to pituitary insufficiency. The spectrum of disorders includes general adrenocortical failure, isolated hypoaldosteronism, or isolated decrease in cortisol and 17-KS such as in adrenal insufficiency following exogenous steroid therapy.

Addison's Disease (Primary Chronic Adrenocortical Insuffi-

ciency) Addison (cited in Ref. 1) directed attention to "anemia, general languor and debility, remarkable feebleness of the heart's action, irritability of the stomach, and a peculiar change in the color of the skin." All manifestations in that description, except for the pigmentary changes, are caused by deficiency in the cortical hormones which is also the basis of weakness and fatigability, weight loss and dehydration, hypotension, small heart, anorexia, nausea, vomiting, diarrhea, and epigastric pain, dizziness, syncopal attacks, nervousness, mental changes, and, occasionally, hypoglycemic symptoms. Some patients may complain of muscle cramps and salt-craving and may have flexion contractures of the hands. Etiologies of Addison's disease include: idiopathic atrophy of the adrenals, possibly on an autoimmune basis (50–60% of cases are in this group); tuberculosis (accounting for 30–40% of cases); rarer causes, such as histoplasmosis, metastatic disease, hemochromatosis, amyloidosis, and vascular accidents.

Laboratory Diagnosis of Chronic Adrenocortical Insufficiency The availability of sensitive methods for measurement of plasma cortisol and urinary corticosteroids makes it unnecessary to depend on indirect tests, but two indirect tests, because of their relative reliability and simplicity, are recommended in screening for adrenal insufficiency. These are: 1) water diuresis test (a failure to excrete over 1,000 ml of the ingested 1,500 ml of water is considered as compatible with adrenal insufficiency); and 2) the serum sodium to potassium ratio is lower than 30 and approaches 20 in adrenal insufficiency, probably a reflection of mineralocorticoid deficiency.

The direct procedures include study of plasma cortisol and responsiveness to corticotropin stimulation, and urinary steroids and the responsiveness to similar stimulation. The following sequence of studies is recommended:

1. In plasma cortisol response to intravenous cosyntropin, an adequate increment in plasma cortisol after cosyntropin effectively rules out adrenocortical insufficiency. The absence of significant increase in plasma cortisol is compatible with adrenocortical insufficiency. In this case, it is useful to repeat the test with repeat injections at 1-hr intervals for 3 doses, at which intervals there should be progressive increases in plasma cortisol in patients with latent adrenal insufficiency. Failure to obtain incremental increases would be compatible with primary adrenal insufficiency. As an alternative, the following procedure may be useful.
2. The repeated 8-hr intravenous ACTH test is performed. Failure of significant incremental increases in urinary 17-OHCS in 17-KGS would be compatible with primary adrenal insufficiency. Incremental increases after repeated challenges would suggest secondary adrenal insufficiency.

Secondary Adrenocortical Insufficiency Secondary adrenocortical insufficiency may occur as part of a multiglandular deficiency of ACTH. The clinical manifestations in adrenocortical insufficiency secondary to panhypopituitarism are similar to Addison's disease except for the lack of pigmentation, but will be complicated by evidence of other hormonal deficiencies, e.g., with hypothyroidism, an associated hypometabolism, coarse skin, alopecia, bradycardia, with hypogonadism, decreased libido, decrease in pubic and axillary hair, amenorrhea, and atrophic vaginal changes in the female. Isolated ACTH deficiency will be similar to Addison's disease except for an absence of pigmentation and a less marked defect in mineral metabolism.

In the laboratory work-up for this type of clinical problem, the following studies are recommended. The vasopressin stimulation test is a relatively simple procedure based on the ability of vasopressin to either act as a corticotropin-releasing factor or to stimulate release of CRF. Increases in plasma cortisol after vasopressin challenge would effectively rule out pituitary ACTH insufficiency. A failure to increase plasma corticol in the face of good response to intravenous cosyntropin would be compatible with pituitary ACTH deficiency. The metyrapone tests, by either intravenous infusion (30 mg/kg in 500 ml of normal saline over a 4-hr period) or ingestion of tablets (750 mg every 4 hr for 24 hr), monitored by urinary 17-OHCS, 17-KGS, or 11-deoxy-17-OHCS, is another recommended study. A more rapid procedure is to give the patient 750 mg of metyrapone with an antacid by mouth at midnight and check the plasma level of 11-deoxycortisol at 8:00 a.m. the next day. A level of deoxycortisol greater than 4 mg/100 ml is compatible with normal pituitary adrenal axis function (1). Pituitary ACTH deficiency should be considered in a patient who exhibits significant adrenal response to repeat ACTH (or cosyntropin) challenges and fails to exhibit a significant increase in the steroid parameters after metyrapone administration. The third procedure, plasma cortisol response to insulin hypoglycemia, is essentially similar to that for GH response (Chapter 13) except that cortisol levels are monitored in this procedure (in most cases it is recommended that both plasma GH and cortisol should be measured during this test, as it is often necessary to determine multiple pituitary function). A normal response is a doubling of the plasma cortisol or an increment of at least 7 μg/100 ml when baseline cortisol is low. Lack of such response, in a patient who responded adequately to cosyntropin, would be consistent with pituitary ACTH deficiency or with lack of hypothalamic CRF response.

Treatment of Adrenocortical Insufficiency

Acute Adrenocortical Insufficiency The immediate treatment goals of treatment of acute adrenocortical insufficiency are to replace fluids to combat dehydration and shock, replace cortisol, and identify the precipitating cause. Vital signs should be monitored continuously or at least every 30 min, and an infusion of 5% glucose in normal saline should be started. Additional solutions may be infused through the tubing. Soluble cortisol (as hemisuccinate) is given intravenously at the dose range of 100–200 mg (in adults) immediately, to be followed by 50–100 mg every 2–4 hr thereafter. Such high doses at these intervals are necessary because of the short biological half-life of this water-soluble cortisol preparation. If there is continued shock, the potent pressor agent angiotensin II (available as hypertensin-Schering) should be employed in preference to norepinephrine or metarminol. If the precipitating cause is identified, appropriate treatment should be instituted at this time.

On the 2nd day, if the patient has stabilized to some degree, cortisone acetate may be substituted by mouth at the dosage of 50 mg/day if oral intake is possible. Otherwise, cortisol hemisuccinate 100–150 mg/day may be given parenterally. With further stabilization, the patient may be continued on a regular diet with adequate sodium chloride, and between 25–37.5 mg of cortisone acetate by mouth daily, as the maintenance dose in chronic adrenocortisol insufficiency. It is recommended that the mineralocorticoid 9α-fluorocortisol be given by mouth at the dose range of 0.1 mg daily. The correct dosage may not be monitored by serum or urine potassium values.

Treatment of Chronic Adrenocortical Insufficiency The therapeutic goals are maintenance of blood volume, restoration of strength, weight, blood pressure, hemoglobin, and blood sugar to essentially normal levels. Cortisol or cortisone acetate is given in replacement dosages, 25 mg daily. Patients who have laboratory or clinical evidence of mineralocorticoid insufficiency are given 0.05–0.2 mg of 9α-fluorocortisol daily, the adequacy of the dosage being monitored by serum or urine electrolytes. Excessive dosages of this mineralocorticoid may result in edema, headache, hypertension, contractures of tendons, and hypokalemia.

Because of the nature of this chronic disorder, the patient should carry a "dog-tag" indicating the diagnosis. Intercurrent stresses or infections may require increased steroid dosages.

Treatment of Secondary Adrenocortical Insufficiency The management of the adrenocortical insufficiency component of this disorder requires replacement doses of cortisol or cortisone acetate. Mineralocorticoid replacement is required very rarely. The other target gland deficiencies should be treated with replacement doses of thyroxin or triiodothyronine (for thyroid), testosterone propionate or cypionate (for male gonadal insufficiency), and estrogens (for female gonadal insufficiency).

Diseases of Adrenocortical Hyperfunction

Hypercortisol and hyperaldosterone disorders are discussed in this section. Biosynthetic defects in the adrenals are discussed in a separate section.

Cushing's Syndrome This disorder is relatively rare, but there are series which suggest a prevalence of 1 in every 1,000 autopsies. It is described as 3–4 times more common in women than in men. The peak incidence is described at between 20–40 years, but the disease has been found in younger as well as older patients. The syndrome is caused by excess adrenal hormones, mainly cortisol, whether because of nonpathological states such as chronic stress or because of three groups of pathological processes, viz, excessive pituitary ACTH with adrenocortical hyperplasia; autonomous adrenocortical neoplasia; or ectopic production of ACTH with consequent adrenal hyperplasia. The adrenals of approximately 10% of patients with Cushing's syndrome show no overt pathology, 60% show hypertrophy and hyperplasia, and 30% show tumors (of which one-half are benign and somewhat less than half are malignant).

Cushing's Syndrome Caused by Excess ACTH Most of these patients have a defect in the regulation of the hypothalamus-pituitary axis as the hypothalamic corticotropin-releasing factor (CRF) mechanism is not responsive to feedback inhibition by circulating cortisol. About 10% of this group have ACTH secreting tumors, either small basophilic adenomas or larger chromophobe adenomas. Patients with bilateral adrenal hyperplasia who were treated by bilateral adrenalectomy may develop chromophobe or basophilic adenomas, some appearing years after the adrenalectomy. These patients secrete large amounts of ACTH and may show considerable amounts of pigmentation as a result. In the patients with adrenocortical hyperplasia, the zona glomerulosa is usually spared of marked histological changes.

Cushing's Syndrome Caused by Adrenocortical Neoplasia Approximately 30% of patients with Cushing's syndrome have autonomous adrenal tumors, in most cases benign adenomas, and, less frequently, carcinomas. The cortisol produced by these tumors suppresses ACTH activity, and, as a consequence, the contralateral adrenal as well as non-tumorous adrenal tissue contiguous with the tumor becomes atrophic.

Cushing's Syndrome Caused by Ectopic ACTH Production Over 100 cases of this syndrome have been reported and with a variety of nonadrenal malignant neoplasms. This disorder has been most frequently reported in association with anaplastic small cell bronchogenic carcinoma. It has occurred in association with pancreatic tumors, malignant thymomas, thyroid and ovarian carcinoma, bronchial adenoma, as well as with other malignant neoplasms.

Clinical Picture in Cushing's Syndrome The major manifestations are caused by hypercortisolemia. These include changes in carbohydrate, protein, and fat metabolism leading to muscle wasting, centripetal redistribution of body fat, with cervicodorsal fat pat, moon-facies, and pendulous abdomen. The skin is thin, with atrophic subcutaneous tissues, and superimposed on this is an erythrocytosis, hence, the plethoric appearance. Purple striae in the abdomen, back, and breasts also appear. Increased capillary fragility is the basis of easy bruisability and abrasions. The hypercortisolemia is also the basis of decreased osteoblastic activity and decreased bone matrix with resulting osteoporosis. This may give rise to back pain and deformities in the spine. Demineralization of the skull is also a feature in the syndrome.

Approximately 90% of these patients exhibit glucose intolerance, but they are not prone to ketoacidosis. An increase in arteriosclerosis in these patients has been ascribed to hyperlipidemia, but hypertension may also be a factor. Hirsutism and acne are caused by an increased production of androgenic 17-ketosteroids by the hyperplasic adrenals. Approximately less than 10% of patients with Cushing's syndrome may show an elevation of aldosterone with resultant hypokalemic alkalosis.

It has been suggested by Forsham (1) that the presence of three or more of the following symptoms strongly suggest Cushing's syndrome: extreme weakness and muscle wasting, obesity with centripetal fat distribution, marked growth arrest in children, red and linear striae, ecchymoses in the presence of normal platelet counts, hypertension, osteoporosis, and hyperglycemic glucose tolerance tests. Sudden onset of symptoms would suggest an adenoma or adenocarcinoma; slower progression should suggest bilateral adrenal hyperplasia.

Laboratory Diagnosis of Cushing's Syndrome The typical patient with Cushing's syndrome will show a leukocytosis with relative lymphopenia, and neutrophilia and eosinopenia. Most of these patients will also have an erythrocytosis with hematocrits of 50% or greater. Either an elevated fasting or postprandial blood sugar is also suggestive, as is a diabetic type glucose tolerance curve. About 10–15% of patients with Cushing's syndrome (especially associated with ectopic ACTH or adenocarcinoma of the adrenal) have a hypokalemic alkalosis despite normal aldosterone levels.

Definitive tests in hypercortisolemia syndromes include: 1) plasma cortisol levels (samples drawn at 8:00 a.m. and at 5:00 p.m. are higher than 25 μg/100 ml, and reveal lack of normal circadian variation); 2) one dose overnight dexamethasone suppression test (the 8:00 a.m. plasma cortisol after receiving 1.0 mg of dexamethasone the previous 11:00 p.m. is below 5 μg/100 ml in normal subjects, and 10 μg/100 ml in obese subjects. Patients with Cushing's syndrome show plasma cortisol levels of 10 μg/100 ml); and 3) urine-free cortisol measurement (3) is quite useful in diagnosis of hypercortisolism. In Cushing's syndrome the levels in urine exceed the normal value of 60–150 μg/24 hr by severalfold. (Additional studies in the differential diagnosis of hypercortisolemic syndromes are presented in Table 15.1.)

Treatment of Cushing's Syndrome Bilateral adrenocortical hyperplasia causing Cushing's syndrome is most effectively treated by bilateral adrenalectomy. After extirpation of the glands, replacement therapy with cortisol or cortisone acetate is imperative. Higher doses are required initially postoperatively, followed by maintenance doses of cortisol, 30 mg/day (or of cortisone acetate in equivalent doses). Addition of 9α-fluorohydrocortisone (0.05–0.1 mg daily) is often required for mineralocortocoid replacement. Approximately 10% of patients treated by surgery may be found a few years later to have basophilic or chromophobe adenomas of the pituitary which may be locally invasive, affecting the visual fields. Hyperpigmentation is a frequent accompaniment in this disorder (Nelson's syndrome).

Cushing's syndrome caused by adrenocortical adenoma is treated surgically, either by resection of the tumor or by unilateral adrenalectomy. Because of atrophy of the remaining non-tumorous adrenal tissue, short-term ACTH stimulation is occasionally employed. The patients may need low dose cortisol replacement until the remaining adrenal tissue becomes active.

In the presence of pituitary overactivity, irradiation, cryosurgery, or yttrium implants may be helpful. Pituitary tumors are treated by surgical hypophysectomy. Replacement therapy of the target endocrine gland functions is imperative (thyroid, adrenals, and gonadal).

Medical management of Cushing's syndrome may be employed in functioning adrenocortical carcinoma. Effective agents include aminoglutethimide, o,p, DDD (1,1-dichloro-2-(O-chlorophenyl)-2-(p-chlorophenyl)ethane, amphenone, and metryapone. These agents block adrenocortical hormone synthesis.

Diseases of Mineralocorticoid Excess

A small number of patients with Cushing's syndrome may exhibit manifestations of aldosterone excess, viz., hypokalemic hypochloremic alkalosis and some elevation in urinary aldosterone. In some of these patients there is also an elevation of the nonaldosterone mineralocorticoids, corticosterone, and deoxycorticosterone, a result of hypernormal adrenocortical biosynthetic pathways.

Primary Hyperaldosteronism In 1955, Conn (9) described a syndrome consisting of arterial hypertension, hypokalemic alkalosis, and muscle weakness, associated with vasopressin-resistant polyuria which he proved to be caused by an excess of aldosterone produced by an adrenocortical

Table 15.1. Laboratory Differentiation of Cushing's Syndrome

Test	Normal	Hyperplasia	Adenoma	Carcinoma
17-Hydroxycorticosteroids (17-OHCS)	2.5–8 mg/24 hr	↑ (14)	↑ (25–30)	↑↑ (50+)
ACTH stimulation	↑↑ (2–4x)	↑↑↑ (4x)	↑↑↑ (4x)	No increment
Dexamethasone suppression				
Light (2 mg/day for 3 days)	↓ (0.5x)	No change	No change	No change
Heavy (8 mg/day for 3 days)	↓ (0.5x)	↓ (0.5x)	↑ (2x)	↑↑↑ (10x)
17-Ketogenic steroids	8–18 mg/24 hr			
ACTH stimulation	↑↑ (2x)	↑↑ (2–3x)	↑↑ (2–3x)	No increment
Dexamethasone suppression				
Light	↓ (0.5x)	No change	No change	No change
Heavy	↓	↓	↑ or normal	No change
17-Ketosteroids	7–15 mg/24 hr	↑ (20)	↑ or normal	↑↑↑ (6x)
ACTH stimulation	↑ (2x)	↑ (2x)	↑ (2x)	No increment
Dexamethasone suppression				
Light	↓ (0.5x)	No change	No change	No change
Heavy		↓ (0.5x)	No change	No change

tumor. The current estimate is that aldosterone-producing tumors, in contrast to hyperplasia, are now the most common form of adrenocortical origin. Aldosterone tumors are usually benign, solitary canary-yellow, containing cells resembling the zona glomerulosa. These tumors may also secrete increased amounts of corticosterone and DOC.

Major clinical manifestations of primary hyperaldosteronism include hypertension, hypokalemia, polyuria, polydipsia, alkalosis, albuminuria, paresthesias, and periodic paralysis. Edema is present only as a complication of hypertension; sodium retention in this state permits an increased glomerular filtration, and there is an escape from "sodium-induced edema." Hypokalemia is often a late sign of this problem, and it may be antedated by hypertension by years (10). There is a relative paucity of retinal arterial disease seen in these patients. Severe headaches may be a manifestation of hypertension.

Decreased total exchangeable potassium is present in all patients with aldosteronism, despite occasional normal serum potassium values. Hypokalemia is more likely to occur when the sodium intake is normal or high, and may be normalized when the sodium intake is low. Hypokalemia is responsible for a fluctuating muscle weakness, postural hypotension, and a peculiar type of tetany (positive Trousseau's and Chvostek's signs) seen more frequently during potassium repletion. Renal concentration defects may result from hypokalemic tubular nephropathy.

Secondary Hyperaldosteronism Excessive and occasionally inappropriate overproduction of aldosterone is observed in some edematous states such as hepatic cirrhosis, nephrosis, and congestive heart failure, occasionally during salt deprivation, in hypovolemia, and in malignant hypertension. Secondary hyperaldosteronism is regularly associated with nephrosis, cirrhosis, and almost invariably with malignant hypertension, other edematous states showing variable increases. Decreased intravascular volume in edematous states induces a release of renin which increases the production of angiotensin, with subsequent activation of the zona glomerulosa to produce increased amounts of aldosterone; subsequent hypernatremia exacerbates the edema. Increased aldosterone secretion during salt deprivation is a compensatory mechanism to aid in retaining sodium. Aldosteronemia in malignant hypertension is secondary to a rise in renin secretion; the most common etiologies in this type of hypertension are intrarenal vascular obstruction and intrarenal lesions not involving large renal occlusion.

The clinical picture seen in secondary hyperaldosteronism is similar to that in the primary form complicated by the underlying cause, e.g., edema and hepatic disease. Nervous, high-strung women may have a cyclic edema with increased aldosterone levels noted during the edematous phases. A defect in the hypothalamic control of ADH is presumed to be responsible for the edema (11), but a disturbance in capillary fragility permitting loss of fluid to the interstitium is undoubtedly an important contributory factor.

Non-Aldosterone Hypermineralocorticoid Syndromes These include the biosynthetic defects in the adrenal cortex such as 17α-hydroxylase and 11β-hydroxylase deficiency. 17α-Hydroxylase deficiency is associated with increased corticosterone and DOC causing hypertension and hypokalemic alkalosis; hypogonadism is caused by decreased androgen release secondary to the biosynthetic defect in the adrenal. 11β-Hydroxylase deficiency is characterized by hypertension and hypokalemic alkalosis caused by accumulation of DOC; virilization noted in this state is caused by increased androgen release secondary to the biosynthetic defect in the adrenal.

Laboratory Tests in Diagnosis of Hypermineralocorticoid States The oral or intravenous sodium chloride loading tests may be monitored by the serum potassium levels; in patients with hyperaldosteronism, the high sodium intake is followed by a decrease in serum potassium to 3.5 mEq/liter or lower. The spironolactone test is best done in patients with hypokalemia. The administration of spironolactone to patients with hyperaldosteronism and hypokalemia is followed by an increase in serum potassium of greater than 1 mEq/liter.

Tests Involving Measurement of Urinary or Plasma Aldosterone In the first test, plasma aldosterone levels are measured after sodium loading procedures (2 liters of normal saline in 3 hr) and are compared to levels in a baseline plasma sample. In hyperaldosteronism, the sodium loading procedure fails to induce a reduction in plasma aldosterone levels. (Urinary excretion of aldosterone may be measured in this procedure also.)

In the second test, deoxycorticosterone (DOC) suppression test, injection of 5 mg of DOC acetate four times daily or oral intake of 0.1 mg of 9α-fluorocortisol four times daily is followed by a decrease in plasma aldosterone levels in normal subjects. Initially high values in secondary aldosteronism decrease to normal ranges, but the high levels in primary aldosteronism are essentially unaltered.

In the third test, plasma renin activity (PRA) responses to challenges in posture and salt intake are helpful in distinguishing aldosteronism associated with high PRA (secondary) and with low PRA (primary).

The fourth test, adrenal venography and cannulation for aldosterone levels in adrenal veins, is usually employed in patients with aldosterone excess. The affected adrenal and location of the tumors may be identified. It is well to note, however, that most aldosteronomas are less than 3 cm in diameter.

Treatment of Hyperaldosteronism Aldosterone-producing tumors are resected surgically. These patients may suffer a temporary hypoaldosteronism soon after surgery. Mild cases of normokalemic primary hyper-aldosteronism with mild hypertension are treated with spironolactone. Rare cases of ACTH-dependent aldosteronism associated with adrenal hyperplasia are treated with ACTH suppressive doses of dexamethasone.

CLINICAL SYNDROMES CAUSED BY BIOSYNTHETIC DEFECTS IN ADRENAL CORTEX

This group of clinical disorders is most simply considered in the context of the biosynthetic scheme presented in Figure 15.1. The clinical manifesta-tions are caused by effects of the accumulation of compounds proximal to the biosynthetic defect; greatest accumulation occurs in the compound (or compounds) which is the immediate substrate for the blocked reaction. In view of the biosynthetic blocks in the adrenal cortex, it is expected that there should always be a decreased level of cortisol in such patients. Indeed this occurs often, the plasma cortisol or urinary 11-oxy-17-OHCS being low or at the lower normal limits, but in most cases there is a compensatory reaction whereby a large amount of substrate aids in in-ducing some enzymatic conversion. The most common forms of the biosynthetic problems involve steps late in the sequence, viz., 21-hydroxy-lase deficiency and 11β-hydroxylase deficiency. Other deficiencies, e.g., 17α-hydroxylase, Δ^5,3β-ol dehydrogenase, and demolase, occur less fre-quently and are rapidly fatal unless diagnosed early. All of these defects are associated with adrenocortical hyperplasia; the hypocortisolemia in-duces increased ACTH release and continued stimulation of the adrenal cortex.

Adrenocortical Hyperplasia Caused by C-21 Hydroxylase Deficiency

This is the most common form of adrenocortical hyperplasia caused by biosynthetic defect, and it may be congenital in origin with manifestations quite early in development (CAH) or may become overt postpubertally. The defect may be partial (more frequent) or "complete" (e.g., salt-losing form of CAH), in which insufficient amounts of aldosterone are produced. The difference between the affinity of 17-hydroxyprogesterone and pro-gesterone for 21-hydroxylase may well explain presence of aldosterone production in the non-salt-losing form. The scheme in Figure 15.3 depicts accumulation of 17-hydroxyprogesterone and 21-deoxycortisol; 17-hy-droxyprogesterone may serve as a precursor of weak 17-KS androgens, but there is also retrograde piling up and accumulation of compounds formed from alternate pathways, e.g., C-19-androgens from the androgen pathway. The androgen effects depend on age of the individual at the time critical levels are achieved; malformations around the urogenital sinus and external

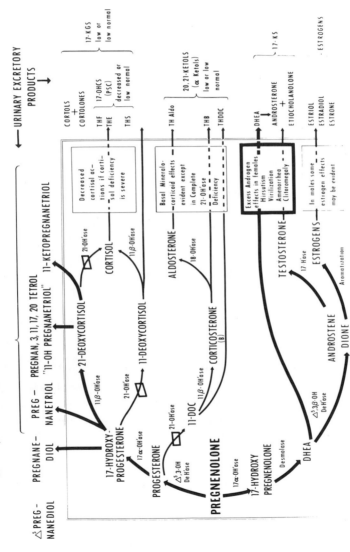

Figure 15.3. Clinical features and pattern of corticosteroid metabolites found in adrenocortical 21-hydroxylase deficiency. Pregnanetriol and 11-ketopregnanetriol, among others, are increased in this defect. Clinical manifestations are listed in the rectangular boxes. Urinary end products are depicted outside the double-lined large rectangle. (Reprinted from Bacchus (3) with permission of the publisher.)

genitalia may occur in early onset of the defect. If the critical levels are achieved later, then the manifestations include hirsutism, clitoromegaly, and amenorrhea. Figure 15.3 also reveals that the major urinary steroids which accumulate in this defect are pregnanetriol, 11-ketopregnanetriol, pregnanolone, and pregnan-3,11,17,20-tetrol (see Figure 15.3).

Adrenocortical Hyperplasia Caused by 11β-Hydroxylase Deficiency

A lack or decrease of the 11β-hydroxylating enzyme results in accumulation of 11-deoxycortisol (S) and its reduction product THS, which are biological inactive. The defect also leads to an accumulation of 11-deoxycorticosterone, a powerful mineralocorticoid, hence the occurrence of hypertension (hypertensive congenital adrenal hyperplasia (HCAH)) and hypokalemic alkolosis. Hirsutism, pseudohermaphroditism, and macrogenitosomia also occur, the results of androgenic derivatives of the precursors and of steroids from alternate biosynthetic pathways. Pigmentation also occurs because of increased ACTH. The compounds which accumulate in this defect include tetrahydrodeoxycortisol, its 20-reduced derivative pregnan-3,17,20,21-tetrol, and 17-ketosteroids from enhanced alternative pathways (Figure 15.4).

Adrenocortical Hyperplasia Caused by 17α-Hydroxylase Deficiency

This syndrome first described by Biglieri, Herron, and Brust (11) is caused by a deficiency in 17α hydroxylation reactions, resulting in absent or decreased formation of 17-hydroxypregnenolone and of 17-hydroxyprogesterone in the adrenals and in the gonads. The former defect leads to decreased formation of the gonadal hormones (androgens and estrogens), and the defective formation of 17-hydroxyprogesterone is the basis of hypocortisolemia. The pathway to DOC and corticosterone is quite active (Figure 15.5). These active mineralocorticoids induce hypertension and hypokalemic alkalosis. The glucocorticoid action of corticosterone partly substitutes for the cortisol lack. The decreased gonadal hormones are responsible for manifestations of hypogonadism as the enzymatic defect is also present in the gonads. The compounds which accumulate (Figure 15.5) include DOC and its reduction product THDOC, corticosterone (B), and its tetrahydro derivative THB. Trace to low levels of 17-KS and estrogens are formed.

Adrenocortical Hyperplasia Caused by
Δ^5,3-Hydroxydehydrogenase (Δ^5,3β-ol Dehydrogenase) Deficiency

This syndrome, originally described by Bongiovanni (12), is caused by a defect in the conversion of pregnenolone to progesterone; also because of this defect 17-hydroxypregnenolone is not converted to strong androgens and estrogens (Figure 15.6). These patients die early because of severe

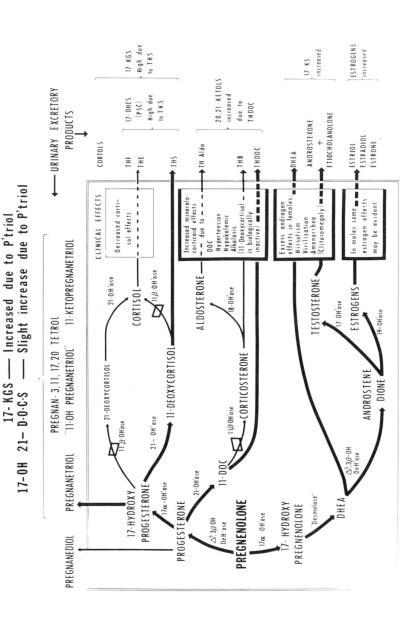

Figure 15.4. Clinical features and corticosteroid metabolites in adrenocortical 11β-hydroxylase deficiency. Clinical manifestations are presented in the small boxes. Urinary end products are depicted outside the double-lined rectangle. (Reprinted from Bacchus (3) with permission of the publisher.)

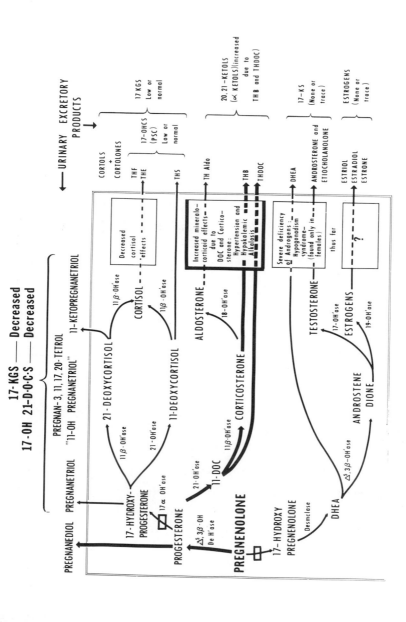

Figure 15.5. Clinical features and pattern of corticosteroid metabolites in adrenocortical 17α-hydroxylase deficiency. Clinical features are listed in the small rectangular boxes. Urinary excretion products are depicted outside the double-lined rectangle. (Reprinted from Bacchus (3) with permission of the publisher.)

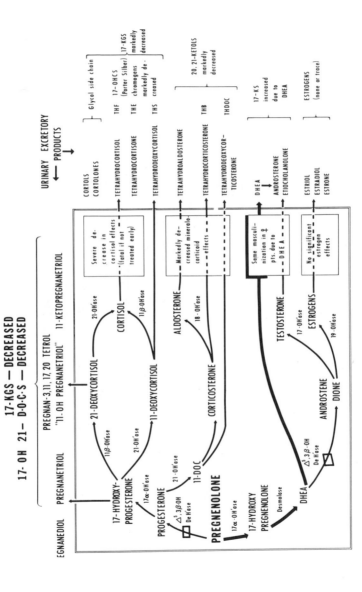

Figure 15.6. Clinical features and pattern of corticosteroid metabolites in adrenocortical Δ⁵,3β-ol dehydrogenase (3β-hydroxysteroid dehydrogenase, HSD) deficiency. Clinical features are listed in the small rectangles, and urinary excretion products are outside the double-lined rectangle. (Reprinted from Bacchus (3) with permission of the publisher.)

adrenal crisis, i.e., deficiency in cortisol and aldosterone. Males with this syndrome show incomplete sexual differentiation with hypospadias. The enzymatic defect also occurs in the testes. Female patients with this syndrome show mild virilization caused by the accumulation of dehydroepiandrosterone. In this enzymatic defect, the following steroids accumulate: derivatives of 17-hydroxypregnenolone, such as Δ^5-pregnenetriol and pregnenetriolone, as well as of dehydroepiandrosterone and its derivatives, DHA sulfate, androsterone, and etiocholanolone.

Adrenocortical Hyperplasia Caused by Defect in Conversion of Cholesterol to Steroid Hormones (Desmolase Defect)

The ovaries and testes are also involved and the adrenal glands are lipid-filled and enlarged. This syndrome was reported by Prader and Gurtner (13). No survivals are reported, the patients dying of severe adrenocortical insufficiency in early infancy. Because of lack of gonadal hormones, genotypic males are born with pseudohermaphroditism, i.e., the intrauterine Müllerian duct system is presented indefinitely.

Adrenocortical Hyperplasia Caused by 18α-Hydroxylase Defect

An 18α-hydroxylase deficiency with decreased aldosterone production and salt loss has been reported. The syndrome is not fully characterized. A defect in 18-hydroxydehydrogenase with elevated levels of 18-hydroxycorticosterone has been reported in one patient with excess salt loss.

There have been reports of adrenogenital syndromes presumably caused by acquired biosynthetic defects in tumors of the adrenal. Diagnosis and procedures are similar to those for adrenocortical tumors in general. The accumulation of abnormal metabolites is not suppressible by exogenous corticosteroids in the neoplastic conditions.

Treatment of Adrenal Hyperplasia Caused by Biosynthetic Defects

The common feature in all of the defects in non-neoplastic glands is excessive production of ACTH in response to decreased cortisol suppression of CRF (and ACTH). In 17α-hydroxylase deficiency, the component of hypogonadal manifestations is added because this defect is also present in the gonads.

The basic therapy in all forms of these biosynthetic defects is administration of doses of dexamethasone sufficient to suppress the excess ACTH release. Doses of dexamethasone (0.5–0.75 mg) or of prednisolone (5–7.5 mg) given preferably at bedtime adequately suppress the excess ACTH. Urinary 17-KS or plasma or urinary levels of the distinctive end products are employed in monitoring therapy. The hypogonadal manifestations in 17α-hydroxylase deficiency are treated with gonadal hormones appropriate to the sex of the patient.

IDIOPATHIC HIRSUTISM

Idiopathic hirsutism is commonly found especially in women in the reproductive years and in the menopause. Only slightly elevated levels of plasma testosterone are noted in most patients, however. Many patients reveal a significant decrease in plasma testosterone after dexamethasone suppression. Others may show decreased testosterone after long-term estrogen therapy. Increased testosterone levels after HCG stimulation exceed those seen in normal women. Recent data (14) reveal that androstenedione levels are elevated out of proportion to the testosterone levels, and the increased androstenedione after ACTH pulses exceeds that in normal subjects. It is now evident, therefore, that an element of increased adrenal androgen production is operative in these patients. The usefulness of corticosteroid suppression in this disorder now seems logical. The possibility that some of these patients possess increased amounts of cytosol receptor and, therefore, an end-organ hyper-responsiveness to androgens is to be seriously considered.

FEMINIZING ADRENOCORTICAL TUMORS

This condition is rare; less than 100 have been reported. The basic mechanism is the over-production of large amounts of estrogen by adrenal carcinoma or adenoma; 17-KS are also elevated. As expected, these elevated levels do not suppress with dexamethasone.

LABORATORY DIAGNOSIS OF ADRENOCORTICAL HYPERPLASIA WITH BIOSYNTHETIC DEFECTS

Since all of these problems are characterized by hyperplasia induced by ACTH, then dexamethasone suppression tests will be helpful in all cases. The steroids which are elevated differ with each defect and are used to monitor the effectiveness of suppressibility.

The compounds expected to accumulate in these syndromes have been discussed above (Figures 15.1, 15.3–15.6), but will be referred to in connection with the specific problems.

Urinary 17-Ketosteroids

The 17-KS are elevated in the C-21 hydroxylase deficiency and 11β-hydroxylase deficiency, and, therefore, the 17-KS levels may be used to monitor suppressibility with dexamethasone. In a patient with virilization, hypertension, and hypokalemic alkalosis, an elevated 17-KS suppressible by dexamethasone would strongly suggest 11β-hydroxylase deficiency.

Similarly, in a patient with virilization, without hypermineralocorticoidism, an elevated 17-KS suppressible by dexamethasone would be consistent with 21-hydroxylase deficiency. Specific identification of metabolites characteristic of the biosynthetic defect is possible and recommended. Studies on 17-KS excretion will not be particularly helpful in the identification of defect in 17 hydroxylation as 17-KS should be decreased in this condition. An increase in 17-KS in Δ^5,3β-ol dehydrogenase deficiency reflecting increased levels of dehydroepiandrosterone, androsterone, and etiocholanolone may be helpful in suppression studies in that defect.

Specific Identification of Defects

In the presence of C-21 hydroxylase deficiency, the metabolites found in excess are pregnanetriol, 17-hydroxypregnenolone, and, occasionally, 11-ketopregnenolone. In normal individuals, pregnanetriol excretion ranges from 0–3 mg/24 hr; 17-hydroxypregnenolone, 0–1.0 mg/24 hr with only traces of 11-ketopregnanetriol. In the presence of 21-hydroxylase deficiency, these values increase to 10–70 mg, 10–20 mg, and 5 mg/24 hr, respectively. The entire group of these compounds may be quantitated by a method for total 17-hydroxy-21-deoxycorticosteroids (3). This value is normally 0.8–3.0 mg/24 hr; in CAH, the values are increased by 10-fold or more; in the postpubertal form of this disorder, the levels are increased 3- to 5-fold.

In C-11 hydroxylase deficiency, the following compounds, in addition to 17-KS, are found in increased amounts in the urine: THS and its C-20 reduced derivative, pregnan-3,17,20,21-tetrol, as well as THDOC. The elevated THS and THDOC levels characteristic of 11β-hydroxylase deficiency are suppressible with dexamethasone, which also is used in the therapy of this condition.

In the presence of 17-hydroxylase deficiency, the major compounds found in large amounts in the urine are THB and THDOC. The elevated levels of THB and THDOC are suppressible by dexamethasone.

When there is a defect in Δ^5,3β-ol dehydrogenase, transformations along the corticosterone or the cortisol series are not possible to any significant extent. Therefore, the compounds which accumulate include Δ^5-pregnentriol and Δ^5-pregnanetriolone.

SUMMARY OF DIAGNOSTIC PROCEDURES

The clinical features of disorders of the adrenal cortex are described in the context of the biogenesis and biological activities of adrenocortical steroid hormones. The procedures for clinical investigation of the adrenal cortex and the pituitary adrenal axis are also presented.

The following clinical laboratory tests for steroid metabolites are recommended in the diagnosis of adrenocortical disorders. These procedures are described in detail in another publication (3). In suspected adrenocortical hypofunction, when the patient is in shock, the plasma cortisol level, which should be elevated in shock because of non-adrenocortical disorders, is determined. After recovery, maintain the patient on dexamethasone (2 mg/day) and fluorocortisol (0.1 mg/day) and perform plasma cortisol studies before and after intravenous infusion of cosyntropin (0.25 mg intravenously).

When patients are not in shock, after obtaining an abnormal water diuresis test, plasma cortisol levels are determined before and after the intravenous injection of cosyntropin. The absence of an increase in plasma cortisol after a single cosyntropin challenge would be consistent with adrenocortical insufficiency. This study would be supplemented by repeat challenges with cosyntropin (every 60 min for 3 doses); if the adrenal hypofunction is secondary to pituitary disease, progressive increments in plasma cortisol levels are noted after each successive infusion of cosyntropin. An alternative, but more cumbersome procedure involves urinary steroid response to a single 8-hr ACTH challenge. In a suspected pituitary hypofunction, repetitive (3 days) 8-hr ACTH tests are performed.

The levels of plasma cortisol before, and after, the intramuscular injection of 10 units of vasopressin will establish the integrity of the pituitary adrenocortical axis. Plasma cortisol after a hypoglycemic challenge provides similar information. An alternative procedure is to study the levels of plasma or urinary 11-deoxycortisol or THS respectively, before and after the administration of metyrapone.

In suspected adrenocortical hyperfunction, the following clinical laboratory steroid tests are recommended. First, plasma cortisol levels at 8:00 a.m. and 5:00 p.m. should be determined. High levels without a circadian variation are compatible with hypercortisolemia. Second, plasma cortisol levels after "overnight dexamethasone suppression test" should be measured. A value of plasma cortisol >10 $\mu g/100$ ml, or greater than ½ of the previous 8:00 a.m. specimen, would be consistent with Cushing's syndrome. Third, these tests may be supplemented by the more cumbersome methods for measurement of urinary steroids before and after dexamethasone suppression.

In suspected biosynthetic defects in the adrenal, determination of plasma cortisol levels at 8:00 a.m. and 5:00 p.m. should be made. These values may be lower than normal in adrenal biosynthetic defects. High levels of plasma 11-deoxycortisol (i.e., 17-OHCS in CCL_4 extract of plasma) are consistent with, or diagnostic of, 11β-hydroxylase deficiency. Urinary 17-hydroxy-21-corticosteroid levels in baseline 24-hr urine, and after 3 days of dexamethasone suppression, should be determined. The above urine samples should also be screened for pregnanetriols and for THS. Elevation of pregnanetriols, with subsequent suppression, would be consistent with adrenal 21-hydroxylase deficiency. Elevation of THS, with subsequent suppression with dexamethasone, would be consistent with adrenal 11-hydroxylase deficiency. Elevated DOC, corticosterone, THDOC, or THB would be consistent with 17-hydroxylase deficiency. Elevated 17-KS, in the absence of increased levels of THS along with increased levels of pregnenetriols in the urine, would be compatible with $\Delta^5,3\beta$-ol dehydrogenase (3-hydroxysteroid dehydrogenase) deficiency.

LITERATURE CITED

1. Forsham, P. H. 1969. The adrenal cortex. *In* R. H. Williams (ed.), Textbook of Endocrinology, pp. 287–379. W. B. Saunders Co., Philadelphia.
2. Bondy, P. K. 1969. The adrenal cortex. *In* Diseases of Metabolism, pp. 827–855. W. B. Saunders Co., Philadelphia.
3. Bacchus, H. 1972. Endocrine profiles in the clinical laboratory. *In* M. Stefanini (ed.), Progress in Clinical Pathology. Vol. 4, pp. 1–101. Grune & Stratton, Inc., New York.
4. Davis, W. W., and L. D. Garren. 1966. Evidence for the stimulation by adrenocorticotropic hormone of the conversion of cholesterol esters to cholesterol in the adrenal *in vitro*. Biochem. Biophys. Res. Commun. 24:805–810.
5. Baxter, J. D., and P. H. Forsham. 1972. Tissue effects of glucocorticoids. Am. J. Med. 53:573–590.
6. Feldman, D., J. W. Fundar, and I. S. Edelman. 1972. Subcellular mechanisms in the action of adrenal steroids. Am. J. Med. 53:545–560.
7. Katz, F. H., M. Lipman, A. G. Frantz, and J. W. Jailer. 1962. The physiological significance of 6β-Hydroxycortisol in human corticoid metabolism. J. Clin. Endocrinol. Metab. 22:71.
8. Ulstrom, R. A., G. Colle, J. Burley, and R. Gunville. 1960. Adrenocortical steroid metabolism in newborn infants. II. Urinary excretion of 6β-hydroxycortisol and other polar metabolites. J. Clin. Endocrinol. Metab. 20:1080–1094.
9. Conn, J. W. 1955. Primary aldosteronism, a new clinical entity. J. Lab. Clin. Med. 45:3–17.
10. Conn, J. W. 1965. Hypertension, the postassium ion and impaired carbohydrate tolerance. N. Engl. J. Med. 273:1135–1143.
11. Biglieri, E. G., A. M. Herron, and N. Brust. 1966. 17α-Hydroxylation deficiency in man. J. Clin. Invest. 45:1946–1954.
12. Bongiovanni, A. M. 1962. The adrenogenital syndrome with deficiency of hydroxysteroid dehydrogenase. J. Clin. Invest. 41:2086–2092.
13. Prader, A., and H. P. Gurtner. 1955. Das Syndrome des Pseudohermaphroditismus masculismus bei kongenitaler Nebenierren-rinden-hyperplasic ohne Androgeniiberproduktion: adrenaler Pseudohermaphroditismus musculinus. Helv. Paediat. Acta 10:397–412.

14. Givens, J. R., R. N. Andersen, J. B. Ragland, W. L. Wiser, and E. S. Umstot. 1975. Adrenal function in hirsutism. I. Diurnal change and response of plasma androstenedione, testosterone, 17-hydroxypro-gesterone, cortisol, LH and FSH to dexamethasone, and 1/2 unit of ACTH. J. Clin. Endocrinol. Metab. 40:988−1000.

16

Adrenal Medulla and Chromaffin System

Clinical disorders of the chromaffin system are caused by the excessive catecholamine synthesis taking place in the brain (1), sympathetic nerve endings (2) of chromaffin tissues (3) including the adrenal medulla, the paraganglia, the organ of Zuckerkandl, and ectopic nests of neural tissue. The cells of the chromaffin system in which catecholamines are produced are derived from neural crest anlagen which evolves either as sympathetic ganglia or as chromaffin cells. Because of this common origin, chemical distinction between ganglioneuromas, neuroblastomas, and pheochromocytomas on the basis of excretion of catecholamine metabolites is difficult. The chromaffin system is located along the sympathetic chain with major components located intra-abdominally, the largest discrete organ being the adrenal medulla. Rarely, tumors of this system may be found in an intrathoracic location. Chromaffin rests in the organ of Zuckerkandl or, associated with the urinary bladder, may produce increased amounts of catecholamines. Epinephrine is the most important catecholamine produced by the adrenal medulla, whereas norepinephrine is the major secretion of the postganglionic nerves and is the major catecholamine in fetal life. Dopamine is a catecholamine produced in the brain, lungs, liver, and the intestinal tract.

BIOSYNTHESIS OF CATECHOLAMINES

The cells of the chromaffin tissue produce the catecholamines from the amino acid tyrosine, which is present in plasma and tissues, as well as in ingested proteins. An alternative source is the amino acid phenylalanine

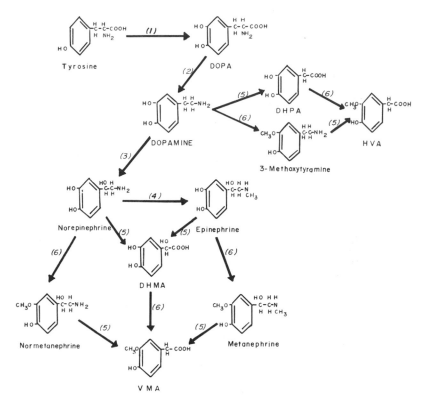

Figure 16.1. Biosynthesis and metabolism of catecholamines. Enzymes *1* through *4* are involved in the biosynthetic scheme; *5* and *6* are the degradative enzymes. The amino acid substrate is L-tyrosine, which is obtained from dietary sources, stored protein, or hydroxylation of phenylalanine. The enzymes are: (*1*) tyrosine hydroxylase, (*2*) aromatic L-amino acid decarboxylase, (*3*) dopamine β-oxidase, (*4*) adrenal medulla phenylethanolamine *N*-methyltransferase; (*5*) monoamine oxidase, and (*6*) catechol-*O*-methyltransferase. (Reprinted from Bacchus (7) with permission of the publisher.)

which may be hydroxylated to tyrosine in the presence of a hydroxylase. The steps in the biosynthesis of dopamine, norepinephrine, and epinephrine are presented in Figure 16.1 (4).

In the initial step in the biosynthetic sequence, the mitochondrial enzyme tyrosine hydroxylase converts tyrosine to dihydroxyphenylalanine (dopa). Cytoplasmic aromatic amino acid decarboxylase converts dopa to dihydroxyphenylethylamine (dopamine) which is the first biologically active catecholamine in this sequence. Dopamine is hydroxylated at the β-carbon to form norepinephrine. The enzyme phenylethanolamine *N*-methyltransferase (5), which is present almost exclusively in the adrenal medulla, is responsible for the methylation of the amino group of norepinephrine to form epinephrine. These hormones are stored in chromaffin granules, whose typical staining characteristics depend on the reaction with chromium salts.

METABOLISM OF CATECHOLAMINES

Catecholamines circulate in the plasma in the free form in which state small amounts may be excreted. Circulating catecholamines have a short biological half-life, rarely exceeding two or three circulation times. They may either bind to receptor sites and induce their biological effects or become inactivated. The major excretion pathways of these substances require the processes of catechol-O-methylation and oxidative decarboxylation (Figure 16.1). A portion of the methylated amines is excreted in the free form or is conjugated with sulfuric or glucuronic acids. The bulk of the 3-methoxy derivatives undergoes deamination following which it is oxidized to 3-methoxy-4-hydroxymandelic acid (vanilmandelic acid, VMA) which is excreted in the free form. If oxidative deamination occurs first, both norepinephrine and epinephrine are converted to 3,4-dihydroxymandelic acid (DHMA), which is subsequently O-methylated to VMA. The quantitatively more significant step is O-methylation and this is followed by deamination; in either event the end product is VMA. A similar sequence of reactions converts dopamine to homovanillic acid (HVA).

BIOLOGICAL EFFECTS OF CATECHOLAMINES

Dopamine, norepinephrine, and epinephrine exert marked effects on the vascular system. Epinephrine, from the adrenal medulla, significantly influences intermediary metabolism. The effects of the different catecholamines are separable on the basis of α- and β-adrenergic effects. Norepinephrine exerts pure α-adrenergic effects which are constriction of veins and arteries with resulting increase in peripheral vascular resistance and venous tone. Epinephrine possesses both α- and β-adrenergic effects, the latter including increased inotropic and chronotropic effects on the heart, increase in coronary blood flow, dilation of the large arteries supplying skeletal muscle, and relaxation of bronchial musculature. The metabolic actions on glycogenolysis and lipolysis are also generally classified among the β-adrenergic effects. Dopamine, classified according to the above effects, dilates the systemic arteries and increases cardiac output and renal blood flow.

The metabolic effects of epinephrine include glycogenolysis and lipolysis. Epinephrine activates liver and muscle phosphorylase leading to glycogenolysis. Skeletal muscle glycogenolysis leads to formation to lactic acid. In adipose tissue, epinephrine activates the membrane adenylate cyclase which increases the formation of cAMP. This mechanism underlies lipolysis and release of free fatty acids from the adipose cells.

CLINICAL DISORDERS OF CHROMAFFIN SYSTEM

The common anlage for the sympathetic ganglion cell and the chromaffin cell is the neuroblast. Tumors arising from these cell types are neuroblastomas, ganglioneuromas, and chromaffinomas or pheochromocytomas. Chromaffin tissues are located in the adrenal medulla, along the sympathetic chain as paraganglia, occasionally in the organ of Zuckerkandl along the abdominal aorta, and in chemoreceptor cells such as the carotid body.

Pheochromocytomas arise slightly more commonly in the right adrenal than in the left, about 10% are bilateral, and 10% occur in extra-adrenal locations. Only 3% of pheochromocytomas are malignant. Because of the absence of reliable cytologic criteria, the diagnosis of malignancy is made only when chromaffin tumors are found in sites where chromaffin tissues are not normally found.

Clinical Features of Pheochromocytoma (6)

All symptoms and signs are related to excessive secretion of catecholamines. Headache, perspiration, palpitations, pallor, and nausea are the most prevalent symptoms. Tremors, weakness, nervousness and anxiety, epigastric or chest pain, flushing and warmth, and numbness or paresthesias constitute the next most frequent constellation of symptoms. Rarely, patients may complain of dizziness or fainting, convulsions, and syncope. These symptoms often occur as episodic spells increasing gradually in severity. The spells are sudden in onset and may occur more frequently at night or shortly after arising in the morning. A very characteristic feature is that they may follow the same pattern, rarely lasting over 1 hr with each attack.

The most important clinical findings include: 1) hypertension, which may be paroxysmal, or, if persistent, it is labile (most patients with persistent hypertension show evidence of grade III or IV hypertensive retinopathy); 2) cardiac hypertrophy, and eventually congestive heart failure (a cardiomyopathy is associated with pheochromocytoma, but myopathic changes in other organs have been reported also); 3) cerebral components of pheochromocytoma essentially similar to these of other hypertensive patients; 4) renal complications that include arteriolonephrosclerosis in patients with persistent hypertension.

Associated clinical findings may include an elevated metabolic rate, hyperglycemia (in 60% of patients), and increased serum free fatty acids.

Because of prolonged excessive vasoconstriction, there is a decreased erythrocyte mass and hypovolemia.

Clinical Investigation of Pheochromocytoma

Diagnostic studies include indirect tests designed to stimulate or suppress the biological effects of excess catecholamines or direct measurements of metabolites of the catecholamines in the body fluids.

The indirect studies involve the use of pharmacological agents to either alter the effects of the catecholamines or to affect the secretion or uptake of these compounds. The phentolamine (regitine) test is done while the patient is hypertensive. Phentolamine (an α-blocking agent) is given intravenously in a dose range of 1.0–5.0 mg. It is recommended that the lower initial dose be used because the hypotensive effect in a patient with pheochromocytoma may last long enough to produce cerebral or myocardial infarction. A fall in blood pressure of 35/25 mm Hg lasting at least 4 min is indicative of a pheochromocytoma. The test is estimated to be 75% accurate, but occasionally false positive results are obtained, especially in patients under sedation, with azotemia, or being treated for hypertension.

The histamine provocative test is done in patients who are normotensive. Histamine is used to provoke an attack. It is, therefore, essential to have an α-blocking agent available for immediate use in the event of large unexpected rise in blood pressure, and this may serve as a confirmatory test (phentolamine test). The patient is kept at bed rest for a few hours before the test. An intravenous infusion of 5% glucose in water is started, and blood pressure readings are obtained for several minutes until a stable baseline is established. From 25–50 μg of histamine are injected through the intravenous needle. Marked elevations in blood pressure occur within 1 or 2 min of the injection of histamine in patients with pheochromocytoma. This test rarely gives false negative results. It is occasionally useful to collect 2-hr urine specimens just before and after the injection of histamine for catecholamine determinations if the test is positive. The phentolamine test should be performed if histamine activates an elevated blood pressure.

The tyramine test depends on direct release of catecholamines from nerve endings. The test is performed by giving a rapid intravenous bolus of tyramine in doses up to 2 mg. In patients with pheochromocytoma, the response is an increase in blood pressure within 40–60 sec, reaching a peak at 60–90 min. If the increase is excessive, or if it lasts longer, it may be reversed by the administration of phentolamine. False negative results are rare.

With definitive chemical tests (7), in all cases, it is recommended that for 2–3 days before, and during the collection of plasma and urine for the chemical tests, the patient should avoid use of certain drugs and foods. These include vasopressors, tetracyclines, α-methyldopa, monoamine oxidase inhibitors, coffee, vanilla, bananas, and citrus fruits. Plasma or urine catecholamines are determined. Normal levels will depend on the procedure employed. Urine vanilimandelic acid is a measure of catecholamine end products (see Figure 16.1 and Table 16.1). Urinary metanephrines may be fractionated into metanephrine and normetanephrine if the total "metanephrines" are elevated (Table 16.1). Adrenal venography is a recommended procedure to aid in locating the site of tumor of involvement. At the time of the procedure, samples of blood are taken from the adrenal vein on the right, the renal vein on the left, and the inferior vena cava for determination of catecholamines. Occasionally this procedure is followed by hemorrhage into the adrenal gland.

Pheochromocytoma Variants

Familial pheochromocytoma is presumed to be transmitted as an autosomal dominant disorder. These patients are more likely to have extra-adrenal and multiple tumors. Multiple endocrine adenomatosis may also include pheochromocytoma. The triad of hyperparathyroidism, medullary carcinoma of the thyroid, pheochromocytoma (bilateral adrenal lesions), and amyloidosis has been described.

Another form of familial pheochromocytoma occurs in von Recklinghausen's neurofibromatosis and in von Hippel-Lindau's disease (cerebellar and retinal hemangioblastoma). There is a 5–20% incidence of pheochromocytoma in patients with neurofibromatosis.

Pheochromocytoma has been found in children, the youngest reported being 1 month old. There is a higher than chance incidence of pheochromocytoma in children with cyanotic congenital heart disease.

In the Riley-Day syndrome (familial dysautonomia), catecholamines are elevated, reflecting the defect in dopamine β-oxidase, hence, an accumulation of dopamine (see Chapter 4). There are several clinical features in these patients suggestive of pheochromocytoma, but urinary VMA is decreased, whereas HVA is elevated.

Pheochromocytoma in pregnancy is occasionally confused with preclampsia and eclampsia. Delivery in such patients is fraught with complications. Surgery for the tumor and cesarean section for delivery are recommended.

Treatment of Pheochromocytoma

The recommended treatment for pheochromocytoma is removal of the tumor or, occasionally, the adrenal gland containing the tumor. In all cases, an abdominal approach is recommended so that the surgeon may explore for multiple or ectopic tumors.

Table 16.1. Clinical and Laboratory Procedures in Disorders of Catecholamine Metabolism

Procedure	Normal values	Abnormal values
Phentolamine test (regitine)	No significant change in blood pressure	Blood pressure reduction of >35/25 mm Hg lasting for several minutes to hours (in pheochromocytoma)
Histamine provocative test	No significant blood pressure elevation	Blood pressure elevation 60–35 mm Hg and cold pressor test (in pheochromocytoma)
Tyramine test	No significant blood pressure elevation	Blood pressure elevation of >20–80/40 mm Hg (in pheochromocytoma)
Urinary VMA	1.8–7.0 mg/24 hr	Markedly increased in pheochromocytoma
Urinary "metanephrines"	1.3 mg/24 hr	Markedly increased in pheochromocytoma
Urinary catecholamines	20–100 mg/24 hr	Increased in tumors of neural crest origin (neuroblastoma: ganglioneuromas) as a reflection of increased dopamine release; catecholamine levels >300 mg/24 hr found in most patients with pheochromocytoma

Special considerations are required for preparation for surgery. These depend on the manifestations of the excess catecholamines in the patient. If the patient has severe sustained hypertension with overt or incipient congestive heart failure, a course of preoperative treatment with phenoxybenzamine is indicated. Starting dose is 10–20 mg daily, which may be increased as indicated. Phentolamine may also be used, but this requires more frequent dosages. Severity of associated renal disease should be evaluated, in order to determine efficacy of contemplated surgery. Propanolol therapy is occasionally required to block excessive β-adrenergic manifestations. Most patients with pheochromocytoma have reduced plasma volume, and this should be corrected preoperatively by the use of plasma. A course of phenoxybenzamine is also helpful in this regard. Special care is regarded in anesthetic preparation. Scopolamine and short-acting barbiturates are employed as preanesthetic agents, and succinylcholine as a muscle relaxant agent. Atropine and similar agents, and derivatives of curare, should be avoided. Methoxyflurane is recommended as anesthetic agent.

Because excess catecholamine stores may not be completely depleted, agents which cause sudden release of catecholamines should be avoided for about 1 week postoperatively. Plasma or urine catecholamine should be checked to determine whether all responsible chromaffin tissue was removed. Medical management of pheochromocytoma is required either as preoperative preparation, as discussed above, or as palliative management when surgery is inadvisable or contraindicated. Phenoxybenzamine (10 mg every 12 hr by mouth as the starting dose, increased as required) is the recommended management. Phentolamine is effective, but its short duration of action makes it useful for paroxysmal attacks only. Excessive adrenergic manifestations may be palliated with propranolol. The drug α-methyltyrosine has been used at the National Institutes of Health with success.

LITERATURE CITED

1. Udenfriend, S., and P. Zaltzman-Nirenberg. 1963. Norepinephrine and 3,4-dihydroxyphenylalanine turnover in guinea pig brain in vivo. Science 142:394–396.
2. Musacchio, J. M., and M. Goldstein. 1960. Biosynthesis of norepinephrine and norsynephrine in the perfused rat heart. Biochem. Pharmacol. 12:1061–1063.
3. Udenfriend, S., and J. B. Wyngaarden. 1956. Precursors of adrenal epinephrine and norepinephrine in vivo. Biochim. Biophys. Acta 21:48–51.
4. Wurtman, R. J. 1965. Catecholamines. N. Engl. J. Med. 273:637–646, 693–700, 746–753.
5. Axelrod, J. 1962. Purification and properties of phenylethanolamine N-methyltransferase. J. Biol. Chem. 237:1657–1660.
6. Odell, W. D., G. A. Bray, de Quattro, D. A. Fisher, M. A. Goldberg, H. B. McIntyre, M. A. Sperling, and R. S. Swerdloff. 1972. Catecholamines: A symposium. Calif. Med. 157:32–62.
7. Bacchus, H. 1972. Endocrine profiles in the clinical laboratory. In M. Stefanini (ed.), Progress in Clinical Pathology. Vol. 4, pp. 1–101. Grune & Stratton, Inc., New York.

17 _____Testes

The testes serve two functions, a reproductive function (spermatogenesis) and a hormonal function (synthesis and secretion of testosterone by the interstitial cells of Leydig). The process of spermatogenesis is the development and maturation of the germ cells in the epithelium of the seminiferous tubules; the developmental stages progress from spermatogonia, the spermatocytes, the spermatids, to mature spermatozoa (1, 2). Both functions of the testes, spermatogenic and hormonal, are under control of the anterior pituitary through the gonadotropic hormones. Follicle-stimulating hormone (FSH) acts on germinal epithelium to promote full spermatogenesis, whereas interstitial cell-stimulating hormone (ICSH) (identical with LH) stimulates the Leydig cells to secrete androgens and estrogens. The release of both gonadotropins is presumably under control of the same hypothalamic peptide (3) but this mechanism now seems unlikely. FSH has been found in the pituitary in prepubertal individuals (4), but available methodology has not shown circulating levels of FSH at this stage of growth. The histological pattern of the prepubertal testis is stable until age 6 years, after which time minimal growth changes occur. At age 9–16 years, pituitary gonadotropin secretion stimulates testicular maturation. FSH acts on the seminiferous tubules to induce and maintain normal spermatogenesis, and ICSH acts directly on the interstitial mesenchymal elements, with resulting secretion of estrogens and testosterone; these elements are then in the process of developing into mature Leydig cells. ICSH has been found in prepubertal urine (5). Testosterone, the male hormone released in the above process, also stimulates seminiferous tubule growth. The physiological role of testicular produced estrogens is not known. Androgen secretion from the fetal testis abolishes the intrinsic hypothalamic cyclicity in regard to gonadotropin secretion. Hence, in the male, there is a steady release of pituitary gonadotropin during adult life.

Cessation of gonadotropin secretion postpubertally results in secondary atrophy of the testes; this may occur, for example, in panhypopituitarism. In general, there is a negative feedback mechanism in the operation

403

of the pituitary-testicular axis, i.e., a decreased level of testosterone is followed by an increase in the gonadotropic hormones. Similarly, in the presence of increased gonadal activity, there occurs a decrease in gonadotropin release. The mechanism of the ICSH feedback, dependent on testosterone (and estrogens?), is reasonably clear-cut, but the mechanism of seminiferous tubule regulating feedback is not well understood. The release of "inhibin" by the testes may provide for feedback inhibition of FSH release.

ENDOCRINE ACTIVITY OF TESTIS

The Leydig cells of the testis perform steroidogenesis similar in several respects to the processes in the ovaries and the adrenal cortex. The end product of testicular steroidogenesis is testosterone. ICSH (LH) releases membrane adenylate cyclase which leads to production of cAMP. This activates conversion of cholesterol to Δ^5-pregnenolone in the Leydig cell mitochondria. Starting with pregnenolone, these are two possible pathways to the formation of testicular hormones. These are presented in Figure 17.1 in which it is noted that either 17α-hydroxylase or $\Delta^5,3\beta$-ol dehydrogenase enzymes may act on the substrate in the initial reaction sequence. The intermediate androstenedione is formed either from dehydroepiandrosterone or from 17α-hydroxyprogesterone, the latter being predominant in man. Androstenedione is reduced to testosterone by hydrogenation (17β-hydroxyl) at C-17. Testosterone, the definitive androgen produced by the testis, is not a 17-KS. The two 17-KS from this gland, androstenedione and dehydroepiandrosterone (DHEA), exhibit weak androgenic activity. Testicular estrogens are formed by the androstenedione by hydroxylation followed by aromatization (Figure 17.1). Biosynthetic defects with accumulation of intermediate components similar to defects in the adrenal have not been demonstrated in the testes. In normal male subjects, the plasma testosterone ranges between 0.35–1.1 μg/100 ml (8), over 95% coming from the testis.

There are some data which suggest that there is a circadian variation in testicular hormone production. It is now known that testosterone production does not decrease with advancing age, but may be decreased in debilitating illness or with nutritional deficiency; these latter states presumably decrease the production of the gonadotropic hormones (6).

Testosterone is transported in the plasma weakly bound to carrier proteins SHBG (sex hormone-binding globulin); presumably the affinity characteristics are responsible for the rapid clearance of testosterone. Testosterone is converted in the liver to 17-KS by the process of 17-dehydrogenation. This process also takes place in the target organs of testosterone action. Recent studies (7, 8) have shown that testosterone is converted

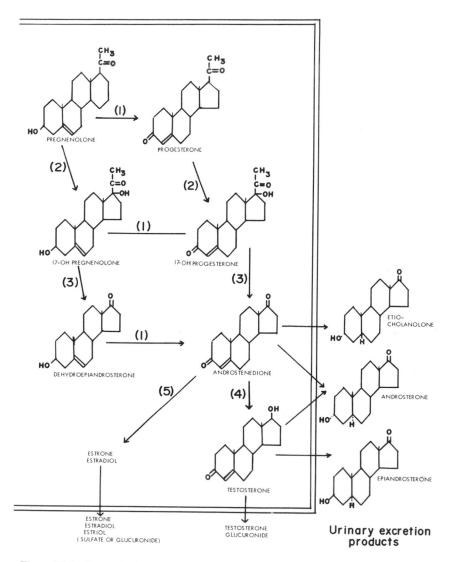

Figure 17.1. Biosynthetic steps in testicular hormone production and their urinary metabolites. The substrate cholesterol is converted to Δ^5-pregnenolone by the "desmolase" reaction. Enzymes *1–3* on the biosynthetic scheme from pregnenolone are: (*1*) Δ^5,3β-ol dehydrogenase; (*2*) 17α-hydroxylase; (*3*) 20-ketoreductase followed by the "desmolase" reaction; and (*4*) 17β-hydroxysteroid dehydrogenase. Testosterone is excreted as testosterone glucuronide or may be converted to the 17-KS depicted in the scheme. The urinary end products are shown outside of the rectangular enclosure in which the biosynthetic steps are presented. (Reprinted from Bacchus (6) with permission of the publisher.)

in the target organs to dihydrotestosterone which serves as the major androgenic substance at the various target cells.

The 17-ketosteroids derived from testosterone are excreted as glucuronide and sulfate conjugates. Of total 17-KS in the urine, 70% comes from adrenocortical sources, and 30% from the testes. The reduced end products, androsterone, epiandiosterone, and etiocholanolone, are end products mainly of testosterone. DHEA in the urine is derived mainly from the adrenal; however, there are interconversions whereby DHEA is reduced to androsterone.

ACTIONS OF TESTOSTERONE AND ANDROGENIC DERIVATIVES

Testosterone (probably via dihydrotestosterone) stimulates the development of secondary sex characteristics exemplified by these effects at puberty: 1) increase in size of penis and scrotum and increased pigmentation of these organs, appearance of rugal folds in scrotal skin; 2) hair growth at base of penis is one early sign of puberty, and this is extended to pubic hair growth into the diamond-shaped male escutcheon; anal, axillary, and body hair also are caused by androgenic hormone action; 3) a spurt in linear growth; 4) development of the prostate and seminal vesicles is androgen dependent, as are their secretory activities; and 5) the voice pitch is lowered, and a more aggressive male psyche, with increased libido and sexual potency, are androgen effects also.

Testosterone also has potent activity in protein anabolism—reflected by positive nitrogen, potassium, calcium, and phosphorus balance; animal studies have confirmed both increased protein anabolism and decreased protein catabolism caused by to testosterone. This hormone also plays an important role in muscle carbohydrate metabolism, as well as in nucleic acid synthesis.

After completion of the pubertal changes, any cessation of male hormone secretion (e.g., trauma or castration) is followed by a very slow regression of the secondary sex characteristics. For example, it may take 10–20 years before the deficiency is detected clinically. Manifestations of sudden androgen withdrawal include irritability, hot flashes, mental depression, and decreased libido and sexual potency. In certain individuals, these latter signs are minimal.

If testicular failure occurs before puberty, the androgen-induced changes fail to develop. The patient exhibits features of sexual infantilism, delay in epiphyseal closure with continued long bone growth, and the resultant eunuchoidal habitus. There are also a lack of adult male hair distribution, sparse or absent facial hair, and lack of temporal hair recession. The patient also exhibits decreased muscle mass and strength, as well as a high pitched voice.

In the differential diagnosis of hypogonadal syndromes, considerable emphasis is placed on history and physical examination, as well as on the results of the following laboratory procedures: sperm count, testicular biopsy, chromosome analysis, urinary or plasma levels of gonadotropic hormones, and levels of plasma testosterone, and occasionally of urinary 17-KS (6).

Clinical and Laboratory Features of Male Hypogonadism

Table 17.1 presents a classification of male hypogonadal syndromes (6) along with laboratory findings which aid in differential diagnosis (6). Treatment of these syndromes is outlined in Table 17.2.

In addition to the causes of hypogonadism listed in Table 17.1, there are other causes of decreased gonadal activity. Decreased potentia and libido occasionally associated with adrenocortical insufficiency are ascribed to the generalized weakness caused by the adrenal disease. Diagnosis of this disorder will depend on adrenocortical function tests which have been discussed in another section. In myxedema of sufficient severity, there may occasionally occur changes as severe as in panhypopituitarism, with consequent hypogonadism; here also the diagnosis will require studies on the underlying thyroid defect.

Two special types of problems related to testicular dysfunction are male infertility and gynecomastia.

Male Infertility

Occasionally, presumably normal patients are seen for infertility problems not ascribable to the spouse. If the overt hypogonadal syndromes listed in Table 17.1 are excluded in the differential diagnosis, definitive work-up in such patients should include: sperm count, testicular biopsy (in many cases), and plasma (or urine) FSH and LH levels. The scheme in Figure 17.2 presents a method analysis of male infertility (6).

Gynecomastia or glandular enlargement of the male breast is a normal occurrence in most males at some time during their development, e.g., pubertal gynecomastia. Other causes of breast enlargement (lipoma, carcinoma, adiposity, neurofibromatosis, or chronic infection) should be differentiated from gynecomastia. Most benign gynecomastia is bilateral, but it may also occur unilaterally. Histological patterns distinguish between two forms of gynecomastia, i.e., changes in parenchymal cells with ductal hyperplasia and lobular formation are found in patients receiving estrogen therapy for prostatic carcinoma and changes in interlobular and periductal tissue with increase in collagenous fibers and adipose tissue are associated with cirrhosis of the liver, rheumatoid arthritis (on steroid therapy), diabetes mellitus, chronic glomerulonephritis, or bronchogenic carcinoma. In general, when ductal changes predominate, the agents mainly responsible are testosterone, estrogen, or adrenal steroids, with prolactin playing a permissive role. When stromal changes are predominant, prolactin activity

Table 17.1. Laboratory Diagnosis of Male Hypogonadal Syndromes[a]

Disorder[b]	Clinical features	Sperm count	Plasma or Urine			
			17-KS	Testosterone	FSH	LH
Hypergonadotropic						
Klinefelter's	Gynecomastia, small testis	0	Normal	Low normal	High	High
Reifenstein's	Hypospadias; gynecomastia	0	Normal	Low	High	High
Functional prepubertal "castrate"	Short stature; "empty scrotum"	0	Low	Low	High	High
Male Turner's	Mental retardation, cryptorchidism; gynecomastia; short	0	Low	Low	High	High
Sertoli cell only syndrome	Gynecomastia absent	0	Normal	Normal	High	Normal
Adult seminiferous tubule failure; mumps orchitis, idiopathic, or in myotonic dystrophy	Normal development; no overt physical findings except in myotonic dystrophy where there are myotonia, baldness, and lens defects	Decreased or absent	Normal (low in mumps orchitis)	Normal (low in mumps orchitis)	High	Normal (high in mumps orchitis)
Adult Leydig cell failure	Hot flashes, decreased libido	Normal	Normal or low	Normal or low	High	High

Hypogonadotropic

Hypogonadotropic eunuchoidism

Complete or typical (Kallman's)	Eunuchoid features, small testes, anosmia or hyposmia	0	Normal or low	Low	Low	Low	Low
Incomplete	Cleft palate, craniofacial dyssymmetry	0 or low	Normal	Low	Low or normal	Low or normal	Low or normal
Delayed puberty	Slow maturation only	0 or low	Normal	Low	Low or normal	Low or normal	Low or normal
Fertile eunuch	Eunuchoidal	Low	Normal	Low	Low to normal	Low to normal	Low or normal
Prepubertal panhypopituitarism	Lack of growth: sexual infantilism	0 or low	Normal	Low	Low	Low	Low
Postpubertal pituitary failure panhypopituitarism	Decreased libido, impotence: regression of secondary sex characteristics	0 or low	Normal	Low	Low to normal	Low to normal	Low to normal

[a] Extragonadal causes of hypogonadism include myxedema, Cushing's syndrome, and adrenal insufficiency.

[b] Chromatin pattern or buccal smear is negative in all except occasionally in Klinefelter's syndrome, where it may be negative. The chromosome karyotype is XY in all except in Klinefelter's, where it may be XXY, poly(X + Y), or mosaic, and in male Turner's syndrome, where it may be XY or poly(X + Y).

Table 17.2. Treatment of Male Hypogonadal Syndromes

Disorder	Treatment
Hypergonadotropic Klinefelter's	Testosterone therapy is started at age 11–12 years; testosterone cyclopentylpropionate, 50 mg is given intramuscularly every 3 weeks; the dose is increased to 100 mg every 3 weeks after 6 months; 50-mg increments are given at 9-month intervals until the adult dose range of 500 mg every 3 weeks is achieved; doses as high as 1,000 mg every 3 weeks have occasionally been used; this therapy results in improvement in muscular development, facial and body hair, and the complexion becomes ruddier; oral androgen therapy is not recommended because of possibility of hepatotoxicity; gynecomastia may require surgical therapy
Reifenstein's	As above; hypospadias should be treated surgically
Functional prepubertal castrate	Full androgen replacement as above to full sexual maturation
Male Turner's	Androgen replacement; orchidectomy is now recommended because of neoplastic potential of the dysgenetic gonads
Sertoli cell only syndrome	Hormone therapy is not needed; infertility is permanent
Adult seminiferous tubule failure: mumps orchitis; idiopathic myotonic dystrophy	Supportive therapy during acute phase only; therapy is unsatisfactory; no known treatment

Condition	Treatment
Adult Leydig cell failure	Maintenance androgen therapy is given: 300–500 mg of testosterone enanthate intramuscularly every 3–4 weeks; therapeutic success will depend on underlying causes, e.g., in vascular or neurogenic disorders, androgen therapy is useless
Hypogonadotropic	
Hypogonadotropic eunuchoidism: complete or typical (Kallman's)	HCG 4,000 IU 3 times weekly for 6–9 months; this allows Leydig cells to develop and become more sensitive to HCG; dose is then reduced to 2,000 IU 3 times weekly for 3 months; the Leydig cells are induced to secrete testosterone, penile size is increased, and pubic, body, and facial hair appear; potentia is increased; after development is well advanced, therapy is discontinued for 3–6 months; any evidence of regression should prompt a secondary course of treatment; rarely tertiary courses are required; failure to reinstitute therapy promptly in face of regression may result in irreversible damage to seminiferous tubules, as hyalinization develops if the stimulus (endogenous or exogenous) is removed for appreciable time. Menotropins as adjunct therapy. One course of therapy as above is usually sufficient
Incomplete delayed puberty	Treatment not often indicated; social or psychological factors may necessitate a 6-week course of HCG 4,000 IU 3 times weekly; if no response is noted, then the patient probably has Kallman's
Fertile eunuch	One or two courses of HCG as above
Prepubertal panhypopituitarism	Androgen replacement, along with replacement of adrenal and thyroid hormones
Postpubertal panhypopituitarism	Usually androgen replacement; if fertility is desired, HCG and menotropins may be tried

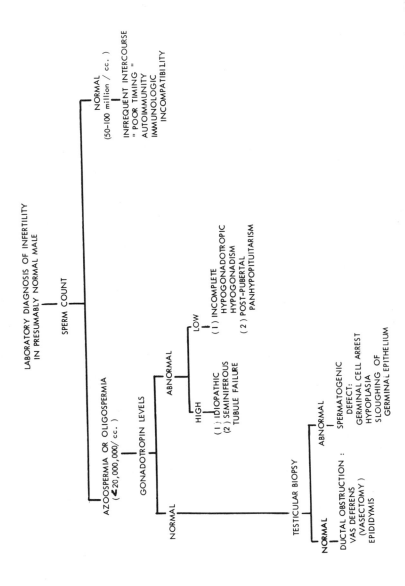

Figure 17.2. Scheme for clinical laboratory work-up of male infertility. (Reprinted from Bacchus (6) with permission of the publisher.)

is primarily responsible. The probability of end-organ hyper-responsiveness should also be considered.

The most well recognized cause of gynecomastia is pubertal (gynecomastia). This disappears within a matter of months up to 2 years after its inception in most patients. It is estimated that as many as 10% of these patients may have persistent gynecomastia (unilateral or bilateral). Other causes of gynecomastia include malnutrition and refeeding. It is known that malnutrition may be accompanied by pituitary hypofunction, and that refeeding permits a spurt in gonadotropin secretion, hence a "second puberty." Included in this category are patients with gynecomastia associated with pulmonary tuberculosis, diabetes mellitus, hepatic cirrhosis, and congestive heart failure treated with cardiac glycosides. Whether the same mechanism is responsible in all of the above types is open to question.

There are data on abnormal testosterone and corticosteroid metabolism in hepatic cirrhosis which may be related to the pathogenesis of this phenomenon. Recent data support the view that an accumulation of 17β-estradiol caused by decreased hepatic degradation is probably responsible for the gynecomastia of chronic liver disease. Other causes include various drugs such as estrogens, testosterone, chorionic gonadotropin (HCG), phenothiazines, meprobamate, hydroxyzine, reserpine, and spironolactone among others. Undoubtedly, some of these induce gynecomastia by interfering with the release of PIF from the hypothalamus (e.g., reserpine and phenothiazines).

Various tumors, testicular in origin, including choriocarcinoma, embryonal and trophoblastic, as well as interstitial cell adenomas, have been implicated as causes of gynecomastia. Other neoplastic processes implicated are Hodgkin's disease and bronchogenic carcinoma. The mechanism in the latter probably involves production of an ectopic gonadotropin by the tumor. Other causes include hypothyroidism, hyperthyroidism, and idiopathic factors.

Analysis of factors involved in the pathogenesis of gynecomastia should include consideration of: 1) competition between androgens and estrogens for sex hormone-binding globulin (SHBG) factors affecting circulation SHBG, and relationship of bound hormones to the receptor protein in breast tissue; 2) influence of reduction of testosterone to dihydrotestosterone (more powerful androgen) on the differential SHBG affinity for androgens and estrogens; 3) influence of SHBG on reduction of testosterone; and 4) influence of binding affinity of gonadal hormones to hypothalamic feedback by 17β-estradiol.

Laboratory tests (6) in evaluating gynecomastia should include: skull x-ray to detect intracranial lesions; chest x-ray to detect problems such as tumors or adenopathy; plasma or urine 17β-estradiol; plasma FSH and LH; and plasma LH (cross-reaction with HCG).

Two groups of testicular tumors (6) are of interest in the field of endocrinology, as they may be either hormone secreting or may affect hormone secretion by the anterior pituitary. These are germinal and non-germinal tumors.

Germinal tumors include: seminoma; embryonal carcinoma, pure or with seminoma; teratoma, pure or with seminoma; teratoma with embryonal carcinoma, with or without seminoma; and choriocarcinoma, pure or with either embryonal carcinoma or seminoma, or both.

Presence of these tumors is reflected by increased plasma or urine HCG. Plasma LH determinations give elevated values as the procedure fails to distinguish between LH and HCG especially in the presence of large amounts of the latter. Measurement of HCG and LH in the plasma is of both diagnostic and prognostic usefulness. Follow-up of therapy is monitored by changes in these hormonal parameters. In some patients with seminomas, there may occasionally occur elevations in pituitary gonadotropins, suggesting production of "ectopic pituitary gonadotropins." In several patients with increased levels of HCG, an elevation of estrogens is also found. This is ascribed to stimulation of the pathway to estrogens in the Leydig cells by gonadotropin.

Non-germinal tumors originate in Leydig cells and are steroid-hormone producing. They are classified on the basis of the types of hormones secreted. Virilizing tumor produces testosterone reflected by elevation of plasma and urine testosterone and of urine 17-KS. If this tumor appears prepubertally, the patients exhibit features of precocious development of the penis, muscles, and hair growth, with associated increased linear growth. It is occasionally difficult to separate these patients from those with congenital adrenocortical hyperplasia. The simplest differential procedure is the dexamethasone suppression test (see Chapter 15). Patients with elevated 17-KS and testosterone caused by adrenocortical hyperplasia exhibit decreases of these hormones to normal or subnormal values, after dexamethasone administration, whereas those with Leydig cell tumors will not. The validity of this concept is being questioned.

The feminizing type of Leydig cell tumor produces estrogens and is only found in adults. Estrogen excess produces impotence, gynecomastia, and decrease in hair growth.

Various chromosomal defects affecting testicular gonadogenesis, as well as other disorders of male sexual differentiation, are discussed in Chapter 20.

LITERATURE CITED

1. Paulsen, C. A. 1974. The testes. *In* R. H. Williams (ed.), Textbook of Endocrinology, pp. 323–367. W. B. Saunders Co., Philadelphia.

2. Lipsett, M. B., and R. J. Sherins. 1974. The testes. *In* P. K. Bondy (ed.), Diseases of Metabolism, pp. 1553–1584. W. B. Saunders Co., Philadelphia.
3. Schally, A. V., A. Arimura, A. J. Kastin, H. Mitsuo, Y. Baba, T. W. Redding, R. M. Nair, and L. Debeljuk. 1971. Gonadotropin releasing hormone. One polypeptide regulates secretion of luteinizing and follicle stimulating hormone. Science 173:1036–1037.
4. Odell, W. D. 1968. Gonadotropins: Present concepts in the human. Calif. Med. 109:467–485.
5. Odell, W. D., G. T. Ross, and P. L. Rayford. 1967. Radioimmunoassay for luteinizing hormone in human plasma or serum. Physiological studies. J. Clin. Invest. 46:248–255.
6. Bacchus, H. 1972. Endocrine profiles in the clinical laboratory. *In* M. Stefanini (ed.), Progress in Clinical Pathology. Vol. 4, pp. 1–101. Grune & Stratton, Inc., New York.

18
The
Ovaries

The ovaries serve two functions in the human female: 1) the function of reproduction through the periodic release of ova, and by accommodation of the processes of fertilization, implantation, gestation, and delivery of the product of conception; and 2) production of estrogens and progesterone (1, 2). The estrogens support growth of the secondary female sex characteristics, and, in association with progesterone, prepare the uterus for implantation and development of the fertilized ovum. Breast development and other female characteristics, as well as aspects of intermediary metabolism, are also dependent on these hormones.

Both functions of the ovaries are under the control of the hypothalamic-hypophysial system. Hypothalamic nuclei release gonadotropic releasing factors, e.g., LRF, and inhibiting factors, e.g., PIF, which control the pituitary-ovarian axis. The hypothalamic factors respond to circulating levels of the ovarian hormones.

Development and release of the ova are dependent on cyclic control by the pituitary hormone FSH. A fund of 5–6 million germ cells is present in the ovarian cortex at birth, and most of these cells are never stimulated to maturity. The processes of development of the primordial germ cell and its movement toward the center of the ovary where it becomes surrounded by other cells and develops an antrum are not dependent on pituitary factors. This antrum formation progresses in several cells simultaneously, but only one of these goes on to form a mature Graafian follicle at each ovulatory cycle. FSH is necessary for follicular ripening; involved in this process is an accumulation of fluid within the antrum as the cell mass is pushed toward the periphery, the follicle forming a bulge on the surface of the ovary. The pituitary hormone LH now causes lysis of the follicle wall by altered vitality of the granulosa cells of the follicle and by weakening the mucopolysaccharide cement between the granulosa cells, releasing the ovum. The spurt in LH release is stimulated by a slight but sharp rise in estradiol

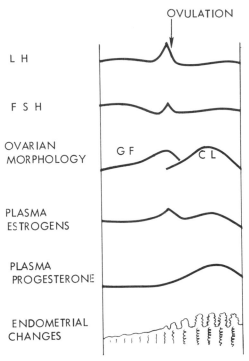

Figure 18.1. Hormonal and endometrial events during the menstrual cycle. Ovulation is precipitated by a positive feedback whereby a spurt of estrogen release triggers release of LH. This lyses the connective tissue around the ovum, with subsequent ovulation.

which occurs 1–2 days earlier, an example of positive feedback control. Fertilization, if it occurs, usually takes place in the lumen of the Fallopian tube, after which the fertilized ovum floats free for 5–6 days before implantation. Several physical and chemical factors influence ovum implantation and blastocyst formation on certain areas of the endometrium. After release of the ovum, the corpus luteum forms at this site and assumes the secretion of progesterone.

There are characteristic changes in urinary and plasma FSH and LH at the time of ovulation (1). A rise in plasma FSH in midcycle and a more marked rise in LH lasting 1–2 days occur just before ovulation. An increase in total estrogens also occurs at this time. These findings are schematized in Figure 18.1.

MENSTRUAL CYCLE

In the absence of fertilization of the released ovum, certain regressive changes follow the incipient progestational changes. There occurs a breakdown of the endometrium with resulting menstrual bleeding which starts at about 14–16 days after ovulation, to continue about 4–5 days. This process of menstruation is unique to primates. The average age for onset of the first menstrual period, or menarche, is approximately 13 years in temperate climates and somewhat earlier in warmer latitudes; there are ethnic and geographic differences in the time of menarche. Initial bleeding episodes may be anovulatory, the ovulatory cycles becoming regular after months or years after the menarche. The postovulatory phase of the menstrual cycle is termed the progestational or luteoid phase, terms that refer to the endometrial changes occurring at this time. After the spurt in serum LH and FSH at time of ovulation, the levels of these gonadotropins drop to slightly lower levels than in the preovulatory or folliculoid phase. This slight decrease lasts until the time of menstruation. During the luteal phase, there are moderately increased levels of pregnanediol, a reflection of increased secretion of the progestational hormone, progesterone. Similarly, during the postovulatory phase, the levels of urinary estrogens are increased, with a slight spurt about midluteal phase (Figure 18.1).

During the luteal phase and perhaps even 1 or 2 days before ovulation, progesterone produced by the corpus luteum converts the proliferative endometrium to secretory structures. Progesterone also increases the vascularity of this secretory endometrium which is now prepared for implantation and blastocyst formation. The peak activities in this regard occur from days 22 to 23 of the normal menstrual cycle. If there is no implantation of a fertilized ovum, then the corpus luteum atrophies, and decreased estrogen and progesterone secretions are followed by sloughing of the endometrium, i.e., menstruation.

STEROID SYNTHESIS IN OVARIES

The ovaries are active in steroidogenesis; several of the steps are identical with those in the testes and the adrenal cortex. Pituitary LH releases ovarian cell membrane adenylate cyclase which permits the cleavage of cAMP from ATP. cAMP actuates processes which culminate in the desmolase reaction which cleaves the side chain of cholesterol, releasing Δ^5-pregnenolone (Δ^5-pregnen-3β-ol-20-one) and isocaproic aldehyde. Pregnenolone has two alternative routes toward estrogen synthesis (Figure 18.2). 1) The Δ^4 pathway: in the presence of the Δ^5,3β-ol dehydrogenase system (actually a two-step reaction, first the dehydrogenation of 3β-ol structure, followed by an isomerase which shifts the double bond from $\Delta^{5,6}$ to $\Delta^{4,5}$) pregnenolone is converted to progesterone. This product is now hydroxylated at C-17 by α-hydroxylase, with the production of 17α-hydroxyprogesterone. The presence of the 17α-OH group permits more ready enzymatic cleavage of the side chain with the resultant end

420   Habeeb Bacchus

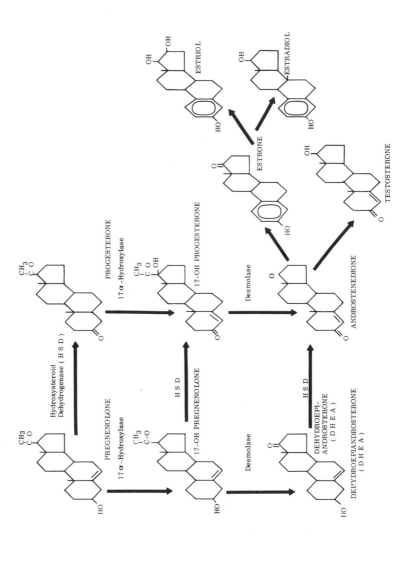

Figure 18.2. Biosynthetic steps in ovarian hormone production and their urinary metabolites. The substrate Δ^5-pregnenolone is produced from cholesterol by the "desmolase" reaction. (Reprinted from Bacchus (1) with permission of the publisher.)

product being androstenedione (Δ^4-androstene-3,17-dione). 2) The Δ^5 pathway in which 17α hydroxylation of pregnenolone to 17α-hydroxypregnenolone (Δ^5-pregnen-3β,17-diol-20-one) is the first step. The side chain is then cleaved off, with the resultant formation of dehydroepiandrosterone (Δ^5-androsten-3-ol-17-one). The action of the Δ^5,3-ol dehydrogenase system then converts DHEA to androstenedione.

Androstenedione is now hydroxylated to 19-hydroxyandrostenedione. This step permits aromatization of ring A with the formation of estrone ($\Delta^{1,3,5}$-estratrien-3-ol-17-one) which is then reduced at the 17-ketone group to form estradiol ($\Delta^{1,3,5}$-estratrien-3,17-diol) and estriol ($\Delta^{1,3,5}$-estratrien-3β,17α,16α-triol). Androstenedione may also be converted to testosterone by reduction of the ketone group at C-17, and this pathway provides minimal amounts of this androgen in the ovaries. Some degree of cell specificity is evident in ovarian steroidogenesis. Androgen production is more active in the ovarian stroma; indeed, this is presumed to be the source of increased androgens in the Stein-Leventhal syndrome. Granulosa and thecal cells are necessary for optimal production of estrogens. The Δ^5 pathway is more active during the follicular phase when less progesterone is needed, and the Δ^4 pathway, which provided progesterone more efficiently, as well as estrogens, is predominant in the luteoid or postovulation phase.

The degradation pathways of the ovarian hormones are largely reductive processes. Δ^5-Pregnenolone and progesterone are reduced to pregnanediol. The intermediate 17α-hydroxypregnenolone may be excreted as pregnenetriolone or as pregnanetriol. 17α-hydroxyprogesterone is excreted as pregnanetriol (pregnan-3β,17 α,20α(or)β-triol). Excretion is facilitated by conjugation of these compounds with glucuronic acid. DHEA is excreted as DHEA sulfate, as androsterone or etiocholanolone, conjugated to either glucuronic acid or to sulfate. Degradation and excretion of estrogens involve mainly the conversion to estriol which is a biologically inactive metabolite. The bulk of estriol excretion is as the sulfate conjugate. Estradiol and estrone may be conjugated with sulfate or with glucuronic acid at C-3. This not a major pathway of estrogen excretion, however. The liver is the major, but not exclusive, organ where these degradative steps occur.

STEROIDOGENESIS DURING PREGNANCY

Should fertilization of the ovum take place, the zygote traverses the oviduct toward the endometrium. The progress through the oviduct is hastened by high estrogen levels, and this effect of estrogens is being used clinically for pregnancy control. The site of implantation of the zygote, now at least at morula stage, on the endometrium usually is an area protected from physical trauma. Implantation takes place within 4–6 days after fertilization. Blastocyst formation is followed by the start of production of HCG, a glycoprotein hormone. This hormone is detectable as early as 9 days after implantation and reaches peak levels at 60–80 days of gestation after which the HCG levels drop considerably to lower levels. The initial persistence and steroidogenesis in the corpus luteum are undoubtedly dependent on the production of HCG. Steroidogenesis in the corpus luteum reaches its peak at 3–4 weeks after fertilization, and decreases thereafter, despite continuing elevation of HCG. The role of HCG in pregnancy was previously presumed to be support of the corpus luteum. The observation that oophorectomy early in pregnancy fails to terminate it makes it likely that the corpus luteum is not necessary for continuation of the pregnancy (1).

New data provide a rationale for the increased HCG secretion beyond active corpus luteum steroidogenesis. HCG is quite active in the support and steroidogenesis in the fetal adrenal cells. This organ provides steroid substrates for the placental fetal unit.

After 90 days of gestation, the HCG levels drop and plateau at a lower level. Simultaneously, the cells of the fetoplacental unit are fully capable of producing the steroid hormones necessary for the pregnancy. The placenta also produces the following peptide hormones.

Chorionic somatomammotropin is also termed placental lactogen (HPL), and is secreted by the syncytiotrophoblast cells until the end of pregnancy. This hormone has several similarities to human growth hormone (HGH) in structure, as well as in biological activity. The production rate is estimated to be over 1 g daily, over 99% of which is in the material compartment where it induces lipolysis and provides free fatty acids for maternal metabolism, sparing carbohydrate and protein for fetal metabolism. This action probably contributes to the "fasting metabolism state" in pregnancy (see section on diabetic pregnancy).

Production of a placental thyrotropin has been reported and it has been shown to have biological activity, but this is questionable.

STEROIDOGENESIS IN FETOPLACENTAL UNIT

Close metabolic relationship between the maternal and fetal compartments is exemplified by the interplay of steroidogenic tissues during gestation (1, 3). The syncytiotrophoblast is active in the production of estrogens and progesterone, but there are now data to show that the placenta is an incomplete steroidogenic tissue. The steroidogenic cells of the fetus, the adrenal cortex, gonads, and liver are derived from the mesoderm. Development of the adrenal cortex in the fetus shows that there are probably two relatively discrete areas of the gland both from morphological and biosynthetic aspects.

By 5–6 weeks of gestation, the adrenal is made up of relatively undifferentiated cells, loosely connected to each other and surrounded by a thin fibrous capsule. By 6–7 weeks, the gland divides into a thin outer zone and a wide inner (fetal) zone. Cell maturation proceeds differently in these two areas. The fetal (inner) zone cells show maturation changes without any evidence of mitosis. The outer zone is actively mitotic, and new cells are formed with evidence of slow maturation. There is reason to conclude that the outer zone eventually evolves into the adult adrenal cortex, whereas the inner wide fetal zone which developed earlier eventually disappears after having functioned during gestation and in early neonatal life. The fetal zone is known to completely involute by 6 months after birth.

There is good evidence that cholesterol from the maternal compartment is the precursor for steroidogenesis in the placenta. The fetal compartment is capable of significant conversion of acetate to cholesterol, with activities greatest in the liver, adrenal tissue, and gonadal tissue, in that order. However, it is likely that precursors for steroidogenesis beyond cholesterol may reach the fetus from the maternal or placental compartment.

There are significant differences between the biosynthetic potentials of the placenta and the fetus (Table 18.1). Those data make it clear why pregnanediol is a reflection of placental activity, whereas the formation of estriol sulfate is largely dependent on the activity of the fetal adrenal (and liver). The fetal zone of the adrenal cortex is the major site of steroid synthesis in early gestation. Structural "maturation" in this gland occurs by 6–7 weeks of gestation, and increased estrogens are detectable at 15–16 weeks. By this time, the adult zone of the adrenal cortex has not yet differentiated structurally. The fetal zone is geared for the Δ^5 pathway and for sulfurylation of these steroids. These compounds constitute the major steroids in fetal and neonatal body fluids until the fetal zone involutes (by 6 months of age) and the adult zone takes over (Figure 18.3).

The fetal adrenal uses placentally produced progesterone for further steroid synthesis, e.g., formation of corticosterone via 21-hydroxylase and 11β-hydroxylase reactions and formation of cortisol via 17α-hydroxylase, 21-hydroxylase, and 11β-hydroxylase reactions. The cortisol to corticosterone ratio is low in gestation and in neonatal life (around 5.5), but this doubles within 1 week of birth and, by age 2 years, reaches the adult ratio of approximately 15:18.

The fetal steroid excretion pattern differs from the adult in the

Table 18.1. Steroidogenic Enzymes in Placenta and Fetal Adrenal

Enzyme system	Reaction	Placenta	Fetal adrenal
Hydroxysteroid dehydrognase	Converts Δ^5,3-ol to Δ^4,3-ketone	Active	Minimal to absent
17α-Hydroxylase	Hydroxylation at C-17 permitting cleavage by 17:20 desmolase	Minimal	Active
17:20 Demolase	Cleavage of side chain of C-21 steroids to form 17-ketosteroids	Active	Active
Sulfokinase	Sulfurylation of steroids at C-3, e.g., DHEA, DHEAS	Absent	Active
16α-Hydroxylase	Hydroxylation at C-16, e.g., estradiol estriol	Absent	Present in fetal liver and adrenals
Steroid sulfatase	Removal of sulfate at C-3	Present	Absent

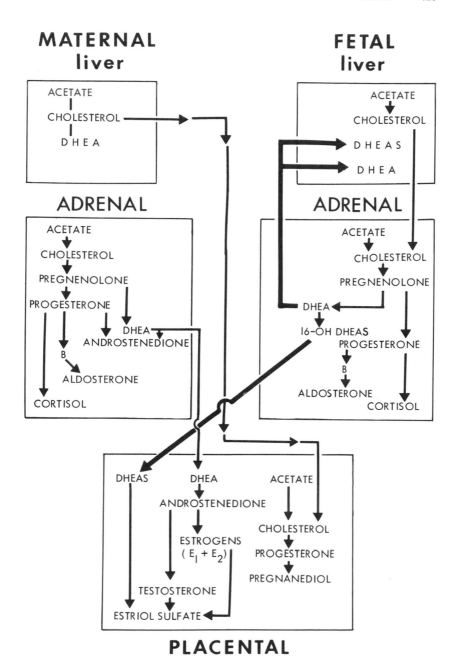

Figure 18.3. Steroidogenesis in the maternal-placental-fetal unit. Certain key enzymatic reactions which take place in the fetal adrenal are responsible for formation of the bulk of sulfurylated steroids and for formation of estriol (see text for details).

following respects: a relatively greater excretion of sulfurylated steroids, especially of the 16-hydroxylated series; a relatively increased excretion of corticosterone series; utilization of 6β hydroxylation and oxidation of 11β-hydroxysteroids so that cortisol may be excreted as 6β-hydroxy-cortisone derivatives, and reduction of the Δ^4,3-acetone structure of cortisol is less than that of cortisone.

Control of Steroidogenesis in Fetal Life (4)

Up to 20 weeks of gestation, development of the fetal adrenal cortex is dependent on HCG and, after 20 weeks, on ACTH from the fetal pituitary. Development of the adrenal cortex beyond the 20-week stage is halted in anencephalic fetuses. There are data to indicate that fetal Leydig cell activity and the onset of testosterone synthesis are dependent on HCG. The bulk of placental HCG goes to the maternal compartment, but it has been shown that the HCG concentration in the fetal compartment at 11–12 weeks is 30 times the threshold for physiological response (5). There is definite proof of HCG uptake by the fetal compartment (6).

It is clear that HCG and ACTH affect different enzyme systems in the adrenal of the fetus. Morphological studies showed that ACTH given intra-amniotically induced changes in the fetal adrenals different from those induced by HCG. Chemical data reveal that HCG in the newborn results in increased DHEA excretion, whereas ACTH injection resulted in increased cortisol production mainly.

OTHER ENDOCRINE CHANGES IN PREGNANCY

Both fetal and maternal endocrine glands are important in fetal development. The hypothalamic-hypophysial system is essential to development of the target endocrine glands, the latter failing to develop in the absence of that system. The thyroid in the fetus becomes active at about the 12th week of gestation; absence of fetal thyroid function results in decreased somatic and neural maturation. Masculine differentiation is absolutely dependent on the presence of the fetal testis. The fusion and differentiation of the Wolffian system and degeneration of the Müllerian system are dependent on testicular hormones. The fetal testis is capable of synthesis of testosterone, and the inception of this process precedes the differentiation of the Wolffian system.

ENDOCRINE CHANGES IN MATERNAL SYSTEM IN PREGNANCY

As levels of estrogens increase during the course of pregnancy, there is a parallel increase in plasma PBI, a reflection of an increase in TBG. Toward the end of pregnancy, there is normally a PBI level of around 11 μg/100 ml, and T_4 is increased similarly. There are increases in plasma and urinary

17-hydroxycorticosteroids during pregnancy, without any evidence of hypercorticism; this is at least partly caused by a progressive increase in plasma CBG. This binding protects the steroid from immediate hepatic inactivation and may be at least in part responsible for changes in the pathways in corticosteroid excretion in pregnancy (7). Later, high progesterone levels may displace cortisol from CBG.

ENDOCRINE CHANGES IN PARTURITION

The placenta probably has a predetermined life span (e.g., the aromatization of steroid ring A decreases with placental aging). The aging placenta becomes more sensitive to the effects of neurohypophysial oxytocin, but this hormone is not absolutely necessary for fetal expulsion. All factors that initiate labor are not fully understood, but it is likely that decreasing levels of progesterone as well as the sensitivity to oxytocin are important initiating factors in this process. The fetal adrenals are probably involved in timing of the gestation period. Premature delivery is associated with hyperplasia of the fetal adrenal, and prolonged gestation with hypoplasia of this gland (8). During delivery, the levels of 17-OHCS increase markedly and drop sharply at the termination of labor. The excretion of HCG continues for about 1 week after parturition; the presence of HCG any longer would suggest retained placental tissue.

ENDOCRINE CONTROL OF MAMMARY GROWTH AND LACTATION

Maximal breast development and growth result from a combination of estrogen, progesterone, and the pituitary hormones, prolactin and growth hormone. Estrogens stimulate development of the duct system in the breast, and progesterone stimulates lobul-alveolar formation. Milk secretion in the fully developed breast is caused by increased levels of prolactin. The relationship between estrogens, progesterone, and prolactin in the initiation of lactation has been explained by the double threshold theory of Folley (9). According to this concept, there is a critical low level of estrogen that activates the release of prolactin. This lactogenic effect of estrogen can be inhibited by high levels of progesterone, and this is presumed to be the inhibitory influence to lactation during pregnancy.

Prolactin is released by the anterior pituitary, but this process is controlled by an interplay between the circulating levels of estrogens, progesterone, and PIF from the hypothalamus. In general, there is a reciprocal relationship between prolactin and gonadotropin. Ovulation is suppressed during the initial phases of lactation, and when ovulation recurs lactation often decreases. Active suckling and physical manipulation induce the release of neurohypophysial oxytocin which induces milk ejection.

CLINICAL INVESTIGATION OF OVARIAN DISORDERS

Endocrinological assessment of the ovaries utilizes studies based on 1) the biological effects of the ovarian hormones and 2) excretion of ovarian hormones of their end products.

Studies of the biological effects of ovarian hormones studies include:

1. Cornification of vaginal epithelium—a reliable index of ovarian estrogen production; absence of these characteristics on vaginal smear would suggest decreased estrogen effect.
2. Endometrial cytology—an endometrial biopsy gives information in the endometrial responsiveness to estrogens and progesterone, depending on the phase of the cycle.
3. Cervical mucus test—the quantity and consistency of the cervical mucus, as well as the arborization pattern of the dried mucus ("fern test"), are an indication of the presence of estrogen.
4. Progesterone withdrawal bleeding—the induction of menstrual bleeding by administration of progestational agent is regarded as evidence for prior estrogen "priming" of the endometrium.
5. Buccal smear examination for nuclear sex chromatin pattern—essential in certain problems associated with amenorrhea and hirsutism.
6. Chromosome karyotype and analysis—necessary in some patients with equivocal gonads and for determining genetic sex as well as the presence of mosaicism.

Studies on hormones and end products in biological fluids include:

1. Urinary excretion of estrogens and pregnanediol—measures of estrogen and progesterone production, respectively.
2. Tests of adrenocortical activity—often necessary in the study of certain ovarian disorders. The tests include urinary 17-OHCS, 17-KGS, and 17-KS, as well as the levels of pregnanetriol, tetrahydrodeoxycortisol, and similar compounds, depending on the physical features presented.
3. Thyroid function tests—indicated in certain cases of amenorrhea and hypermenorrhea syndromes.
4. Ovarian and adrenocortical stimulation tests—performed to determine whether they operate under control of their appropriate tropic hormones or function autonomously as in the presence of neoplasm. Such tests include:

a) Dexamethasone suppression test in which the patient is given 0.5 mg of dexamethasone 4 times daily for 3 days (light dose). Parameters measured include plasma cortisol and plasma testosterone. If there is cortisol suppression but no decrease in the increased plasma testosterone, then the source of the androgen is extra-adrenal. The validity of this concept is being questioned.

b) Dexamethasone plus diethylstilbesterol suppression which follows the above test. While dexamethasone is continued (0.5 mg 4 times daily), diethylstilbesterol 5 mg twice daily is given for 10 days.

c) Dexamethasone suppression (of adrenals) plus HCG stimulation. The dosage of dexamethasone is continued as above, and the patient is given HCG injections (4,000 units) intramuscularly every 2 days for 3 doses.

In the three procedures listed above, plasma or urinary testosterone and/or urinary 17-KS are measured before and after the challenges. There are suggestions that data from these perturbations are not as helpful as hitherto assumed.

ENDOCRINE DISORDERS OF OVARIES

These disorders are considered under the headings of hypofunctional (Tables 18.2 and 18.3), hyperfunctional syndromes (Table 18.4), syndromes of unknown pathogenesis (such as Stein-Leventhal syndrome and idiopathic hirsutism), and disorders of unknown pathogenesis affecting ovarian function. Under this last grouping are included: polycystic ovarian disease (Stein-Leventhal syndrome) and its variants, as well as idiopathic hirsutism and certain virilizing syndromes. Comparisons will be made with adrenal disorders which may also present with similar signs and symptoms.

Polycystic Ovarian Disease (Stein-Leventhal Syndrome)

Studies from various centers suggest clinical and chemical variants of this disorder (10–12). Sterility, primary or secondary amenorrhea, oligomenorrhea, hirsutism, obesity, or several of these symptoms are the usual presenting manifestations. The most characteristic finding is that of globular enlargement, usually bilateral, of the ovaries. When visualized by culdoscopy, laparascopy, or laparotomy, they are found to have a white glistening surface which is ascribed to condensation of collagen at the surface, giving the appearance of a "thickened capsule" covering several small follicular cysts. Hyperplasia and luteinization of the thecal elements, as well as an increase in the interstitial components, are prominent.

These ovaries are quite active in estrogen and androgen synthesis, and the plasma levels of androstenedione and testosterone are above normal, as is the response to gonadotropin stimulation. A defect in gonadotropin regulation of the ovary is suggested by the finding of normal levels of FSH and high levels of LH in the plasma. The occasional finding of Δ^5-pregnenetriolone in patients with this disorder suggests possible adrenocortical participation in the pathogenesis. The improvement observed after use of exogenous corticosteroids in approximately 30% of these patients is consistent with this concept. Despite clinical success with the use of

Table 18.2. Intrinsic Ovarian Disorders Causing Hypofunction

Intrinsic ovarian disorder	Etiology	Clinical features	Diagnostic tests
Gonadal dysgensis and variants	Chromosomal XO and occasional mosaicism	Phenotypic female; classic Turner's syndrome: webbed neck, short stature, cubitus valgus, microthelia, low hair line in back; external genitalia female; occasional coarction of aorta; Mullerian fusion occurs but structures are very immature; amenorrhea; in patients with + chromatin pattern, the congenital defects are not marked; differential diagnosis includes patients with amenorrhea caused by absence of vagina and uterus and ovaries	Chromatin pattern +; chromosome karyotype XO; urinary or plasma pituitary gonadotropins are high
Testicular feminization	Incomplete descent of testes (abdominal, inguinal, or scrotal); testicular hormone production normal, but there is target organ nonresponsiveness	Chromatin negative patients with primary amenorrhea, mature appearance, but genotypically XY; scant axillary and pubic hair; no Wolffian duct stimulation	Chromatin pattern−; chromosome karyotype XY; urinary or plasma gonadotropins high; plasma testosterone probably normal
Premature senescence of ovaries	Unknown	Secondary amenorrhea cessation of menses before age 40 years; severe menopausal symptoms	Plasma and urine pituitary gonadotropic hormones elevated

Table 18.3. Ovarian Disorders Caused by Defects in Gonadotropin Secretion by Hypothalamic-Hypophysial System

Disorder	Etiology	Clinical features	Diagnostic tests
Destructive lesions of pituitary or hypothalamic nuclei	Infection, neoplasms, hemorrhage; most common tumor in children is craniopharyngioma	Altered menses may be early sign of pituitary tumor; features depend upon location: anterior suprasellar location may cause visual defect and hypogonadotropinism; mediolateral area damage causes obesity; posterior location of suprasellar tumor affects release of anterior and posterior pituitary hormones	Depending on area of involvement: plasma and urinary gonadotropins should be decreased; other tropic hormones, see test under anterior pituitary
Postpartum pituitary necrosis	Thrombosis in portal system supplying anterior pituitary	Failure of reappearance of menses after delivery; failure to lactate; slow or no regrowth of pubic hair, axillary hair, sparse body hair; atrophic changes in vagina and uterus, breasts; thyroid and adrenal insufficiency later	Urinary estrogens decreased; pituitary gonadotropins in urine and plasma low; plasma cortisol response to vasopressin absent
Panhypopituitarism	Neoplasms, infections, hemorrhage	Children who fail to mature normally; adults with secondary amenorrhea; in addition, will have features of lack of other tropic hormones (thyroid and adrenal)	Plasma and urine pituitary gonadotropins decreased; also see section on anterior pituitary

Table 18.4. Syndromes of Ovarian Hyperfunction

Disorder	Etiology	Clinical features	Diagnostic tests
Sexual precocity			
Constitutional	Premature release of gonadotropins in adult sequence; may be genetic	Occurrence of menarche before age 10, or evidence of feminization before age 8 or 9 Breast development, pubic and axillary hair growth; menstruation; accelerated linear growth and advanced bone age; premature epiphyseal closure eventually shorter than normal	Urine and plasma pituitary gonadotropins elevated Urine estrogens elevated
Organic lesion (cerebral)	Cerebral lesions abolish hypothalamic inhibitory influences	Similar manifestations as in constitutional disorders; usual locations of lesions are tuber cinereum, posterior hypothalamic mamillary body and pineal destruction; other causes are meningitis, encephalitis, internal hydrocephalus, and trauma	Urine and plasma pituitary gonadotropins; urine estrogens increased
Precocious pseudopuberty		In pseudoprecocious puberty, there is no increase in gonadotropic hormones, ovulation does not occur	
Ovarian	Ovarian tumors (rare)	Isosexual precocity; absence of ovulation and cyclic menstrual bleeding; presence of adnexal mass	Plasma and urine gonadotropins are low or absent; estrogens increased

Adrenal	Adrenal tumor (non-virilizing, estrogen producing—very rare)	Similar to above	As above
Amenorrhea caused by ovarian disease	Non-neoplastic: persistent follicle cyst; polycystic ovary, ovarian hyperthecosis, stromal hyperplasia	Expression depends on age of host: precocity, anovulatory amenorrhea, menometrorrhagic postmenopausal bleeding	Plasma and urine gonadotropins decreased; Urinary estrogens increased
Androgenic	Arrhenoblastoma: Sertoli-Leydig cell tumor	Defeminization before masculinization; amenorrhea, loss of breast fullness, followed by acne, hirsutism, clitoral hypertrophy, beard formation, deepening of voice	Urine 17-KS normal; testosterone elevated
	Hilus cell tumors (rare) benign		Urine 17-KS normal; testosterone probably high
	Luteoma of pregnancy Gynandroblastoma, Brenner tumor		

adrenal suppression (by dexamethasone), recent data suggest that dexamethasone suppression is not necessarily confined to the pituitary-adrenocortical axis. It is now suggested that dexamethasone suppressibility of plasma androsterone and testosterone may be independent of adrenal suppression.

Idiopathic Hirsutism

Idiopathic hirsutism refers to excess growth of facial, body, pubic, and axillary hair in female patients. These findings are ascribed to increased androgen secretion from the adrenals or ovaries or to end-organ hypersensitivity to normal amounts of androgens. Several factors are undoubtedly involved in this "hyper-response." These include levels of SHBG, its differential affinity for androgens and estrogens, and the effect of binding on conversion of testosterone to dihydrotestosterone, the most active androgen. Local cutaneous factors may be involved in the latter reaction.

Virilization

Virilization is characterized by the following features: increased muscle mass, deepening of the voice caused by changes in the larynx, enlargement of the clitoris, and an increase in sexual hair. In these patients, the menstrual periods are either absent or irregular. Onset of these symptoms in the adult female should suggest the presence of a neoplasm in either the ovary (e.g., arrhenoblastoma) or in the adrenal cortex (e.g., adrenocortical carcinoma). Occasionally, the postpubertal form of virilizing adrenal hyperplasia is detected at this age to be a cause of this syndrome. Several of the factors described under idiopathic hirsutism may also be involved in this disorder.

Laboratory Diagnosis of Virilization and Hirsutism

The clinical signs reflect increased androgenic effects, whether caused by increased androgen levels or the hyper-response to normal amounts of the hormones. Accordingly, the parameter that is emphasized in the work-up of such patients is plasma testosterone. The scheme in Figure 18.4 presents an approach to the diagnosis of these problems. The dexamethasone and diethylstilbesterol procedures provide useful information on the degree of autonomy of the glands. It is listed that urinary 17-KS and 17-KGS are also helpful. Flow sheets for differential diagnosis of such problems were presented previously (1, 2).

Treatment of Hirsutism In patients with hirsutism in whom the basis is identified, e.g., Cushing's syndrome or masculinizing ovarian tumors, surgical therapy results in resolution of the excessive hair growth in most patients. Hirsutism caused by virilizing adrenocortical hyperplasia improves in about 35–50% of the patients after several months of dexa-

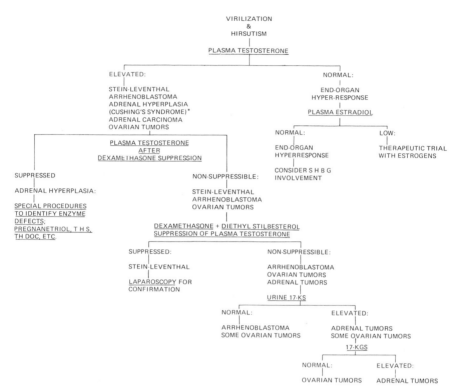

Figure 18.4. Scheme for laboratory diagnosis of virilization and amenorrhea utilizing measurement of plasma testosterone before and after dexamethasone and/or diethylstilbesterol suppression. Supplementary studies may include quantitation of 17-KS, 17-KGS, and other adrenocortical metabolites in the urine.

methasone suppression therapy. Hirsutism associated with the Stein-Leventhal syndrome rarely improves after wedge resection despite permanent or temporary restitution of menstrual cyclicity. Patients with Stein-Leventhal syndrome and with "idiopathic" hirsutism may reveal patterns of suppressibility of previously elevated plasma testosterone after challenges with dexamethasome, with and without diethylstilbesterol. A regimen of dexamethasone (0.5 mg/day) along with a high estrogen oral contraceptive has resulted in decreased hair growth in 40–50% of patients in our series.

Laboratory Diagnosis of Amenorrhea

The schemes presented in Figures 18.5 and 18.6 outline the laboratory methods for the work-up of primary and secondary amenorrhea. The employment of the dexamethasone suppression procedure is included largely because of evidence of its practical value despite some data suggest-

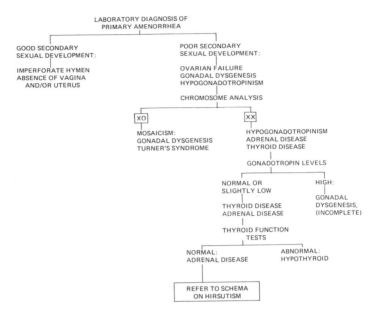

Figure 18.5. Scheme for laboratory diagnosis of primary amenorrhea. Absent gonad-otropins (FSH and LH) indicate work-up for hypothalamic-pituitary disease. (Reprinted from Bacchus (2) with permission of the publisher.)

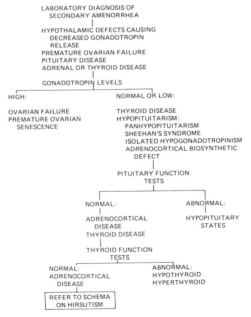

Figure 18.6. Scheme for laboratory diagnosis of secondary amenorrhea. The scheme on work-up of hirsutism would be useful if the amenorrhea is associated with signs of increased androgen effects. (Reprinted from Bacchus (2) with permission of the publisher.)

ing that dexamethasone suppressibility does not necessarily define adrenal involvement in pathogenesis. Despite the widespread and established usefulness of these physiological perturbations in the differential diagnosis of these problems, there are now suggestions that the only definitive diagnostic methods should involve cannulation of venous effluents from the ovaries and adrenals for blood samples for hormone measurements. In view of the expense and hazards of these invasive procedures and the relative reliability of the methods outlined above, it is unlikely that hormone determinations on gland effluents will be practical for widespread use.

LITERATURE CITED

1. Bacchus, H. 1975. Essentials of Gynecologic and Obstetric Endocrinology, pp. 37–67. University Park Press, Baltimore.
2. Bacchus, H. 1972. Endocrine profiles in the clinical laboratory. *In* M. Stefanini (ed.), Progress in Clinical Pathology. Vol. 4, pp. 1–101. Grune & Stratton, Inc., New York.
3. Villee, D. B. 1969. Development of endocrine function in the human placenta and fetus. N. Engl. J. Med. 281:473–484.
4. Villee, D. B. 1972. The development of steroidogenesis. Am. J. Med. 53:533–544.
5. Bruner, J. A. 1951. Distribution of chorionic gonadotropin in mother and fetus at various stages of pregnancy. J. Clin. Endocrinol. 11:360.
6. Lauritzen, C., and W. D. Lehrmann. 1967. Levels of chorionic gonadotropin in the newborn infant and their relationship to adrenal dehydroepiandrosterone. J. Endocrinol. 39:173–182.
7. Plager, J. E., K. G. Schmidt, and W. S. Stanbetz. 1958. Increased unbound cortisol in the plasma of estrogen tested subjects. J. Clin. Invest. 18:208–221.
8. Anderson, A. B., K. M. Lawrence, and A. C. Turnbull. 1969. The relationship in anencephaly between the size of the adrenal cortex and the length and gestation. J. Obstet. Gynaecol. Br. Commonw. 76:196–199.
9. Folley, S. J. 1956. The Physiology and Biochemistry of Lactation. Oliver & Boyd, Ltd., Edinburgh.
10. Stein, I. F., and M. L. Leventhal. 1935. Amenorrhea associated with bilateral polycystic ovaries. Am. J. Obstet. Gynecol. 29:181–191.
11. Axelrod, L. R., and J. W. Goldzieher. 1962. Polycystic ovary. Steroid biosynthesis in normal and polycystic ovarian tissue. J. Clin. Endocrinol. Metab. 22:431–440.
12. Kirschner, M. A., and C. W. Bardin. 1972. Androgen production and metabolism in normal and virilized women. Metabolism 21:667–688.

19

The
Parathyroids

The parathyroid glands, through secretion of parathyroid hormone (PTH), serve essential functions in maintenance of the internal milieu, ranging from regulation of hormone secretion to participation in remodeling of the skeletal system. There is good evidence to indicate that these glands may have evolved in vertebrates which left the calcium-rich ocean to live on dry land. The actions of parathyroid hormone are closely related to and influenced by activities of other hormones, such as calcitonin from the C cells of the thyroid, 1,25-dihydroxycholecalciferol from the kidneys, as well as by pituitary and gonadal hormones. This discussion is based on considerations presented previously (1–4). In this chapter, the participation of calcitonin and the vitamin D metabolites will be considered in detail as it is impossible to consider the various actions of PTH without an understanding of the relationships of those substances to the parathyroid function.

In man, four or five small parathyroid glands are located just beneath the thyroid gland substance. Despite this association, the embryological derivation of the parathyroids from the third and fourth branchial arches is distinct from the origin of the thyroid gland. In rare instances, parathyroid tissue may be found in ectopic sites, such as within the thyroid gland and the mediastinum. The major cell type in the gland is the chief cell of which there are two subgroups, the dark cells that contain glycogen and are actively secretory and the lighter chief cells that are presumably quiescent in this function. Oxyphil cells and wasserhelle (water clear) cells are presumably developmentally related to the chief cells, but do not produce PTH under normal conditions.

PTH is a polypeptide hormone which is made up of 84 amino acids. The complete structures of the hormone in ovine, porcine, and human tissue have been elucidated. Biological activity of the PTH molecule resides in the peptide made up of amino acids 1–29. New findings indicate that the hormone is synthesized as a relatively larger peptide on the polysomes. This pre-proparathyroid hormone is attached to the site of synthesis by the amino acid methionine. The proparathyroid (pro-PTH) is also larger than PTH. Intracellular cleavage of pro-PTH releases PTH which is stored in the cytosol of the cell. There are convincing data that the additional amino acids present in pre-pro-PTH and in pro-PTH are attached to the NH_2-terminal end of the PTH molecule. After the 84 amino acid peptide is released into the circulation, there is further cleavage so that the biologically active component is smaller than the secreted PTH. Species of PTH of molecular weights 11,500, 7,500, and 4,500 are now known, and these fragments are quantitated by the current radioimmunoassay methods. The COOH-terminal fragment is the predominant hormonal species in the blood stream. Partly based on this finding, it is suggested that the disappearance of the NH_2-terminal fragment exceeds that of the COOH-terminal. It is now also clear that the larger fragment lacks the critical structure for biological activity. As stated above, biological activity resides in the peptide 1–29 of the molecule. It is also known that the presence of alanine at the NH_2-terminal is essential for full biological activity of PTH.

Immunological activity is dependent on several smaller fragments, and this factor is responsible for considerable confusion as to the significance of levels of PTH assayed and of the meaning of several kinetic studies in parathyroid disorders. There are some data to suggest the possibility of biologically active PTH isohormones. In view of the above considerations, it is clear that caution is necessary in interpretation of data based on radioimmunoassay, at least until more information on the nature of the circulating fragments is available and antibody specificity is defined.

There is no significant storage of PTH in the gland, and studies based on hormone secretory rates indicate that, under normal conditions, the glands replenish their content of hormones by biosynthesis 3–15 times/hr in order to support normal rates. Maximal stimulation is accommodated by biosynthetic rates sufficient to replenish the entire gland content every few minutes.

BIOLOGICAL ACTIONS OF PTH

PTH is intimately involved, along with factors such as calciferols and calcitonin, in the maintenance of calcium kinetics in the body. Calcium ions play a vital role in normal neuromuscular function, blood coagulation, numerous enzymatic reactions, cell membrane function, and regulation of secretion of several hormones. Insoluble calcium plays a vital role in the maintenance of skeletal structure. Specific functions of PTH in bone, renal, and gastrointestinal mucosal functions are now clearly identified.

PTH Action on Gastrointestinal Mucosal Cell

PTH is known to induce an increase of calcium absorption by the intestinal mucosal cell. While some studies suggest a direct action of the hormone in this process, there are now highly suggestive data that this action of PTH is mediated by the stimulation of production of 1,25-dihydroxy-cholecalciferol (1,25-DHCC) in the kidneys. This hormone (1,25-DHCC) induces the synthesis of mucosal calcium-binding protein.

PTH Action on Bone

PTH is known to have distinct effects on bone. The initial action, osteocytic osteolysis, is of rapid onset and serves to release calcium from bone mineral into the blood. This mechanism of activity involves the release of membrane adenylate cyclase in the osteocytes. The second action of PTH on bone is to promote extensive bone remodeling, a process mediated through the stimulation of osteoclast replication and cellular activity. This action is also activated by the PTH-induced release of membrane adenylate cyclase. PTH also induces an increase of intracellular calcium, and this action may be important in the release of adenylate cyclase from the inner membrane of the cell. During the process of osteocytic osteolysis and of bone remodeling, there is a release of hydroxyproline and hydroxylysine from the bone matrix. Continuous exposure to large amounts of PTH is followed by extensive morphological changes and bone remodeling. This may result in marked dissolution of bone mineral and severe weakening of skeletal structure.

PTH Action on Renal Tubule Cell

The earliest response of the kidneys to PTH is an increased phosphate clearance. This action is noted within minutes of administration of PTH. A marked decrease in tubular reabsorption of sodium in the proximal convoluted tubule is also noted to occur. An associated decreased reabsorption of potassium results from PTH administration. PTH markedly increases the tubular reabsorption of calcium. A 2- to 3-fold reduction of urinary calcium has been reported after administration of PTH in human subjects. The renal reabsorption of calcium approaches 99%, and, in hypocalcemic states, may reach 100%. Despite the release of calcium from bone under PTH influence, there is a decrease in total renal clearance of calcium. The increased urine calcium in hyperparathyroidism is a reflection of the effects of PTH on bone, with an increased filtered load, despite the increased PTH-induced reabsorption of calcium. These factors indicate clearly that the renal conservation of calcium by the kidney is of sufficient magnitude to contribute to calcium homeostasis.

PTH Actions on Other Systems

Through its effects on calcium levels and partition, PTH may affect the activity of the central nervous system, but there are certain actions on the nervous system by PTH which may be independent of calcium. The permeability of the ocular lens to calcium is affected by PTH.

INTERRELATIONSHIPS AMONG METABOLIC ACTIONS OF PTH, CALCITONIN, AND VITAMIN D

There is a close interplay between PTH and the hormones calcitonin (CT) and 1,25-dihydrocholecalciferol in the regulation of calcium and bone metabolism. Effects of this interplay are also noted in the renal handling of other ions including phosphate, sodium, potassium, chloride, and bicarbonate.

Calcitonin

The hormone calcitonin is produced by the C or parafollicular cells of the thyroid gland. These cells are derived from the fourth branchial pouch in higher vertebrates, and their origin is related to the neural crest. Parafollicular cells may also occur in the parathyroids and the thymus. In medullary carcinoma of the thyroid, there is an increased production of calcitonin. This hormone is a 32-amino acid peptide which has been characterized for several animal species. The entire 32-amino acid chain is required for biological activity. Several studies have shown that fragments of the peptide, whether derived from the NH_2-terminal, middle, or COOH-terminal regions, are totally without biological activity.

Despite considerable evidence that calcitonin secretion by the parafollicular cells occurs in several vertebrate species, similar information is lacking in man. The presence of calcitonin in the peripheral circulation of man was unequivocally demonstrated only in patients with medullary carcinoma of the thyroid and in hypercalcemic subjects. The influence of alterations in serum levels on calcitonin secretion in pigs and cattle was clearly demonstrated, hypercalcemia inducing an increase and hypocalcemia a decrease in serum calcitonin. It seems likely that the failure to demonstrate circulating calcitonin in man is caused by relative insensitivity of current assay methods.

Biological Actions of Calcitonin   The principal effect of calcitonin on bone is the inhibition or blockade of resorptive processes in the bone. This is in direct contrast to the action of PTH in this tissue. There are additional data to suggest that calcitonin may also inhibit bone formation, but this is not clearly established. The hormone calcitonin exerts significant effect on the renal tubule so that there is an increased renal clearance of calcium, phosphate, sodium, potassium, and magnesium. These effects are noted at similar dosage levels of calcitonin as are active on bone. However, in spite of elevated levels of calcitonin in the plasma of patients with medullary carcinoma of the thyroid, no renal clearance abnormalities are defined in these patients. This could be related to opposing actions of PTH and CT on the kidneys. CT exerts effects on the gastrointestinal absorption of calcium, but the direction of the effect is dose related. Experimental studies have shown that low doses are followed by decreases, whereas high doses are followed by increased calcium absorption. Kennedy and Talmage (5) showed that the effects of CT on calcium and phosphate are independent of each other. The effects on phosphate excretion are often greater, and the effect is directly proportional to the initial plasma phosphate.

Calcitonin activates the above processes by inducing a release of membrane-bound adenylate cyclase at the appropriate target cell. It is now clear that the renal tubule cells responsive to CT are located in different sections of the kidney from those responsive to PTH.

Vitamin D

Some consideration of vitamin D was presented in Chapter 9. New information on the actions of vitamin D metabolites on gastrointestinal, renal, and bone handling of calcium and phosphate is now available. It has long been apparent that vitamin D or its metabolites are importantly involved in the absorption of calcium and phosphorus. Several studies suggested that metabolic transformation of vitamin D was necessary for many actions ascribed to the vitamin. The intestinal transport of calcium occurs after vitamin D administration. But this increased transport which is maximal at the duodenum is not observed until 24–48 hr after administration of the vitamin. It is now apparent that this delay in the observed action relates to the metabolic transformation of the vitamin to compounds which are biologically active. The biologically active metabolite is now known to be the hormone 1,25-dihydroxycholecalciferol (1,25-DHCC). The synthesis of this hormone from the substrates 7-dehydrochosterol and ergosterol requires the processes of ultraviolet irradiation and enzymatic conversion in the liver and the kidneys. The substrate 7-dehydrocholesterol is present in the skin, whereas ergosterol is a dietary constituent. Ultraviolet irradiation of these substrates is responsible for the introduction of the 5,6- and 7,8-diene structure which is essential to hormonal activity (Figure 19.1).

Conversion of cholecalciferol (D_3) derived from 7-dehydrocholesterol to 25-hydroxycholecalciferol (25-HCC) is mediated by the hepatic enzyme 25-hydroxylase. This enzyme also converts ergocalciferol (derived from ergosterol) to 25-hydroxyergocalciferol. Prolonged irradiation followed by

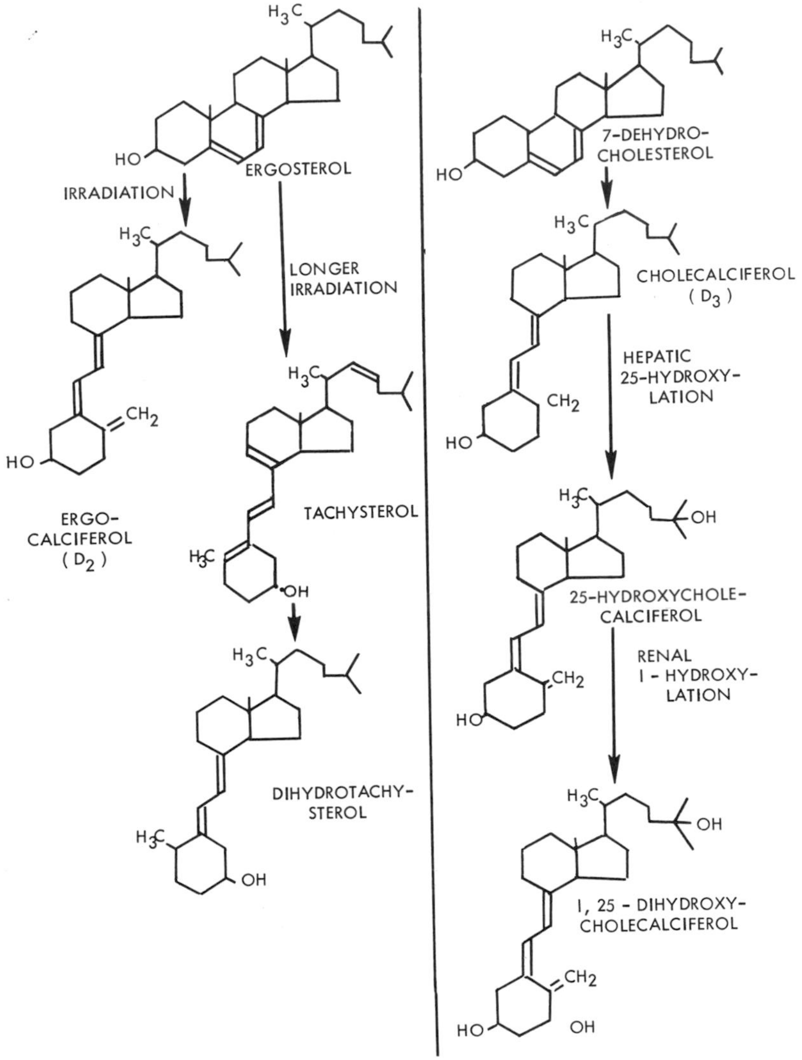

Figure 19.1. Synthetic steps in the formation of 1,25-dihydroxycholecalciferol, the active vitamin D principle. This compound fulfills the requirements for classification as a hormone. Parathyroid hormone exerts a tropic effect on the renal hydroxylation of the intermediate 25-hydroxycholecalciferol.

reduction is responsible for the production of dihydrotachysterol (DHT_2) from ergosterol. DHT_2 is converted by a hepatic 25-hydroxylase to 25-hydroxy-DHT_2. The enzymatic hydroxylation steps in the liver are subject to product inhibition. For example, the accumulation of 25-HCC inhibits the reaction responsible for its production. By this autoregulatory mechanism, the excessive production of 25-DHCC, the first step in the metabolic actions of vitamin D, is blocked. This hydroxylation step is also responsive to hormonal influences; for example, it is suppressed by glucocorticoid hormones.

A transport shuttle utilizing certain plasma proteins to transfer 25-HCC to the kidneys for further chemical change is known. The metabolite 25-HCC is converted to the biologically active hormone 1,25-DHCC by the 1α-hydroxylase in the kidneys (Figure 19.2). Addition of the hydroxyl group at position 1 in the metabolites of D_2 and D_3 is essential for optimal biological activity. The 1α hydroxylation step is regulated by PTH, but an indirect regulation by plasma calcium levels, presumably through PTH, is also known. DeLuca (6) has demonstrated that the renal conversion of 25-HCC to either 1,25-DHCC or 24,25-DHCC is dependent on PTH and calcitonin, respectively.

Biological Actions of Active Vitamin D Metabolites on Gastrointestinal Tract Vitamin D metabolites, the most active of which is 1,25-DHCC, are quite active in the intestinal mucosal cell. The major action of this hormone at this level is stimulation of synthesis of calcium binding or transport proteins. A second action which appears to be independent of protein synthesis may involve direct intestinal cell membrane effects and the stimulation of calcium diffusion into cells. There are considerable data indicating that the action of the 1,25-DHCC is to

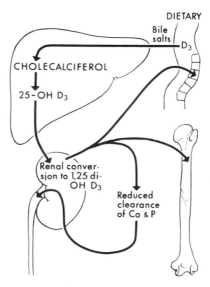

Figure 19.2. Absorption, hepatic and renal transformation, and physiological effects of vitamin D.

stimulate transcription of a messenger RNA which directs synthesis of protein components which act in transport function both in the intestinal mucosal cell and presumably in bone. The intramucosal synthesis of calcium-binding protein is the major method of calcium absorption at this level. It has been suggested that a calcium-dependent ATPase might be linked to the function of the binding protein.

Action on Bone The action of 1,25-DHCC on bone appears to be stimulation of subcellular systems necessary for calcium transport out of bone. It is known that even in the absence of PTH, however, a factor important in the formation of 1,25-DHCC, large pharmacological doses of vitamin D lead to enhanced bone resorption and dissolution of both bone mineral and matrix. There are data to suggest that vitamin D metabolites may be essential cofactors in PTH-induced bone resorption.

Action on Kidneys Vitamin D, probably through its biologically active metabolites, leads to a reduced renal clearance of calcium and phosphate in the presence of intact parathyroid glands. This action is possibly secondary to reduced PTH secretion caused by vitamin D-induced increased serum calcium.

INFLUENCE OF INTERPLAY AMONG PTH, CT, AND 1,25-DHCC ON CALCIUM HOMEOSTASIS

The actions of the hormones 1,25-DHCC, PTH and, presumably, calcitonin are interrelated in the maintenance of calcium and phosphate homeostasis. Although vitamin D does promote intestinal absorption of calcium even in the absence of PTH, this action is considerably enhanced by PTH. That some vitamin actions may be present even in the absence of PTH is confirmed by the therapeutic usefulness of the vitamin in hypoparathyroid patients.

PTH exerts actions on the renal clearance of phosphate even in the presence of severe vitamin D deficiency. In many forms of osteomalacia, the development of secondary hyperparathyroidism is responsible for increased phosphate excretion and eventual phosphate wasting.

In vitamin D deficiency, serum levels of calcium tend to be low or low normal, but serum PTH is usually increased, a reflection of parathyroid hyperplasia. Undoubtedly there is considerable resistance to PTH action in this state, as parathyroidectomy is not followed by significant decreases in serum calcium.

There is considerable interest in the probable relevance of the double loop control of serum calcium levels by PTH and CT, known to exist in several animal species, to human calcium metabolism. There are data showing that CT secretion is directly proportional to serum calcium concentration. An inverse proportion between PTH secretion and calcium concentration has also been shown. In the presence of normal serum calcium concentration, both hormones are continuously being secreted. The secretion of CT is not suppressed until serum calcium decreases by 1 mg/100 ml below normal levels. The secretion of PTH is not suppressed until serum calcium is about 2 mg/100 ml above the normal calcium level. This system presumably serves a measure of fine control of serum calcium, at least in the species studied. It is likely that the patterns relating to PTH in the double loop control concept apply to man, but the relevance of CT levels in fine control of calcium in man is less certain.

Local ionic control of calcium and phosphate transport in the kidney is suggested by several lines of data. The renal clearance of phosphate is, at least in part, dependent on extracellular and renal cellular concentration of calcium. Calcium replenishment in hypoparathyroid subjects is followed by increased renal clearance. Phosphate loads may lead directly to increased renal phosphate clearance in hypoparathyroid patients whose serum calcium concentration is normal.

As described previously, PTH promotes absorption of calcium and phosphate in the gastrointestinal tract, and induces a mobilization of calcium and phosphate from mineralized bone and of hydroxyproline from bone matrix. These effects of PTH on bone and intestinal transport are lost in the vitamin D-deficient state, perhaps in part related to resistance to PTH action caused by hypocalcemia. The effect of PTH on the kidney is not dependent on vitamin D, so that renal phosphate excretion caused by PTH is noted. The effect of PTH on mobilization of bone matrix and mineral is antagonized by an equivalent dose of CT, but the phosphatemic effect of PTH is not altered. Another example of interrelationships among these hormones in mineral metabolism is seen in the effect of CT in lowering the rate of resorption of bone mineral and matrix. This effect of CT is not inhibited in vitamin D deficiency, contrasting markedly to the effect on PTH action.

CLINICAL DISORDERS OF PARATHYROID FUNCTION

The clinical disorders of parathyroid function cover a spectrum ranging from excessive, presumably autonomous production of PTH from the parathyroid gland or from ectopic sources to the underproduction of PTH as well as decreased end-organ responsiveness to the hormone. The hyperparathyroid states include primary hyperparathyroidism, ectopic production of PTH, familial hyperparathyroidism with associated endocrinopathies, and various forms of secondary hyperparathyroidism. The hypoparathyroid states include decreased PTH production caused by parathyroid damage or removal, autoimmune hypoparathyroidism, and end-organ nonresponsiveness to PTH (pseudohypoparathyroidism).

HYPERPARATHYROIDISM

Primary Hyperparathyroidism

Primary hyperparathyroidism is a generalized disturbance of bone, calcium, and phosphorous metabolism resulting from excessive and presumably autonomous production of parathyroid hormone. Around 90% of all cases of primary hyperparathyroidism are ascribable to benign adenomas of single or multiple parathyroid glands. Rarely, malignant neoplasms of the parathyroid may produce excessive amounts of PTH. Parathyroid adenomas may occur in any of the four parathyroids, but are more frequently associated with the two inferiorly located glands. Rarely, parathyroid adenomas may be found in aberrant locations such as in the thymus, the thyroid, the pericardium, or in retroesophageal areas. Most parathyroid adenomas are confined to chief cell proliferation, often with a surrounding rim of normal tissue. Mixed cell populations, or primarily oxyphil cells, may rarely be found in adenomas. Parathyroid hyperplasia is another cause of excessive PTH production; in primary hyperplasia the cells are mainly of the wasserhelle (water-clear) type, but in secondary parathyroid hyperplasia the cell type is mainly the chief cell. Parathyroid carcinoma is an extremely rare slow-growing neoplasm which may occasionally metastasize to the liver and lungs.

In multiple endocrine adenomatosis (MEA), hyperparathyroidism is a frequent feature. Two forms of MEA are recognized. MEA type I consists of hyperparathyroidism caused by adenomas, associated with tumors of the pituitary and the islet cells of the pancreas. Occasionally there are associated gastric hypersecretion and peptic ulcer disease in this form of MEA. The association of hyperparathyroidism with pheochromocytoma and medullary carcinoma of the thyroid is found in MEA type II. The components of these syndromes may occur at different intervals during the course of the disorders.

Ectopic production of PTH has been found in patients with malignant neoplastic disorders not associated with bony metastases. Hypercalcemia is a feature of this disorder, and it is often associated with hypophosphatemia. The chemical findings in the blood resemble those in patients with primary hyperparathyroidism. The most frequently found tumors associated with pseudohyperparathyroidism are squamous cell carcinoma of the lungs. Renal cancers, as well as others, have been found as sites of ectopic production of PTH.

Clinical Manifestations of Hyperparathyroidism

Hyperparathyroidism is characterized by clinical symptoms and signs referrable to several organ systems, and quite frequently the complaints are only retrospectively described after therapy. Many of the clinical manifestations are ascribed to the associated hypercalcemia, although all details of the mechanism are not clear.

Neuromuscular involvement noted in patients with hyperparathyroidism may range from mild personality disturbances to psychiatric disorders. Neurological involvement may include obtundation and coma. In many patients, the sole complaint may be muscle weakness, quite often of the hands.

Renal manifestations of hyperparathyroidism are ascribed to hypercalcemia. These include nephrocalcinosis and nephrolithiasis. Microscopic or gross hematuria may result from calcium phosphate or calcium oxalate calculi. Nephrocalcinosis is caused by microscopic calcium deposits, primarily in the renal tubules. Associated manifestations include polyuria with a renal concentration defect, aminoaciduria, renal tubular acidosis, and occasionally glycosuria. Severe involvement may involve the glomeruli so that renal failure may supervene. The sequelae of renal failure may mask the chemical findings of hyperparathyroidism and serum phosphate may increase.

The gastrointestinal manifestations of hyperparathyroidism include an incidence of peptic ulcer disease higher than in the general population. This is presumably ascribable to the increased gastrin production caused by hypercalcemia. Pancreatitis has been described as occurring in this disorder, but the mechanism is not clear. Constipation is found in most patients with hyperparathyroidism. Elevated blood pressure is found quite frequently in patients with hypercalcemia, but the mechanism of this finding is not yet determined. An association between hyperparathyroidism and gout has been reported. Chrondrocalcinosis (pseudogout) is frequently seen in hyperparathyroidism, and there are suggestions that all patients with pseudogout should be screened for possible hyperparathyroidism. Depositions of calcium in the skin and soft tissues are occasionally palpable. Calcification of the cornea leading to band keratopathy is occasionally found in hyperparathyroidism.

The bone involvement of hyperparathyroidism is especially marked even though bony changes may not be detectable by x-ray studies until late in the course of the disorder. PTH induces osteocytic osteolysis so that dissolution of mineralized bone and matrix may be detected by microscopic and isotope tracer studies on bone turnover. Osteomalacia, osteitis fibrosa cystica, osteosclerosis, and, occasionally, metastatic calcification may be found. The incidence of osteitis fibrosa cystica is significantly less in the United States, but the reason for this is not clear. Involvement of several bones may occasionally be seen on x-ray studies. These include the "salt and pepper" pattern of resorption seen in the skull, subperiosteal bone resorption in the fingers, as well as bone cysts and bone tumors on the long bones or jaws. Absence of the lamina dura on dental x-rays is also reliable evidence of increased parathyroid hormone actions.

Clinical Laboratory Features of Hyperparathyroidism

The most frequent finding on blood chemistry in hyperparathyroid patients is hypercalcemia, however slight the elevation may be. Quite frequently, the serum phosphate level is decreased. Most patients with hyperparathyroidism reveal a serum chloride level greater than 103 mEq/liter. Serum alkaline phosphatase is often elevated, but not invariably so. It is essential in all cases of hypercalcemia that adjustment be made for the relationship to serum protein levels, as elevated proteins may cause a falsely high total serum calcium value. Urinary pH is often alkaline, and a lowered specific gravity is quite frequently found in patients with increased PTH. Urine hydroxyproline elevations in PTH excess reflect the dissolution of bone matrix.

Laboratory Diagnosis of Hyperparathyroidism

With rare exceptions, the detailed diagnostic work-up for hyperparathyroidism is undertaken because of the unequivocal finding of hypercalcemia. In this context, therefore, the differential diagnostic procedures are designed to distinguish the various etiologies of hypercalcemia. Table 19.1 presents the findings in several hypercalcemic states.

In addition to the unequivocal finding of hypercalcemia (on at least

Table 19.1. Laboratory Findings in Hypercalcemic States

	Serum					Urine		
Disease	Ca	Mg	P	Alk PO$_4$ase	TP[a]	Ca	Specific gravity	TRP[a]
Hyperparathyroidism	↑	↑	↓	↑	N[a]	↑	↓	↓
Ectopic PTH	↑	↑	↓	↑	N	↑	↓	↓
Sarcoid	N, ↑	N	N	N	↑	↑	N	↓, N
Milk alkali	N, ↑	N	N, ↑	N	N	N	N	N
Vitamin D excess	↑	↑	↑↓	N	N	↑	N	↓ N
Multiple myeloma	N, ↑	N	N	N	↑	↑	↑ N ↓	
Thyrotoxicosis	↑, N, ↓	N	N	N	N	↑	N	N
Bone metastases	↑	N	N	N	N	N	N	N
Adrenal insufficiency	↑	N	N	N	N	↑↓	N	N
Osteopetrosis	N	N	N	N	N	↑↓	N	N
Immobilization	↑	N	N	N	N	↑	↓, N	N

[a] TP, total protein; TRP, tubular reabsorption of phosphate; N, normal.

three occasions), the following battery of procedures has been formed to provide a very high degree of accuracy in diagnosis of hyperparathyroidism: 1) tubular reabsorption of phosphate; 2) the response of hypercalcemia to a glucocorticoid challenge; 3) determination of the serum chloride to phosphate ratio; and 4) where available, the quantitation of serum PTH, especially in relationship to the serum calcium level. A finding consistent with, but not diagnostic of, hyperparathyroidism is an elevated urine calcium, largely reflecting increased bone resorption. Some of these procedures were described in detail previously (7).

The total serum calcium is measured by standard chemical methods or as part of a battery such as in the SMA 12/60. As stated above, the calcium levels should be considered in relation to the serum proteins. It is essential that the range of serum calcium is firmly established. Normal serum calcium levels are reported to be between 8.8 and 10.4 mg/100 ml, but there are variations among different laboratories. The serum calcium levels determined in normal subjects by the SMA 12/60 method range from 8.8–10.6 mg/120 ml.

Tubular Reabsorption of Phosphate   The test for tubular reabsorption of phosphate takes advantage of the known phosphaturic action of PTH. The following measurements are made, creatinine and phosphate on a single 4-, 8-, 12-, or 24-hr urine sample and serum creatinine and phosphate on blood drawn at approximately the midpoint of the period of urine collection. The tubular reabsorption of phosphate (TRP) is calculated according to the following formula:

$$TRP = 1 - \frac{\text{Urine phosphate (mg/100 ml)} \times \text{serum creatinine (mg/100 ml)}}{\text{Urine creatinine (mg/100 ml)} \times \text{serum phosphate (mg/100 ml)}} \times 100$$

Normal subjects generally absorb in excess of 90% of the filtered phosphate load. Patients with hyperparathyroidism reabsorb less than 85%. It should be noted that high phosphate intakes as well as renal insufficiency may negate the accuracy of the test.

A pharmacological perturbation of this test is occasionally employed as a diagnostic test. In this test, the TRP is determined before and after an infusion of calcium. The premise that the test distinguishes autonomous PTH secretion from normal control is valid, but there are some data indicating that not all forms of hyperparathyroidism are caused by autonomous PTH production. In the actual conduct of the test, a baseline TRP is determined during a 4-hr period (8 a.m. to 12 noon) on day 1. Between 9 p.m. and 12 midnight of day 1, the patient is given an intravenous infusion of calcium at the dose range of 10 mg/kg body weight. On day 2, urine is collected between 8 a.m. and 12 noon, and blood is drawn at 10 a.m. Serum creatinine and phosphate are measured as in the description of the

TRP test, and the TRP on day 2 is calculated. In normal subjects given intravenous calcium, there is a greater than 50% increase in TRP, reflecting a drop in PTH, and, therefore, a nonautonomous source of the hormone. In patients with ectopic or autonomous PTH secretion, there is no significant change in TRP after the calcium infusion. The calcium infusion may induce a moderate to severe hypertension in some patients, and should be employed with due caution.

Another pharmacological perturbation utilizing the TRP involves the infusion of PTH based on the premise that TRP in patients with autonomous PTH production is not altered by exogenous PTH.

Glucocorticoid Provocative Test   This test is based on the observation that the hypercalcemia of sarcoidosis is eliminated by therapy with glucocorticoids. Subsequent studies showed that glucocorticoids also lower the hypercalcemia associated with multiple myeloma, vitamin D intoxication, and some malignant neoplasms, but not in patients with primary hyperparathyroidism or in the presence of ectopic PTH. More recent data suggest that not all patients with primary PTH excess exhibit a resistance to glucocorticoid challenge. In addition, there are some non-parathyroid hypercalcemic states in which there may be resistance to the glucocorticoid action.

The glucocorticoid challenge is performed as follows. One or two baseline elevated serum calcium levels are obtained. The patient is then given 80–100 mg of prednisone (or equivalent doses of cortisone acetate) daily for 10 days. If possible, serum calcium levels are determined daily or at 3–4 day intervals. In face of a suppression to normal calcium levels, the test is discontinued, but is continued for 10 days if an earlier drop is not seen. Failure to drop to normocalcemic levels after 10 days of glucocorticoid challenge suggests an autonomous PTH production, either primary or ectopic.

Serum Chloride to Phosphate Ratio   Based on the observations that PTH in excess induces a phosphate loss with resulting hypophosphatemia and an elevated serum chloride secondary to hyperchloremic acidosis caused by PTH-induced bicarbonate leak (8,9), it was concluded that a test utilizing these biological effects of PTH could be utilized to gauge PTH action.

Palmer, Nelson, and Bacchus (10) showed that the serum chloride to phosphate ratio is extremely useful in the differential diagnosis of hypercalcemia. In the calculation, serum chloride (as mEq/liter) is divided by serum phosphate (as mg/100 ml). Studies on several patients with non-hyperparathyroid hypercalcemic states and on a relatively large series of patients with surgically proved hyperparathyroidism showed that 96% of patients with hyperparathyroidism had Cl/PO_4 ratios over 33. In 92% of patients with non-parathyroid hypercalcemia, the ratio was less than 30

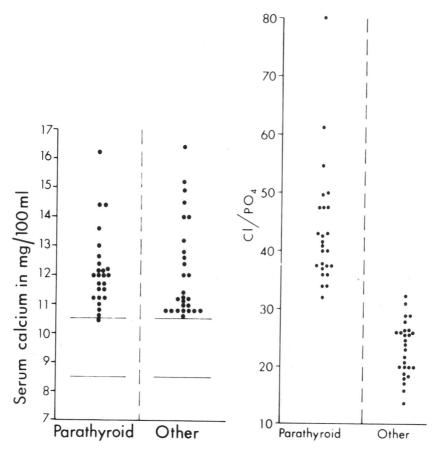

Figure 19.3. Serum calcium and Cl/PO$_4$ in patients with hyperparathyroid and non-hyperparathyroid (other) hypercalcemic states. (Reprinted from Palmer, Nelson, and Bacchus (10) with permission of the publisher.)

(Figure 19.3). This procedure has continued to be employed with at least comparable degree of success at this institution and others (11). It is important to recognize that this test employs known target organ effects of PTH and, in effect, provides an intrinsic biological assay system which can be effectively and inexpensively employed in the diagnosis of hyperparathyroid disease. The application of this procedure in laboratory followup of surgically treated patients is seen in Figure 19.4.

Radioimmunoassay of PTH in Differential Diagnosis of Hypercalcemia Despite several problems with the establishment of reliable radioimmunoassay of PTH as described by Potts et al. (12), this test is quite useful and reliable in the diagnostic evaluation of hypercalcemic states. By the best available method for PTH radioimmunoassay, the mean concen-

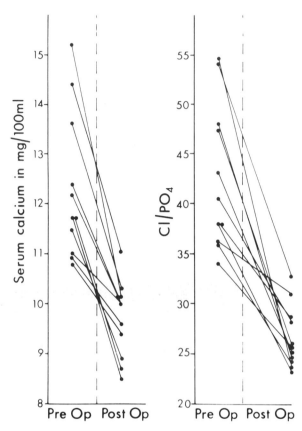

Figure 19.4. Preoperative and postoperative serum calcium and Cl/PO$_4$ ratios in patients with hyperparathyroidism. (Reprinted from Palmer, Nelson, and Bacchus (10) with permission of the publisher.)

tration of PTH in normal subjects is 0.56 ng/ml. In the series presented (12), 8 out of 18 patients with hyperparathyroidism showed levels of PTH above the highest values seen in normal subjects. All patients with hypercalcemia of other cause showed nondetectable PTH levels. When the PTH levels were plotted against serum calcium levels, there was clearer separation of the types of hypercalcemia. Now 14 out of 18 hyperparathyroid patients were clearly separated from normal subjects. By both methods of analysis, there was clear separation between the hypercalcemias from PTH excess as against those of other etiology. It has been pointed out (4), however, that in view of technical difficulty as well as expense, there remains a need for other parameters in the differential diagnosis of hypercalcemia. As shown above, the inexpensive Cl/PO$_4$ ratio may fill this need, with accuracy rate exceeding 96%.

Treatment of Hyperparathyroidism

Surgical removal of the source of excess PTH production is the preferred method of management, but this will depend on whether there are any medical contraindications to surgery. At the time of surgery, all parathyroid tissues should be identified. If an adenoma is identified and confirmed by frozen section, the tumor should be removed. The remaining glands should also be explored for the possibility of a second adenoma. If hyperplasia of the glands is found, all four or five glands should be examined and all but one should be removed in toto. The remaining gland should be partially resected and the remnant with adequate blood supply be left in situ. Parathyroid carcinoma should be widely excised.

Should no overt glandular abnormalities be found in the neck, then exploration for an aberrant site (most commonly the anterior mediastinum) is indicated.

Patients undergoing parathyroid excisional surgery may experience hypocalcemia within hours or months after surgery. This is often transient, but, if found, should be treated. It is therefore necessary to examine the patients for evidence of hypocalcemia (e.g., Chvostek's and Trousseau's signs or the occurrence of carpopedal spasms). Serial follow-up of serum calcium and phosphate is also necessary. Hypocalcemia sufficient to induce symptoms is treated with infusion of calcium gluconate or calcium lactate.

Medical Management of Hyperparathyroidism

It is occasionally necessary to palliate the clinical manifestations of hyperparathyroidism by medical means. These measures are designed to decrease or oppose the effects of hypercalcemia. The methods employing phosphate or ethylenediaminetetraacetate (EDTA) are less than satisfactory, the former causing metastatic calcification and the latter, renal toxicity. Sulfate and citrate in the doses required may precipitate renal toxicity also.

Hypercalcemic crises may be effectively treated with one of the three following methods. The first method is infusion of sodium chloride to assure abundant urinary output and calciuria. One procedure recommends the addition of furosemide to the regimen. Because of the marked tubular sensitivity to this drug in the presence of hypercalcemia, only low doses (10–20 mg) are recommended. Should a vigorous diuresis follow, then vigorous fluid replacement is absolutely essential. Occasionally the vigorous diuresis may be accompanied by hypomagnesemia, and replacement of magnesium may become necessary. The drug mithramycin at the dose level of 25 μg/kg body weight is quite effective in blocking osteocytic osteolysis. Significant decreases in serum calcium, often hypocalcemia, may be noted within 2 days after administration of the drug for 1 or 2 days. The dosage of the drug should be monitored closely and should not be repeated without ascertaining the degree of decrease of calcium. The dosage of this drug should be decreased in the presence of renal insufficiency. The use of glucocorticoids in dosages as in the glucocorticoid challenge test is rarely helpful in hypercalcemic crises caused by primary hyperparathyroidism. A more significant response is seen in patients with non-parathyroid-induced hypercalcemia.

Secondary Hyperparathyroidism

Secondary hyperthyroidism is found in several disorders of diverse etiologies in which there is an elevated and nonautonomous hypersecretion of PTH associated with resistance to the biological actions of PTH. Because of the latter phenomenon, these disorders are characterized by a mild degree of hypocalcemia, often of total calcium and frequently of ionized calcium.

Osteomalacia, pseudohypoparathyroidism, and chronic renal disease are the usual causes of secondary hyperparathyroidism. Several questions remain regarding the mechanisms of the development of secondary hyperactivity of the parathyroids in these disorders. It is known that the secretory capacity in these states may increase by 50- to 100-fold compared to the increase to 5—6 times under a hypocalcemic stimulus. It has been postulated that in chronic renal disease a component of vitamin D deficiency may be present. In pseudohypoparathyroidism, the target cell response is inadequate as demonstrated by a lack of an increase of renal tubule adenylate cyclase.

The scheme in Figure 19.5 depicts the pathogenesis of secondary hyperparathyroidism associated with chronic renal disease. Basic to this concept of pathogenesis is the resistance to vitamin D action. This prevents adequate absorption of calcium and phosphate from the gastrointestinal lumen. Factors contributing to this resistance are the presence of a phosphopeptide inhibitor and an acidosis secondary to chronic renal disease. In addition to the above phenomena, decreased conversion of 25-HCC to 1,25-DHCC, the active hormone, is responsible for a decreased calcium absorption. The resulting lowered serum calcium stimulates the production of PTH. This hormone is known to stimulate the 1α hydroxylation of 25-HCC by the kidneys. Despite the increased PTH levels, because of resistance to its action as well as of renal disease, the phosphaturic action of the hormone is suppressed, with a resultant hyperphosphatemia when the glomerular filtration rate reaches 15 ml/min or less.

The secondary increase in PTH activates osteocytic osteolysis and bone remodeling. These effects on bone evolve in four stages, namely, osteomalacia, osteitis fibrosa cystica, osteosclerosis, and, finally, metastatic calcification. Osteomalacia, the first change in the above sequence, is

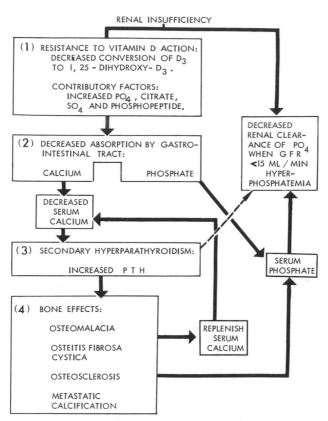

Figure 19.5. Pathogenesis of secondary hyperparathyroidism. The following major pathogenetic mechanisms are presented: resistance to vitamin D action, increased release of parathyroid hormone caused by decreased serum calcium, and decreased responsiveness of the kidneys to PTH.

caused by decreased calcium required for the calcification process. The treatment at this stage of disease progression is the administration of vitamin D. Osteitis fibrosa cystica is found with sustained increased PTH effect on bone, a reflection of increased bone resorption and remodeling. By this stage, there is significant phosphate retention, and therefore vitamin D therapy is dangerous because of possible precipitation of meta-static calcification. The therapy of choice at this stage involves use of agents to decrease phosphate absorption, e.g., aluminum hydroxide inges-tion. Osteosclerosis represents an advanced stage of PTH excess and is characterized by areas of bone remodeling and destruction.

Metastatic calcification is probably a reflection of increased phosphate in the circulation. In addition, the increased PTH action releases more phosphate from bone. The combination leads to the formation of calcium phosphate crystals in soft tissues, including the blood vessels and kidneys. Arterial calcification, readily seen in the interosseous vessels in the feet, is a frequent finding in this degree of secondary hyperparathyroidism. In these latter stages, the treatment of choice is parathyroidectomy. Renal transplantation in patients with the secondary hyperparathyroidism induced after the above fashion is followed by disappearance of resistance to PTH actions, and phosphaturia with decreased renal calcium clearance supervenes. This change is now termed "tertiary hyperparathyroidism." Later, there is re-equilibration of the various factors described above, and the hyperactivity of the parathyroid glands disappears.

HYPOPARATHYROIDISM

The most common cause of hypoparathyroidism is the surgical removal of the glands or trauma to their blood supply during thyroid surgery. Parathyroid atrophy of unknown etiology is occasionally found in children, especially females, and is relatively rare in Blacks. A familial incidence of this disorder, in association with pernicious anemia and adrenocortical insufficiency, has been reported. Idiopathic hypoparathyroidism is also found occasionally with Hashimoto's thyroiditis, moniliasis, and steatorrhea. A generalized autoimmune disorder is the probable mechanism of this syndrome. It has been suggested that, rarely, ^{131}I therapy for thyrotoxicosis may precipitate hypoparathyroidism, but this is highly questionable. Hypoparathyroidism starting in intrauterine life has occasionally been found in infants born of mothers with hyperparathyroidism.

A hypoparathyroid state is seen in the rare X-linked dominant disorder known as pseudohypoparathyroidism, representing an end-organ nonresponsiveness to PTH. The disorder is characterized by hypocalcemia and hyperphosphatemia as well as short stature, round face, and brachydactyly. These patients also exhibit subcutaneous calcification, strabismus, and mental retardation. Impaired taste and olfaction also occur. In these patients, despite an increase in the production of PTH, the biological actions of the hormone are lacking. Exogenous PTH fails to induce an increase in renal cAMP in these patients, a reflection of end-organ refractoriness.

Clinical Manifestations of Hypoparathyroidism

The major clinical manifestations seen in these patients are caused by the decreased circulating levels of ionized calcium. Tetany and convulsions are the most serious sequelae of the hypocalcemia. Latent neuromuscular hyperirritability may be elected by the Chvostek's and Trousseau's signs. Carpopedal spasms may be readily elicited by hyperventilation as well as by calciuretic agents such as furosemide. Phenothiazines and other drugs

Table 19.2. Laboratory Findings in Hypocalcemic States

Disease	Plasma					Urine		
	Ca	Mg	P	Alk PO$_4$ase	TP^a	Ca	Specific gravity	TRP^a
Hypoparathyroidism	↓	N^a	↑	N	N	↓	N	↑
Pseudohypoparathyroidism	↓	↓	↑	N	N	↓	N	↑
Malabsorption	↓	↓	↓	N	N,↓	↓	N	↑,↓
Rickets (simple)	↓	N	↓	N,↑	N	↓	N	↑
Rickets (vitamin D resistant)	↓	N	↓	N,↑	N	↓	N	↑
Pancreatitis	↓	N	↓	N,↑	N↓	↓,	N	N (?)

^{a}TP, total proteins; TRP, tubular reabsorption of phosphate; N, Normal.

which affect the central nervous system may also precipitate acute neuro-muscular manifestations. Posterior column decrease has been reported to result from hypocalcemia.

Osteosclerosis is the most common bony abnormality in hypoparathyroidism. Skull x-ray shows a thickened calvarium as well as calcification of the basal ganglia. Dentition is hypoplastic in these patients. Dry skin is often present in hypoparathyroidism. Monilial infections of the skin are found in the autoimmune form of this disorder.

Laboratory Findings in Hypoparathyroidism

The most important clinical laboratory data found in this disorder are hypocalcemia and hyperphosphatemia. Laboratory findings in several hypocalcemic states are presented in Table 19.2.

Treatment of Hypoparathyroidism

Current methods for management of these hypoparathyroid disorders are not ideal, as progression of certain aspects of hypoparathyroidism, for example, lenticular opacities, may continue despite therapy. The goals of current therapy are essentially to prevent the neuromuscular disorders secondary to hypocalcemia. To serve this goal, the treatment regimen involves the ingestion of 50,000–100,000 units of ergocalciferol daily along with an exogenous source of calcium. Calcium gluconate or calcium lactate wafers are quite widely used, but a convenient form of calcium supplement with higher levels of calcium is achieved by ingestion of 3–4 tablespoons of Neocalglucon daily. These agents are given in an attempt to maintain the serum calcium levels at 8.5–9.5 mg/100 ml. The newer vitamin D derivatives promise to be quite helpful in management of these patients. The use of dihydrotachysterol (1 mg/day) has helped maintain serum calcium at the desired levels. Acute hypocalcemic episodes are treated with intravenous or oral calcium gluconate.

Excessive therapy may precipitate hypercalciuria, nephrocalcinosis, and metastatic calcification. It is, therefore, essential that the patient be followed closely and that serum calcium, phosphate, and urea nitrogen be monitored at intervals.

In the event of excessive vitamin D dosage, the hypercalcemia may be treated with furosemide as outlined previously. In addition, glucocorticoid therapy may be used to suppress the 25-hydroxylase step in the liver which is essential to further biosynthesis of 1,25-DHCC.

LITERATURE CITED

1. Potts, J. T. Jr., and L. J. Deftos. 1974. Parathyroid hormone, thyro-calcitonin, vitamin D, bone and bone mineral metabolism. *In* P. K.

Bondy and L. E. Rosenberg (eds.), Diseases of Metabolism, 7th Ed., pp. 1225–1430. W. B. Saunders Co., Philadelphia.

2. Rasmussen, H. 1972. The cellular basis of mammalian calcium homeostasis. Clin. Endocrinol. Metab. 1:3–20.

3. Parsons, J. A., and J. T. Potts, Jr. 1972. Physiology and chemistry of parathyroid hormone. Clin. Endocrinol. Metab. 1:33–78.

4. Rasmussen, H. 1972. The parathyroid gland. In R. H. Williams (ed.), Textbook of Endocrinology. 5th Ed., pp. 660–773. W. B. Saunders Co., Philadelphia.

5. Kennedy, J. W., III, and R. V. Talmage. 1972. Effects of thyrocalcitonin on bone phosphate without concurrent effects on calcium. In R. V. Talmage and P. L. Munson (eds.), Calcium, Parathyroid Hormone and the Calcitonins, pp. 407–415. Excerpta Medica, New York.

6. DeLuca, H. F. 1975. The kidney as an endocrine organ involved in the function of vitamin D. Am. J. Med. 58:39–47.

7. Bacchus, H. 1972. Endocrine profiles in the clinical laboratory. In M. Stefanini (ed.), Progress in Clinical Pathology, pp. 1–101. Grune & Stratton, Inc., New York.

8. Muldowney, F. P., J. F. Donohue, R. Freaney, et al. 1970. Parathormone-induced renal bicarbonate wastage in intestinal malabsorption and in chronic renal failure. Ir. J. Med. Sci. 3:221–231.

9. Muldowney, F. P., D. V. Carroll, J. F. Donohue, et al. 1971. Correction of renal bicarbonate wastage by parathyroidectomy. Quart. J. Med. 40:487–498.

10. Palmer, F. J., J. C. Nelson, and H. Bacchus. 1974. The chloride phosphate ratio in hypercalcemia. Ann. Intern. Med. 80:200–204.

11. Haenel, L., L. J. Kryston, and L. C. Mills. 1974. Chloride: Phosphate and hypercalcemia. Ann. Intern. Med. 80:270–271.

12. Potts, J. T., Jr., L. J. Deftos, R. M. Burke, L. M. Sherwood, and G. D. Aurbach. 1967. Radioimmunoassay of parathyroid hormone: Studies of the control of secretion of the hormone and parathyroid function in clinical disorders. In Radioisotopes in Medicine: In vitro studies, pp. 207–229. U. S. Atomic Energy Commission, Oak Ridge.

20

Special
Topics

METABOLIC BONE DISEASE

Integrity of the bony skeletal system is dependent on the active process of resorption and formation. A considerable amount of data indicating that these two processes change in the same direction cast doubt on previous dualistic concept that the process of bone resorption and formation is independent and occurs at scattered areas of the entire skeletal system (1, 2). In Paget's disease, both the rates of bone formation and of bone resorption are markedly increased. In parathyroid hormone excess, a net increase in bone mass is often observed, despite the fact that PTH increases bone resorption and inhibits bone formation. There are now considerable histological and kinetic data confirming the fact that new bone is only laid down at sites of previous resorption. This coupled process is determined by the life-cycle of the bone metabolic unit.

Kinetic studies revealed that DNA synthesis in bone cells occurs first in the osteoclasts, then into preosteoblasts, and finally into osteoblasts. The hormone calcitonin has been shown to stimulate this sequence, and calcitonin treatment has been observed to lead to a decrease of osteoclasts within 15 min, with the formation of young osteoblasts taking place within hours of the treatment. In the bone metabolic unit, the only cells which show active mitosis were the mesenchymal cells and their immediate derivatives. The sequence of events in endosteal bone remodeling is now pictured to be first an activation of a new group of mesenchymal progenitor cells, resorption of bone by the daughters of these cells, and sequential new bone formation at the site of prior bone resorption, so that bone formation never occurs without prior resorption. The entire system, consisting of progenitor cells, osteoclasts, preosteoblasts, and osteoblasts, exists as a unit and does not operate as an independent and random population of osteoclasts and osteoblasts. The entire unit operates to achieve, sequentially, bone matrix synthesis and mineralization, and only at the termination of this sequence does this activity cease.

The initial activation process may take place over a period of a few hours to a few days; the resorptive or osteoclastic phase lasts 1 to a few weeks, and the final bone formation phase covers an additional period of 2–3 months. These units function in cortical bone as the Haversian system, and in trabecular bone in a distinct structure located between cement bone and the bone surface. An extensive canalicular-lacunar system connects the osteocytes in each unit with their neighbor osteocytes. The osteocytes of one metabolic unit do not communicate with those of another unit. The units described constitute the functional units for skeletal remodeling and are involved in mineral homeostasis. Osteocytes undergo cyclic activities from bone resorption to bone formation under various hormonal and ionic influences. Normally only a small percentage of the osteocytes within a metabolic unit is engaged in osteocytic osteolysis. But in the presence of parathyroid excess, this quantity increases considerably and rapidly and provides an extremely sensitive and reliable osseous indicator of PTH action.

In continued excess of PTH, there is a shift to the osteolytic stages, resulting in sufficient resorption of lamellar bone so that the unit fuses with adjacent ones to form an osteoclastic pool on the bone surface. The size of the osteoclast pool is determined by the rate of modulation of osteoclastic transformation to osteoblasts and by the period during which the osteoblasts are actively synthesizing new bone matrix. PTH increases net bone absorption by increasing both the activation of progenitor cells and the activity of pre-existing osteoclasts, as well as by decreasing the activity of osteoblasts and reducing the rate of modulation of osteoclasts to osteoblasts. The activation of mesenchymal cells to form osteoclasts is stimulated by PTH (above), T_4, and physical activity, and is inhibited by calcitonin, thyroid hormone, physical activity, and HPO_4.

Most of the activities described above take place at the endosteal bone surface, but bone remodeling also takes place at the periosteal surface, its characteristic feature being that it results in a slight progressive net bone formation throughout life. On the other hand, after age 30 years or 80, there is progressive net absorption of bone on the endosteal surface.

Clinical Disorders of Bone Metabolism

Paget's disease presents several aspects of disturbed bone metabolism. This disorder is characterized by high rates of both bone resorption and bone formation. The osteoclasts in this disorder exhibit various sizes and are markedly multinucleated. Similarly, the osteoblasts show morphological signs of markedly increased activity. These findings suggest that the disease fulfills some of the characteristics of a neoplasm. There is an active proliferation of new progenitor units from the mesenchymal cells, with the progenitor cells showing considerable heterogeneity. Treatment of Paget's disease with calcitonin depresses this active proliferation of progenitor cells and stimulates the modulation of osteoclasts to osteoblasts, resulting in a decrease of bone resorption and a transient increase in bone formation.

Primary hyperparathyroidism is characterized by the effects of excess PTH as described above. The effect of these changes is an increase in the osteoclastic pool size and a decrease in the osteoblast pool size. The clinical sequelae of these changes were described in Chapter 19. In hypoparathyroidism, there is a decrease in bone resorption and formation, and the remodeling process is attenuated. The overall effect is slight positive skeletal metabolic balance.

Medullary carcinoma of the thyroid is characterized by increased levels of calcitonin, the sustained exposure to this hormone resulting in a marked reduction in the proliferation of osteoprogenitor cells. Thus, both resorption and formation are equally reduced; hence, skeletal balance is maintained.

Glucocorticoid-induced osteoporosis is seen in Cushing's syndrome and in patients receiving pharmacological doses of glucocorticoids. These hormones inhibit collagen synthesis in the bone, increase the osteoclast pool, and decrease the osteoblast pool. This combination results in a net resorption of bone. Several features suggest the participation of excess PTH in this process, perhaps a secondary hyperparathyroidism. The major clinical effect of these processes is the production of severe osteoporosis.

Postmenopausal osteoporosis is the result of significant and abruptly increased loss of bone during the 5th and 6th decades in female patients. It is now well established that there is a progressive bone loss with normal aging, but this process is significantly slower in black and white males, and partly so in black females. The etiological basis of postmenopausal osteoporosis is not known, but there is strong evidence that it results from a failure of osteoblastic activity. In view of the relationship between the various events in osteocyte development in normal subjects, it is likely that the defect in osteoblastic activity in postmenopausal osteoporosis is an uncoupling of the normal functional sequence in the bone metabolic unit.

There is as yet no completely satisfactory therapy for this process. It is now clear that estrogen therapy alone results in only a transient increase in bone formation. Nevertheless, replacement therapy is recommended in this disorder and especially in patients with premature ovarian senescence. Adjunctory therapy with calcium supplements, vitamin D, and fluoride promises to be helpful in this disorder. Perhaps the best therapy is prevention by the early use of estrogen even before the menopause is established. (For additional information on clinical disorders of bone metabolism, see also Chapters 9, 14, 15, and 19.)

OBESITY

Obesity is generally defined as an excess of fat content in the body. Assessment of the actual excess is difficult, however, and many methods have been employed to approximate the exact data provided by carcass analysis studies. Dilutional techniques as well as densitometric studies have provided reliable data on lean body mass and fat content, but these methods are impractical for widespread use. Skin-fold thickness in standardized areas of the body provides an excellent method of assessment of obesity. But the method most widely employed clinically remains the weight related to height which is reasonably well correlated with the more accurate methods. Recent studies revealed that, in obesity, there is an increase in both the numbers and sizes of adipose cells. It has been established that the mean adipose cell volume is increased 3-fold in the grossly obese patient, with a close correlation between obesity and the size of the adipose cell. An actual increase in the number of these cells is seen mainly in the grossly obese.

Obesity imposes several mechanical and metabolic complications. The major mechanical complications include arterial hypertension and respiratory embarrassment. It is also likely that degenerative arthritis may be a result of excess weight in some cases. The mechanism of the altered blood pressure relates to the increased circulating blood volume and increased stroke volume in obesity. The respiratory complication is caused by decreased chest cage compliance in the obese patient. Severe obesity is the basis of the Pickwickian syndrome which is characterized by hypoventilation, CO_2 retention, and somnolence secondary to the latter.

There are several metabolic complications noted in obesity, many of which have been considered perhaps to be pathogenetically related to the induction and progression of obesity (3, 4). Hyperinsulinism has been demonstrated repeatedly in clinical as well as experimental obesity. There is a direct correlation between body weight and serum insulin levels. In addition, the insulin response to glucose, tolbutamide, glucagon, and amino acids is markedly increased. This exaggerated response disappears with weight reduction. It has been ascertained that the increased insulin response is more related to body fat than to body weight per se. The general conclusion at this time is that the hyperinsulinism of obesity is secondary rather than causal in the genesis of the syndrome. Factors such as fat, fatty acid, and ketone body-induced insulin resistance in obesity undoubtedly operate.

There is a considerable amount of data consistent with decreased growth hormone (GH) levels in obesity, noted especially after challenges with insulin, arginine, starvation, and sleep. Weight reduction is followed by reversion to normal GH response. The cortisol secretion rate as well as its degradation is increased in obesity. The pathway of degradation is probably also affected (5). In view of these changes, the plasma cortisol level may be high or normal in obese patients. If found, hypercortisolemia in obesity is suppressed to $< 10\ \mu g/100$ ml after overnight dexamethasone suppression (see Chapter 15). These alterations revert to normal on weight reduction. It is concluded that the alterations in GH and cortisol kinetics, as those in insulin levels activity and antagonism, are secondary to the obese state.

Studies of etiology of obesity have resulted in the conclusion that most forms of clinical obesity are probably of multifactorial pathogenesis. There are, however, specific obesity syndromes which have been identified. These include the hypothalamic forms caused by either tumors, trauma, or inflammatory or infectious disease. Insulinoma and Cushing's syndrome represent forms of endocrinopathic obesity. In general, these patients are not massively obese, however. Several studies have implicated underactivity as a major factor in obesity. Genetic forms of obesity include the Lawrence-Moon-Biedl syndrome, hyperostosis frontalis interna, and the Prader-Willi (hypomentia, hyperphagia, hypogonadal obesity) syndrome. Some forms of gorging obesity have been produced experimentally and observed clinically. Behavioral and psychological characteristics of obesity have also been established in several studies.

Experimental obesity has been produced by lesions in the ventral median hypothalamus. Damage to this area is followed by hyperphagia, decreased activity, and increased body weight. Lesions in this area have been induced mechanically, as well as by the use of gold thioglucose. It is of major interest that the uptake of gold thioglucose by this area is insulin dependent (A. F. Debons, personal communication, 1972). This area is also responsive to α- and β-adrenergic influences. This injection of norepinephrine into this area is followed by hyperphagia, whereas the use of an α-blockade agent reduces food intake. An area of the lateral hypothalamus, responsive to adrenergic influences, is also concerned with satiety. Injection of propranolol into this area is followed by rejection of food.

It has been shown that the frequency of food intake is also related to the ability to gain weight. There is increased lipogenesis when food is ingested in one large feeding rather than if isocaloric food is ingested in several small feedings.

Methods of Obesity Control

Several methods have been employed, none with universal success. Specific endocrinopathic forms of obesity are treated by the definitive management of the endocrine disorder, if possible. The sheet anchor of therapy of all other forms of obesity is the judicious restriction of calories in a balanced diet. Failure of diet control is caused by several factors mainly related to impatience and disappointment. It is of importance to recognize that most dietary restriction regimens are rapidly followed by loss in lean body mass (protein) early. Decreased blood glucose and tissue glycogen levels during dietary restriction induce gluconeogenesis from proteins early. Fat yields 9 cal/g, whereas lean tissue yields 0.8 cal/g because of the requirement of 3–4 times its volume in water for storage. Therefore, when caloric loss comes from protein, the reflection of weight loss is much greater than when the caloric loss is from fat.

The use of unbalanced diets in the management of obesity has been successful in many situations, but it is now concluded that the most efficient method probably is the use of balanced diets with caloric restriction and an exercise program. It is prudent in treating a patient with obesity to commit him to moderate rather than to severe caloric restriction, as a major factor in failure is the lack of faithful acceptance of the regimen. The patient should be advised that after a period of restriction a spree of dietary indulgence is followed by adaptive hyperlipogenesis.

Starvation (0 cal) or semistarvation (300–600 cal) diets have been employed in the management of moderate to severe obesity. Several hemodynamic and metabolic changes accompany this regimen including hypotension, sodium and water loss, acidosis, lactic acidemia, ketosis, and hyperuricemia. Postural hypotension is a symptom of the decreased fluid volume. Anorexia and dizziness may accompany the ketosis, and weakness is related to hypoglycemia. Supportive measures to prevent hyperuricemia include adequate fluid intake and the use of allopurinol. Supplemental vitamins are recommended, experimental data suggesting, for example, that vitamin C is involved in the mobilization of fat (6). Laxatives are also recommended to prevent fecal impaction and atony. On this regimen, the patient may lose 0.5–0.9 kg/day. When the fast is terminated, the patient should be given tea with small amounts of carbohydrate initially. Salt intake should be restricted for several days in order to avoid aldosterone-mediated sodium retention and edema.

Small bowel bypass surgery, whereby the absorptive area of the small intestine is restricted, has been employed in the management of morbid obesity. This procedure has met with some measure of success, but the complications may prohibit the wide application of this procedure. The surgical complications include wound evisceration, obstruction, intussusception, anastomotic leaks, and pulmonary infarction. Several severe metabolic complications include malabsorption of vitamins and minerals leading to hypokalemia, hypocalcemia, hypomagnesemia, and iron deficiency. Hypotension, renal calculi, and muscle wasting have been observed. A nonspecific polyarthritis and fatty metamorphosis of the liver have been described in some patients with intestinal bypass surgery.

Drug Therapy in Obesity

Several preparations to achieve appetite control have been produced. The success rate with use of these agents is very limited, however. Several of these agents are also contraindicated in many patients. While pharmacological doses of thyroid hormones lead to weight loss, this effect is achieved only in concert with other toxic manifestations. Amphetamine drugs enhance lipolysis by stimulating catecholamine-induced lipolysis. After depletion of stored epinephrine (within 1—3 weeks), the drugs become useless in diet control. Phenformin may decrease gastrointestinal absorption and aid in the management of obesity. This procedure is a poor alternative to the use of calorie restriction, however.

ENDOCRINE HYPERTENSION

Several hormonal agents may directly or indirectly affect blood pressure by alterations in mineral metabolism, sensitization of the arterial vasculature to endogenous pressor agents, actions as pressor agents, or inducing renal and vascular changes. The occurrence of alterations in blood pressure was discussed in the sections on the various endocrine glands. In this section, the various forms of endocrine hypertension are presented in summary form (Table 20.1).

DISORDERS OF SEXUAL DIFFERENTIATION

Several factors are involved in the normal development of sexual characteristics beyond the stage of earliest gonadal development (Table 20.2). The clear requirement of two normal sex chromosomes for maturation of germ cells is exemplified by the occurrence of afollicular streak gonads in the absence of germ cells. The earliest stage of gonadal development is a thickening of the coelomic epithelium which occurs by the 4th week of embryonic life. Primary sex cords grow down from the coelomic epithelium into the mesenchymal structure of the primordial gonad. Up to this point, gonadal development is essentially identical in both sexes so that this structure is truly an undifferentiated gonad. Germ cells derived from extragonadal elements in the entoderm of the yolk sac caudal to the embryonic disc migrate to the gonad. That these cells are necessary for further gonadal development is shown by the occurrence of gonadal agenesis in their absence. These germ cells at this stage are bipotential in their ability to become either sperm cells or ova. Their eventual location in the undifferentiated gonad and their subsequent development are determined by the X and Y chromosomes. These sex-determining genes influ-

Table 20.1. Endocrine Hypertension Summarized

Gland	Clinical features and mechanisms	Clinical and laboratory diagnosis	Treatment
Posterior pituitary	Mild to severe hypertension from excess vasopressin therapy of diabetes insipidus	History of drug administration	Withdrawal or reduction of vasopressin
Anterior pituitary	Excess GH in acromegaly may predispose to mild or moderate hypertension; perhaps synergism of GH with mineralocorticoid action	Plasma GH levels during hyperglycemic challenge	Therapy of acromegaly (see Chapter 12)
Thyroid gland	Systolic hypertension with wide pulse pressure in hyperthyroidism Mild hypertension in myxedema; perhaps related to bradycardia	Serum T_4 and T_3 levels by radioimmunoassay T_4 and TSH by radioimmunoassay	Therapy of thyrotoxicosis (see Chapter 14) Thyroid hormone replacement
Parathyroid glands	Hypertension is found in over one-third of patients with hyperparathyroidism and is probably ascribable to hypercalcemia; contributory factors may be secondary renal disease and nephrocalcinosis	Serum calcium, phosphate, chloride/phosphate ratio; serum PTH levels	Surgical therapy of hyperparathyroidism; occasionally medical palliative therapy (see Chapter 19)

Islets of Langerhans	Increased prevalence of hypertension in diabetes mellitus probably of multifactorial mechanism, including renal arterial disease, glomerulosclerosis, arteriolosclerosis, and microvascular disease	Glucose intolerance; insulin levels inappropriate to blood glucose levels	Management of diabetes mellitus; preventive management of renal concomitants; antihypertensive drugs (see Chapter 2)
Adrenal medulla and chromaffin system	Paroxysmal or sustained hypertension, tachycardia, sweating caused by catecholamine (CA) secretion; sources of excess CA include: pheochromocytoma (adrenal medulla); paraganglioma (sympathetic ganglia); neuroblastoma (malignant tumor of early ganglion cell origin); ganglioneuroma in sympathetic ganglia; and adrenal medullary hyperplasia	Urinary metanephrines and normetanephrines, catecholamines, and VMA; pharmacological tests; nephrotomograms; adrenal venography (see Chapter 16)	Surgery after preparation with phenoxybenzamine and fluid replacement; if surgery not possible, medical therapy with phenoxybenzamine, phentolamine, and similar drugs
Adrenal cortex	Hypertension in 85% of Cushing's syndrome; etiologies include: (a) adrenocortical hyperplasia caused by pituitary tumors or ectopic ACTH production, (b) adrenal adenoma, (c) carcinoma, and (d) nodular adrenal hyperplasia which may be ACTH-independent	Plasma cortisol or urine 17-OHCS, 17-KGS, and 17-KS before and after dexamethasone suppression; ACTH stimulation to differentiate (b) from (c) (see Chapter 15)	Surgical therapies, bilateral adrenalectomy or removal of adenoma; if surgery not feasible, the use of pharmacological agents: o,p-DDD; metyrapone; aminoglutethimide

continued

Table 20.1. *continued*

Gland	Clinical features and mechanisms	Clinical and laboratory diagnosis	Treatment
Adrenal cortex	Hyperaldosterone states are most common form of endocrine hypertension; hypokalemia and decreased PRA usually caused by aldosterone-producing adenoma (APA) or, in 20%, nodular hypertension	Plasma aldosterone before and after DOC or fluorocortisol suppression, or after saline infusion; studies on PRA	Surgical removal of APA; in nodular hyperplasia, surgical removal lowers aldosterone but hypertension may persist
	ACTH-dependent aldosteronism with hypertension, a familial disorder with features of APA, but suppressible with dexamethasone	As above; also dexamethasone suppression test	Medical therapy with dexamethasone 0.75 mg/day; if a greater dose is required, adrenal ablation is done or aldosterone antagonists are tried
	Hypercorticosteronism caused by corticosterone-secreting tumor; rare, with similar features as APA but aldosterone levels are normal	Corticosterone levels in plasma; tetrahydrocorticosterone (THB) in urine; nonsuppressible if caused by tumor	Surgical removal of tumor; if not feasible, medical therapy with op,DDD; metyrapone; aminoglutethimide
	Congenital adrenocortical hyperplasia 1) 11β-hydroxylase deficiency: with hypokalemic alkalosis and hypertension caused by increased DOC; virilization caused by androgens	Plasma DOC (or urine THDOC) before and after dexamethasone challenge	Dexamethasone or prednisone suppression therapy

2) 17α-hydroxylase deficiency: with hypokalemic alkalosis and hypertension caused by DOC and corticosterone; sexual infantilism caused by decreased gonadal hormones; in both 1) and 2) aldosterone levels are decreased	Plasma DOC and corticosterone (or THDOC and THB in urine) before and after dexamethasone suppression	Dexamethasone or prednisone suppression therapy plus replacement of gonadal hormone appropriate to patient's sex
Other hypertensive disorders with secondary aldosteronism:		
Malignant hypertension	Elevated aldosterone levels See Chapter 14 for differential diagnosis	Antihypertension drugs
Use of oral contraceptive agents which increase substrate for renin action		Discontinue oral contraceptives
Primary hyperreninism caused by tumors of juxtaglomerular apparatus	Plasma aldosterone elevation and PRA nonsuppressible with NaCl infusion or intake	Removal of tumor
Thiazide-induced aldosteronism: excessive natriuresis leads to increased PRA which underlies secondary aldosteronism	Plasma aldosterone elevated but suppressible with saline infusion	Discontinue natriuretic agents
Essential hypertension; some forms may be caused by increased nonaldosterone mineralocorticoids, e.g., 16β-hydroxydehydroepiandrosterone	Mainly a diagnosis by exclusion; finding of specific non-aldosterone mineralocorticoids	Spironolactone therapy is useful in management of all conditions of secondary hyperaldosteronism; other aldosterone antagonists are being developed

Table 20.2. Factors in Sexual Differentiation and Development

Characteristic	Origin	Mechanism of differentiation	Identifying features
Chromosomal sex	Sex chromosomes of parental germ cells	Normal: chromosomal composition of sperm; abnormal: nondisjunction during meiosis in parental germ cells; nondisjunction or lag in early mitotic divisions; chromosomal breakage	Karyotype analysis
X chromatin	Heterochromatic X chromosomes	Partial inactivation and heterochromatization of all chromosomes in excess of one	Buccal, neutrophil, or other somatic cells
Y body	Y chromosome	Distal segment of long arm of Y	As above
Gonadal sex	Ovary or testis	Ovaries: presence of genes on two X chromosomes; testes: presence of genes on Y chromosomes	Histological appearance
Genital ducts	Müllerian (♀) or Wolffian (♂) ducts	Intrinsic tendency to feminize in absence of androgens which stimulate Wolffian system	Morphological appearance

External genitalia	Genital tubercle, urethral and labioscrotal folds, urogenital sinus	As above; masculinization requires androgen stimulation before 12th week; abnormalities: 1) virilized female; adrenal hyperplasia or maternal androgens; 2) incompletely differentiated male: insufficient androgen from fetal testes, or end-organ refractoriness such as caused by absence of cytosol receptor	Examination; urethroscopy; x-ray contrast study
Secondary sexual characteristics	Hypothalamic and suprahypothalamic centers; pituitary FSH, LH, ovaries, testes, adrenals	Suprahypothalamic and hypothalamic centers: gonadotropin-releasing hormones; gonads: responsiveness to FSH and LH; target organs: responsiveness depends on presence of cytosol receptor	Overt secondary sexual characteristics: ♀: breast development, rounded contours, growth of reproductive tract, ovulation, menstruation (all caused by gonadal hormone release under tonic and cyclic control); ♂: sexual hair pattern, voice, muscular development, phallic size (secondary to release of androgens under tonic control)

ence sexual development primarily by directing the primitive bipotential gonad to develop into testes or ovaries. Beyond this stage, most of the other sexual characteristics derive from the bipotential primordial structures which inherently tend to feminize. The female pattern emerges in the course of development unless there is an active influence by masculinizing factors. The absence of one X chromosome apparently fails to affect the intrauterine gonadal structure up to the 3rd month of gestation, although growth subsequent to this time fails to occur. This is apparently caused by the fact that meiotic division, which begins at 2 months of embryonic life, is impossible in the abnormal germ cell; at this time, however, mitotic division is quite normal. It is now clear that two normal chromosomes are necessary for crossing over in meiosis I whereby there is an exchange of genetic material. There are several levels of sexual differentiation, and beyond the influence of the X and Y chromosomes on the bipotential precursors, a wide spectrum of disorders of differentiation is possible.

Sex Chromosomes

The sex chromosomes X and Y possess three kinds of genes. There are multiple sex-determining loci on both the long and short arms of the two X chromosomes which are necessary for normal ovarian differentiation and oogenesis. Full testicular differentiation and spermatogenesis are determined by multiple loci on the pericentromeric region of the short arm of the Y. There are also genes "paired" between X and Y chromosomes which are probably located on the short arm of X and the longer of the arms of Y. But unpaired genes also exist, for example, the traits for hairy ears and tall stature which are located on the Y chromosome. It is estimated that there are 150 loci responsible for a wide variety of sex-linked traits on the X chromosome. It is now known that on the long arm of the X chromosome, genes for the following processes are located: hypoxanthine-guanine phosphoribosyltransferase, phosphoglycerate kinase, glucose-6-phosphate dehydrogenase, hemophilia A, and color blindness.

Biological Functions of Y Chromosome The Y chromosome carries the male determining genes responsible for induction of development of the testes even in the presence of two or more X chromosomes. The male germ-cell determinants essential to spermatogenesis are present on the Y chromosome, with most variation ascribable to changes in the long arm. The factors constituting the testes determiners are located in the short arm of the Y close to the centromere and possibly in the centromeric region of the long arm. It is likely that the long arm of the Y contains loci which are homologous to those of the short arm of the X. The presence of either of these segments on the Y or the X chromosome with a normal X prevents the short stature and most of the somatic changes associated with Turner's syndrome. The traits of hairy ears and of tall structure are transmitted through loci on the Y chromosome.

Biological Functions of X Chromosome   The X chromosome is the eighth longest of the normal karyotype and contains 5% of the total DNA in the haploid set (22+X). Presence of a second X chromosome is required for the differentiation of the primitive gonad into an ovary, so that in the XO individual there is a lack of ovarian differentiation. It is likely that multiple loci for ovarian differentiation are located on both the long and short arms of the X chromosome. The importance of X chromosomes in general body function and metabolism is demonstrated by the fact that these chromosomes contain DNA coding for functions involving every system of the human body.

Chromosomal Errors   Errors in chromosomal constitution can result from faulty replication of the germ cells during the processes of spermatogenesis and oogenesis or from abnormalities in mitotic division of cells in the zygote after fertilization. One abnormality in which the cells contain a number of chromosomes different from that characteristic of the species is termed aneuploidy. This abnormality may result from nondisjunction either during meiotic or mitotic division, or from anaphase lag. In nondisjunction, there is a failure of either a pair of sister chromatids or members of a pair of homologous chromosomes to separate during anaphase. In anaphase lag, there is a loss of a chromosome from one or both daughter cells. This is caused by the failure during metaphase of one chromosome to become properly oriented at the equatorial plane. A gradual increase in aneuploid cells is noted with aging, especially in females. Another chromosomal abnormality is described as mosaicism, in which individuals have two or more cell lines differing in chromosomal constitution, but originating from a single zygote. This may arise from errors in mitosis after fertilization had occurred. Other errors in replication may be noted in embryos derived from gametes of abnormal chromosomal constitution. Occurrence of more than one cell line each of different genetic origin is termed chimerism. Chromosomal abnormalities caused by nondisjunction during meiosis are summarized in Table 20.3.

Structural errors in chromosomes may result from breakage or partial deletion of parts of the chromosome followed by improper reunion of fragments. This may result in either long or short arms. The presence of two long arms is described as Xqi and of two short arms as Xpi. Deletion, detachment, or loss of a portion of the long arm of the chromosome is termed Xq⁻ and, when a similar anomaly affects the short arm, it is termed Xp⁻. Yet other chromosomal aberrations include duplication, in which a deleted segment is incorporated into another chromosome (usually the other member of a homologous pair), and translocation, caused by exchanges of chromosomal segments between two chromosomes.

Table 20.3. Chromosomal Abnormalities Caused by Nondisjunction during Meiosis

	Oocyte	Meiosis (ovum + polar body)	Product of conception[a]	Meiosis (2 sperm)	Spermatocyte
Normal	44 + XX[a]	22 + X + 22 + X (p.b.)	44 + XX or 44 + XY	22 + X + 22 + Y	44 + XY
Maternal nondisjunction	44 + XX 44 + XX	22 XX 22 + 0 (p.b.) 22 + 0 +	44 + XXX 44 + YO 44 + XO	22 + Y 22 + X 22 + Y 22 + X	44 + XY 44 + XY
Paternal nondisjunction	44 + XX	22 + XX (p.b.) 22 + X + 22 + X (p.b.)	44 + XXY 44 + XXY 44 + XO	22 + Y 22 + XY 22 + 0	44 + XY

[a]Standard nomenclature now requires that the first numerical refer to the total number of chromosomes, so that 46, XX is the normal karyotype and indicates 44 autosomes plus XX. Products of conception 46 XX = normal female; 46 XY = normal male; 47 XXX = superfemale; 47 XXY = Klinefelter's syndrome; 45 XO = gonadal dysgenesis (Turner's); 45 YO is incompatible with life.

The X chromatin or Barr body is a distinguishing characteristic of the female sex and is present in the peripheral cells of most mammalian species. It is a planoconvex body with the flattened side in apposition to the inner surface of the nuclear membrane and it gives a positive reaction for DNA. In buccal smears from female subjects, this body is found in over 25% of cells. In the peripheral polymorphonuclear leukocytes of female, 1—15% of the cells have a drumstick appendage to the nucleus that is not seen in males. This drumstick has the same significance as the Barr body. In patients with more than two X chromosomes, the maximum number of X chromatin bodies is one less than the number of X chromosomes, so that in XXX females or XXXY males there is a maximum of two chromatin bodies in diploid nuclei. But in XO and XY individuals, the cells are chromatin-negative. An abnormally small X chromatin body is found in female subjects with one normal X and one X with deletion, for example, in the XXp⁻, or in patients with one ring chromosome, XXr. On the other hand, in the presence of a karyotype with a large isochrome (XXqi), a large chromatin body is found. It is important to recognize that the chromatin body (Barr body) arises from one of the two X chromosomes in the interphase nuclei of female somatic cells. According to the Lyon hypothesis, only one X chromosome per cell is genetically active during the interphase.

Gonadal Differentiation

The earliest stage of gonadal development occurs at the 4th week of gestation when there is a thickening of the coelomic epithelium. Primary sex cords grow down from the coelomic epithelium into the mesenchymal structure of the gonad. This stage of development is essentially identical in both sexes and represents a truly undifferentiated gonad. Gonocytes or germ cells (seen in the dorsal endoderm in the 24-day embryo) then migrate to the gonads, their presence being essential to further gonadal development. Absence of these germ cells results in gonadal agenesis. At this stage, the germ cells are essentially bipotential in their ability to become either sperm cells or ova. By 6 weeks of gonadal development, the total content of gonocytes is around 100,000. Their eventual location in the undifferentiated gonad and their subsequent development are determined by the sex chromosomes (X and Y).

Testicular Differentiation and Spermatogenesis Testicular differentiation takes place between 6 and 8 weeks of gestation, at which time there is appearance of medullary primary sex cords or primitive tubules and formation of a limiting membranous tunica and cleft separating deeper layers from the surface epithelium. This process of differentiation is dependent on the chromosomal constitution which confers inductor capabilities to the germ cells and on receptivity of the mesenchymal elements. In the presence of the Y chromosomes, testicular development proceeds; the cortex disappears, and the medullary portion persists. Primary sex cords form the seminiferous tubules, and the cells of these cords become the Sertoli or sustentacular cells. Mesenchymal cells which surround the tubules become the Leydig or interstitial cells. The fetal testis secretes a Müllerian duct inhibiting substance distinct from ordinary androgens and is probably of peptide or nucleic acid structure. There are data that to suggest that this substance is produced either by the seminiferous tubules or from the Sertoli cells. Androgen effect is necessary for stimulation of the primitive Wolffian ducts to differentiate into epididymis, vas deferens, and seminal vesicles.

Testicular descent takes place at the 28th week of gestation, and, during this process, the testis, gubernaculum, and the epididymis (partly derived from the tubules) migrate as a unit into the inguinal canal preceded by a sac of peritoneum, into the scrotum. The process is completed at about the first 4–6 weeks of extrauterine life, by which time there is elongation of the vas deferens, disintegration of the gubernaculum, and enlargement of the testes. Wolffian ducts become the vasa deferentia, seminal vesicles, and epididymis, and the Müllerian primordia disappear. The prostate is derived from the urethra except for the utricle which is a Müllerian remnant.

The germ cells are quiescent during childhood and fail to differentiate further until late in the prepubescent period. At adolescence, the basement membrane becomes lined with proliferating spermatogonia arising by mitotic division of the primitive germ cells. Mitotic activity in the spermatogonia gives rise to the primary spermatocytes. Formation of haploid secondary spermatocytes by the process of meiosis in the euploid primary spermatocytes then takes place. The secondary spermatocytes give rise to spermatids by a second meiotic division which is analogous to mitosis because the process involves a longitudinal split. The cycle from spermatogonium to spermatid formation in the adult male takes place over a course of 74 days.

Ovarian Differentiation and Oogenesis In the presence of the XX chromosomal constitution (44 autosomes plus XX), the process of ovarigenesis takes place. Ovarian formation from the undifferentiated gonad takes place later than testicular differentiation, and the developmental course is quite different from that of the male. There is rapid oogonial development at 8–10 weeks, but it is not until 14 weeks of gestation that a number of germ cells are surrounded by precapsular cells derived from the sex cords; others not destined to persist undergo degenerative changes. Nuclear maturation takes place at 15–20 weeks, and most oogonia are transformed into oocytes. The thickened cortex with maturing germ cells is now penetrated by vascular ingrowths perpendicular to the surface and divided into secondary sex cords. Capillaries originating in the meso-nephric area separate the cortex from the medulla. The Müllerian pri-mordia grow caudad and meet in the midline, giving rise to the Fallopian tubes, uterus, and upper third of the vagina. Simultaneously, there is regression of the Wolffian system.

The formation of oogonia from primary germ cells ceases by the 28th week of gestation and is never resumed throughout life. Envelopment of the closest oocytes with a single layer of granulosa cells, associated with capillaries, completes the formation of the primary follicle. Perifollicular vascular cells not involved in this process ultimately form the interfollicu-lar stroma. Most of these changes occur at the junction of the cortex and the anatomically minor medulla. The number of primary follicles in the ovaries is greatest at the time of birth, after which event the number rapidly diminishes. In the germ cells that survive, the oocyte exists in the late prophase of its first meiotic division in which stage it may stay until ovulation takes place years later. It has been suggested that this relatively long life span of the female germ cells may be responsible for the increased prevalence of chromosomal anomalies with advancing age. But the quies-cent stage may be quite short in some follicles as any oocyte may enlarge up to 3-fold and resume maturation. The Graafian follicle now matures, and there is proliferation of a multilayer granulosa, antrum formation, and formation of a thecal layer with rich vascular supply. This maturation process may terminate at any step, with regression and eventual replace-ment by connective tissue. It is probable that there is no degeneration of the oocyte in the primary follicle. From the above considerations, it is clear that the cycle of formation, ripening, and atresia of follicles is characteristic of fetal ovarian existence. The medullary remnant is made up of cords, nodules, and rete testis and persists beyond fetal life as the hilus of the ovary. At birth, the female ovaries contain 300,000–400,000 ova, of which only 300–400 will eventually be extruded by ovulation; variable degrees of atresia are the fate of the rest of the ova.

At birth each ovary measures 1 cm in diameter, the major part of its bulk being made up of primary follicles in various stages of preatretic development. The prepubertal ovary contains a hilar area with many blood vessels and some medullary remnants with a peripheral cortex of stroma and follicles at various stages of maturity, but without any corpus luteum or evidence of ovulation. Just before ovulation, the first polar body is extruded, completing meiosis I. The haploid secondary oocyte begins meiosis II but remains in metaphase and does not extrude the second polar body until the ovum is penetrated by the sperm cell.

Mechanisms of Gonadal Differentiation The importance of the normal complement of the sex chromosomes in a karyotype for normal sexual differentiation was described above. In the XO chromosomal constitution, neither testicular nor ovarian differentiation takes place, and the postnatal gonad is represented by a long pale streak of connective tissue in the mesosalpinx, which is devoid of germ cells, follicles, and seminiferous tubules. The role of the Y chromosome in induction of testicular development from the undifferentiated gonad was described above. The role of the second X chromosome in female differentiation is less direct, as, rarely, fertility has been reported in XO females. It is clear that the primitive gonad has an inherent tendency to develop into an ovary if the germ cells persist and prior testicular differentiation has not taken place. This latter event is mediated by the non-steroidal testes determiners on the Y chromosome, concentrated on the short arm. The differentiation of the genital ducts in the female is not contingent on the presence of an ovary, as equally good development of the uterus and Fallopian tubes takes place even in the absence of the gonads. The influence of the fetal testes on duct development is exerted unilaterally and locally. Higher local concentrations of androgen are required for male duct stimulation than for masculinization of the external genitalia and derivatives of the urogenital sinus. The urogenital sinus and genital tubercle, in contrast with the male ductal tissue, develops the enzyme 5α-reductase which converts testosterone to dihydrotestosterone, the more active metabolite. This probably underlies the finding that the urogenital sinus and genital tubercle are sensitive to systemic androgens whereas the Wolffian derivatives are not.

Role of Androgens in Differentiation of External Genitalia

As with the genital ducts, the external genitalia have an inherent tendency to feminize. Testosterone and other androgens play a decisive role in determination of the external genitalia along male lines early in fetal life. Androgens stimulate growth of the genital tubercle and induce fusion of the urethral folds and labioscrotal swellings. They also prevent growth of the vesicovaginal septum, thus preventing separation of the vagina from the urogenital sinus. In females, the genital tubercle gives rise to the clitoris, and with some elongation this becomes the penis in the male. Androgenic stimulation at any time during intrauterine life and after birth causes clitoral hypertrophy. The labia minora in the female are derived from the genital folds which in the male fuse to form the ventral raphe which displaces the urethral opening to the tip of the penis. The labia majora are formed from the genital swellings which in the male fuse in the midline to form the scrotum. Several of the factors at various levels of involvement in sexual differentiation and development are presented in Table 20.4.

Hormonal Sexual Differentiation

Puberty is marked by a reversal of the ratio of androstenedione to testosterone from the prepubescent higher level of the former; this reversed ratio is ascribed to a significant elevation of testosterone noted at puberty. Testosterone is necessary for full maturation of the seminiferous tubules as well as for increase in the muscle mass, growth of the penis, prostate and seminal vesicles, deepening of the voice, and a male pattern of sexual hair.

With the approach of adolescence in the female, the cyclic ripening and involution of follicles are intensified, and fibrous stroma becomes more abundant, with a tendency toward development of the ovarian cysts and hyperthecosis. Before age 9 or 10 years, the ovarian secretion is too little to induce vaginal comification. Rising estradiol levels at the time of puberty induce the development of nipples and mammary ducts, enlargement of the uterus, the rounding of body contours, and cornification of the vulvar and vaginal epithelium.

The adrenal steroid secretions play an important role in sexual differentiation. The role of the fetal zone in fetal steroidogenesis and steroid economy in the fetal placental unit was discussed in a previous chapter. Postnatally, there is involution of this zone with alterations in the steroidogenic pathways to the mature pattern. With the onset of adolescence the adrenal cortex undergoes enlargement largely in the zona reticularis with an increase in the production of androgens and estrogens. These factors contribute to the growth rate, increased muscle mass, growth of sexual hair, and seborrhea, all characteristic of adolescence. It has been suggested that this process of adrenarche may be stimulated by LH. The development of the female libido is suggested to be dependent on adrenal androgens.

There are abundant data that the mechanisms of the various hormonal changes at time of puberty are secondary to a decreased sensitivity of the hypothalamic gonadostat to circulating sex steroids; this results in an increased release of the gonadotropin-releasing hormone and an orderly and sequential increase in pituitary gonadotropins.

The negative or inhibitory feedback relationship between ambient levels of estrogens and the tonic area of the gonadostat probably differentiates during fetal life, whereas the positive or stimulatory feedback mechanism affecting the cyclic center and responsible for the midcycle preovulatory surge of FSH and LH matures during midpuberty in the female. An episodic secretion of LH during sleep is seen in pubertal, but not in prepubertal, children. It is likely that the pituitary content of FSH in girls is greater than in boys, and this is readily demonstrable after a challenge with GnRH. Although the activity of the cyclic center is obliterated by androgen exposure in other species, there are some data to suggest that in primates there is at least a slight potential for cyclic center activity.

No major sexual differences in secretion of testosterone and estrogen are noted until the time of pubescence, but there are indications of greater enlargement and activity in the ovaries than in the testes during childhood.

Table 20.4. Anomalous Sexual Differentiation in the Male

Disorder	Chromosomal constitution and metabolic defect	Clinical features	Associated findings
Disorders of gonadal differentiation			
Seminiferous tubule dysgenesis	Chromatin positive XXY in typical Klinefelter's; also mosaics: XXXY-XXXXY Variant chromatin negative form	Typical Klinefelter's is a most common form of primary male hypogonadism and infertility; Clinical features become manifest during adolescence; patients taller than average; gynecomastia; variable degree of eunuchoidism; atrophic testes, (3 cm) with hyalinization of seminiferous tubules, aggregation of Leydig cells, aspermatogenesis; increased gonadotropins; hypospadias and cryptorchidism rare; mental retardation in one-fourth of patients; in chromatin negative variant, mental retardation incidence is less	Occasional hypothyroidism; slight increase in diabetes incidence Increased incidence of carcinoma of breast in patients with gynecomastia; congenital heart disease in XXXXY
True hermaphroditism	70% are chromatin positive; in many XX cases, there may be Y cell line in mosaicism; others have XY,XXY mosaicism	External genitalia may simulate male or female, and may be ambiguous; most patients have hypospadias (penile to perineal); cryptorchidism is common; genital duct development depends on location of gonads, e.g., lateral (testis on one side and ovary on the other), bilateral (ovotestes), and unilateral (ovotestis on one side and ovary or testis on other side). Two-thirds of patients have breast development; two-thirds may menstruate; ovulation not uncommon, but spermatogenesis is rare	

Familial XY gonadal dysgenesis and incomplete form	XY Karyotype	Female phenotype; normal to tall stature; sexual infantilism; eunuchoid habitus; amenorrhea; somatic features of Turner's are inconspicuous; internal structures are female; clitoromegaly is often present; plasma testosterone is high, secreted by hilar elements of streak gonads	Incidence of neoplasms: gonadoblastoma and dysgerminoma high; bilateral prophylactic gonadectomy is indicated
Pseudo-Turner's or Noonan's syndrome	In both sexes, the karyotype is normal	Characteristic facies; frequently webbed-neck and short stature; congenital heart diseases in order of frequency: pulmonic stenosis and atrial septal defect or both, ventricular septal defect, patent ductus arteriosus, and ventricular hypertrophy; occasionally pectus excavatum and mental retardation; cryptorchidism is common, testes hypoplastic with germinal aplasia; often androgen deficiency at puberty; occasionally normal testicular function and fertility	
Male pseudohermaphroditism caused by Inborn errors of androgen synthesis	All have XY karyotype Defect in testicular and adrenal steroid synthesis	Testes present, but genital ducts and external genitalia undermasculinized; phenotype ranges from female to male with cryptorchidism or hypospadius	
Desmolase deficiency	Defect in testicular and adrenal steroid synthesis	Autosomal recessive; phenotypic female, genital ducts male	
Hydroxysteroid dehydrogenase deficiency	Defect in testicular and adrenal steroid synthesis	Normal male genital ducts, absence of Müllerian structures; may develop male features and gynecomastia at puberty	
17α-Hydroxylase deficiency	Defect in testicular and adrenal steroid synthesis	Phenotypic female with testes, female external genitalia, vagina; male duct development, absence of secondary sex characteristics; sexual infantilism	Hypertension and hypokalemic alkalosis caused by increased mineralocorticoids

continued

Table 20.4. *continued*

Disorder	Chromosomal constitution and metabolic defect	Clinical features	Associated findings
Lyase (17,20-desmolase) deficiency	Decreased formation of testosterone and androstenedione	Male genital duct development; ambiguous genitalia; hypospadias, but male-type urethra	No gynecomastia
17β-Hydroxy-steroid dehydrogenase deficiency	Decreased testosterone and increased androstenedione	At birth: female or ambiguous genitalia; testes in inguinal canal; blind vaginal pouch; at puberty: gynecomastia; presence of male genital ducts; may be familial	May include Reifenstein's syndrome
End-organ insensitivity to androgens: feminizing testes	Failure to masculinize in utero, and end-organ failure to androgens later; caused by defective cytosol receptor	X-linked inheritance; female external genitalia; female sex characteristics at puberty; testes may be located in labia majora, inguinal canal, or in abdomen; immature fetal seminiferous tubules; feminization caused by increased estrogens caused by increased LH; FSH is normal; testosterone levels normal, estrogens high; elevated estrogens prevent occurrence of castration levels of gonadotropins	Testes are predisposed to malignant transformation; variant forms with ambiguous genitalia
With virilization at puberty	XY karyotype; intrauterine deficiency of testosterone during first 12 weeks	External sexual ambiguity from mild hypospadias and normal phallus to phenotypic female with clitoral enlargement and incomplete masculinization of urogenital sinus	Variant: familial perineal hypospadias with ambiguous development

Clinical Disorders of Sexual Development

An interchange of chromosomal fragments between X and Y during their alignment in meiosis I of spermatogenesis in the father is usually the basis of the presence of both testes and ovaries in certain forms of true hermaphroditism and in rare phenotypic males with the XX karyotype without mosaicism. In the male pseudohermaphrodite, the gonads are exclusively testes, but the genital ducts or external genitalia or both exhibit in one or several respects the phenotypic characteristics of the female. In the female pseudohermaphrodite, on the other hand, there are exclusively ovarian gonadal structures, but the genital development exhibits some masculine characteristics.

Anomalous Sexual Differentiation

The clinical features and chromosomal constitution (7–9) of the various forms of anomalous sexual differentiation in the male are presented in Table 20.4. These disorders in the female (7–9) are summarized in Table 20.5. Management of several of the disorders is described in Chapters 15, 17, and 18.

SEXUAL PRECOCITY IN MALES

Male isosexual sexual precocity is defined as the onset of masculinization before age 10 years. This disorder is characterized by an increased testicular size and maturation, increased penile and scrotal growth, appearance of facial and body hair, loss of frontoparietal hair, activation of axillary sweat glands, acne, and increased cutaneous pigmentation. Skeletal changes include increased growth of long bones initially with subsequent slowing of linear growth caused by premature epiphyseal closure. A classification of isosexual precocity in males is presented in Table 20.6 (8).

Constitutional (Idiopathic) Sexual Precocity

Constitutional or idiopathic sexual precocity is an example of true sexual precocity and is caused by premature release of adult levels of gonadotropins and gonadal hormones which results in the appearance of the various features of masculine maturation listed above. This disorder often shows a familial incidence and, although many cases are undoubtedly of genetic origin, the diagnosis is made largely by exclusion of other causes. The clinical manifestations may appear at any time during infancy or childhood, with the order of appearance approximately corresponding to the sequence seen in ordinary adolescence. The appearance of testicular, penile, and scrotal enlargement, pubic hair, deeper or hoarser voice, accelerated linear growth, and an increase in musculature and body weight, are followed by gradual assumption of all physical characteristics of a

Dysgenetic male pseudohermaphroditism	Mosaic XO, XY, or defective Y (XYp⁻); defective gonadogenesis	Ambiguous development of the genital ducts, urogenital sinus, and external genitalia	Increased incidence of malignant gonadal tumors
Variants With degenerative renal disease	XY; chromatin negative	Male pseudohermaphroditism with early onset of primary degenerative renal disease and hypertension; variable development of genital ducts, incomplete masculinization of external genitalia	Predisposed to malignant renal neoplasms
Female genital ducts in otherwise normal men	XY; chromatin negative	Probable failure of Müllerian structures to respond to testicular duct-inhibiting substance or failure of its production; unilateral or bilateral cryptorchidism is found; testis is hypoplastic; uterus may be in inguinal canal; may be an X-linked characteristic	Increased tendency for malignant transformation of hypoplastic testes
Maternal ingestion of estrogens and progestogens	XY; chromatin negative	Probable suppression of hydroxysteroid dehydrogenase by ingested steroids or possible direct teratogenic effect of progestogens; ambiguous genitalia	
	XY		
Others			
Cryptorchidism Anorchia	Developmental defect	Cryptorchidism (vanishing testes); perhaps Leydig cell only syndrome	
Hypogonadism with gynecomastia (Rosewater syndrome)	Familial; mutant gene	Familial hypogonadism; gynecomastia (variable); increased estrogens, decreased gonadotropins	

normal man, except for final height. Significant laboratory parameters are levels of plasma testosterone, urine 17-KS, and plasma or urines FSH and LH above the normal values for the chronological age. Testicular biopsy reveals adult type Leydig cell development and the presence of active spermatogenens.

The natural history of male isosexual precocity, unlike that in the female type, is one of premature aging. The patient, if untreated, therefore undergoes the usual physiological aging process of chronologically older individuals and becomes subject to many of the vascular and other concomitants of the aging process.

True precocity caused by organic causes is secondary to premature release of gonadotropins probably as a consequence of abolition of inhibitory factors from the hypothalamus. The diagnosis of intracranial and cerebral disorders may require neurological, ophthalmologic, x-ray, electroencephalogram, and pneumoencephalographic studies, as well as examination of the cerebrospinal fluid. Occasionally serological tests for toxoplasmosis, syphilis, and tuberculosis may be helpful. Certain clinical features may be especially useful in differential diagnosis. For example, in precocity caused by hamartomas in the tuber cinereum and mammillary body, the onset of sexual maturation is often noted as early as 2 years of age. On the other hand, in most of the other etiologies, sexual precocity is usually a late symptom (6 years or later) and is often preceded by neurological manifestations. In neurofibromatosis, there is a characteristic skin lesion in addition to the sexual precocity disorder.

An incomplete form of true sexual precocity occurs in which the patients show gross signs of precocious male development, but with normal testicular size. On biopsy, this organ shows interstitial cells in pseudohyperplastic clumps, but the tubules appear relatively immature in size and appearance and lack any evidence of spermatogenesis. These findings are caused by an increased secretion of LH but not of FSH.

Management of true sexual precocity requires treatment of the underlying process if this is feasible. Estrogen therapy to oppose the actions of androgens is not recommended as it may induce degenerative changes in the spermatic tubules. Management in the sociopsychological sphere is very important.

Precocious pseudopuberty caused by organic causes is manifested by appearance of similar external findings as in children with true precocious puberty, but the inciting agents, the androgens, are produced in excess caused by primary disturbances in the testes, disturbed activity of the pituitary-adrenal axis, or therapy with HCG or androgen. As there is no activation of the pituitary-testicular axis, there is no spermatogenesis. Therapy is directed to management of the underlying process when feasible, along with sociopsychological counseling.

Table 20.5. Anomalous Sexual Differentiation in the Female

Disorder	Chromosomal constitution and metabolic defect	Clinical features	Associated findings
Disorders of gonadal differentiation			
Gonadal dysgenesis	XO; chromatin negative in 80%		
Turner's syndrome	XO karyotype is caused by nondisjunction or chromosomal loss during somatogenesis in either parent	Absence of second X (X chromosome monosomy) is associated with female phenotype, short stature, sexual infantilism caused by rudimentary gonads and a variety of somatic anomalies; features modified by lesser degrees of chromosome deficiency; somatic stigmata: micrognathia, epicanthal folds, prominent low-set ears, fish-like mouth, and ptosis, shield-chest, microthelia, and short neck with low hairline in back are prominent; webbing of the neck is found in 40%; cubitus valgus, puffiness of fingers, congenital lymphedema of hands and feet, short 4th metacarpal, high-arched palate, skeletal abnormalities, keloid formation, hypoplastic nails, pigmented nevi, recurrent otitis and hearing loss are also found	Coarctation of aorta is found in 10–20% of cases who have webbed neck; renal abnormalities in 40%; unexplained hypertension is also found

Bonnevie-Ullrich variant		In addition to classic features above, these patients have lymphedema of distal extremities, pleural and pericardial effusions and ascites, all ascribed to defects in lymphatic system
X chromatin positive variants	XO:XX; XO:XXX; XO:XX·XXX mosaicism	Most common is XO:XX mosaicism with fewer associated abnormalities; few menstruate and are fertile; one gonad is streaked or hypoplastic
	XXqi and XO:XXqi Xqi is more commonly from paternal X XXpi	Somatic abnormalities of classical form are not as prominent
		Sexual infantilism; normal or near normal height, minor somatic stigmata of Turner's
	XO:XXr	Short stature, absence of webbed neck and coarctation of aorta; sex characteristics may develop at puberty; may have dysfunctional bleeding
	XXp⁻ and XO:XXp⁻ (deletion of short arm of X)	May lack clinical stigmata of typical Turner's syndrome; streaked ovaries may be present in XXp⁻; in mosaic form, menstruation may occur
	XXq⁻ and XX:XXq⁻ (deletion of long arm of X)	Streak gonads, primary amenorrhea, and sexual infantilism

continued

Table 20.5. *continued*

Disorder	Chromosomal constitution and metabolic defect	Clinical features	Associated findings
Familial gonadal dysgenesis		Normal stature, sexual infantilism, bilateral streak gonads, normal female internal and external genitalia; primary amenorrhea and hypergonadotropinism	Occasionally hirsutism and clitoromegaly; gonadal tumors are rare in XX dysgenesis
True hermaphroditism	XX; XY and XX:XXY mosaicism	See Table 20.2	
Female pseudohermaphroditism	XX; positive X chromatin		
Congenital virilizing adrenocortical hyperplasia		See Chapter 15 on adrenocortical biosynthetic defects	
21-Hydroxylase deficiency	Defective cortisol synthesis; increased androgens and estrogens	Complete form: virilization, hirsutism, hyponatremia and hyperkalemia. Incomplete form: no electrolyte disturbances	
11β-Hydroxylase deficiency	Defective cortisol synthesis; increased androgens, estrogens, and deoxycorticosterone	Virilization, hirsutism, amenorrhea, hypertension, and hypokalemic alkalosis	

Hydroxysteroid (3β) dehydrogenase deficiency	Defective cortisol synthesis; increased dehydroepiandrosterone	Less virilization than above; salt loss may be found
17α-Hydroxylase deficiency	Defective synthesis of cortisol and gonadal hormones; increased mineralocorticoids	Sexual infantilism, hypertension, and hypokalemic alkalosis
Desmolase (20α) defect	Decreased adrenal and gonadal hormones	Sexual infantilism; adrenal insufficiency crisis
Exposure to androgens and progestogens		Masculinization of external genitalia female babies caused by maternal ingestion of testosterone or progestogens
Malformation of intestinal and urinary tract	Defect in embryonic development	Ambiguous genitalia
Vaginal agenesis		
Postpubertal virilism and infertility		Virilization, amenorrhea and infertility; postpubertal form of adrenal hyperplasia with biosynthetic defects (?)

Table 20.6. Classification of Isosexual Precocity in Males

I. Constitutional sexual precocity (idiopathic)

II. Precocity caused by organic causes (complete and incomplete)
  A. Tumors in tuber cinereum and posterior hypothalamus
  B. Tumors which destroy the pineal; hamartomas in tuber cinereum or mammillary body
  C. Astrocytoma, neurofibroma, ependymoma, craniopharyngioma, suprasellar teratoma, optic gloma
  D. Non-tumorous processes: encephalitis, meningitis, internal hydrocephalus, tuberous sclerosis, diffuse cerebral atrophy
  E. Trauma with cerebral disorder
  F. Mongolism with polydactyly
  G. Hypothyroidism
  H. McCune-Albright syndrome (polyostotic or monostotic fibrous dysplasia, occasionally with fractures and skin pigmentation)

III. Organic precocious pseudopuberty (in which there is no spermatogenesis)
  A. Excessive secretions
    1. By testes (Leydig cell tumors rare; 17-KS and testosterone are increased)
    2. By adrenal cortex (hyperplasia and tumors)
  B. Medicational
    1. Chorionic gonadotropins (HCG)
    2. Androgens

SEXUAL PRECOCITY IN FEMALES

Female isosexual precocity is defined as the onset of menses at less than 10 years of age, or the occurrence of thelarche (breast development) and pubarche (development of pubic hair) at less than 8 years of age. Early thelarche as part of sexual precocity should be distinguished from the disorder premature thelarche which is the precocious development of breasts (with pale areolae) without concurrent pubarche. This is a benign disorder which is caused by end-organ hypersensitivity to minimal amounts of estrogen. Isosexual precocity is more common in girls than in boys. A review of over 500 cases (1) revealed that 75–90% of cases of sexual precocity in girls are of idiopathic origin, but it is possible that a few of these may actually be caused by undetected small central nervous system lesions. A classification of sexual precocity in the female is presented in Table 20.7 (8).

Constitutional Sexual Precocity

Constitutional or idiopathic sexual precocity in the female is characterized by the premature release of adult amounts and sequence of pituitary FSH and LH. This pattern results in Graafian follicular development, ovulation,

Table 20.7. Classification of Sexual Precocity in Females

I. Constitutional sexual precocity
II. Precocity caused by organic causes (complete and incomplete)
   A. Tumors in tuber cinereum and posterior hypothalamus
   B. Tumors which destroy pineal (rarely a cause of female precocity)
   C. Hamartomas in tuber cinereum or mammillary body
   D. Astrocytoma, neurofibroma, ependymoma, suprasellar teratoma
   E. Optic glioma
   F. Non-tumorous process: encephalitis, meningitis, internal hydro-cephalus, tuberous sclerosis, diffuse cerebral atrophy
   G. Trauma with cerebral disorder
   H. Mongolism with polydactyly
   I. Hypothyroidism
   J. McCune-Albright syndrome
   K. Corticosteroid treatment of congenital adrenal hyperplasia (caused by sudden release of hypothalamic releasing factors)
III. Organic precocious pseudopuberty
   A. Excessive secretions by
      1. Ovaries; granulosa, theca cell tumors, follicular cysts, teratomas, chorionepitheliomas
      2. Adrenal cortex; hyperplasia, tumors
   B. Ingestion of exogenous estrogens

---

and secretion of the gonadal hormones. As a result, there is premature initiation of breast, pubic and axillary hair development, and menstruation. In normal subjects, the normal developmental sequence is thelarche followed by pubarche and menarche, but in patients with sexual precocity menarche may antedate the other two landmarks. While an element of end-organ hyper-responsiveness may be present in constitutional precocity, it is likely that most of the cases are of genetic orgin. Most of the patients ovulate, and the presence of this process effectively rules out etiologies such as autonomous ovarian or adrenal sources, or medications, as basis of the clinical manifestations. Increased gonadal hormones in patients with constitutional precocity stimulate linear growth, so that the patients are temporarily taller than their contemporaries, but this rapid growth is soon terminated by estrogen-induced epiphyseal closure. These patients are shorter than normal adults eventually. The diagnostic criteria for constitutional sexual precocity are: 1) thelarche, 2) pubarche, 3) menarche, 4) advanced bone age, 5) adult levels and sequence of FSH LH and estrogens, 6) normal adrenocortical functions, 7) absence of neurological manifestations, and 8) absence of adnexal masses.

The natural history of the disorder continues with the development of short adult women whose sexual and reproductive functions are quite normal. Treatment is directed mainly to the emotional and social adjustments of the girl with this diagnosis, as these patients are often abused sexually. The use of depomedroxyprogesterone to suppress gonadotropin secretion and estrogen actions may arrest the progression of the disorder, but this is not widely employed.

Among the types of sexual precocity due to organic causes (Table 20.7), there is presumed to be a loss of hypothalamic inhibitory influences on the pituitary resulting in the release of adult amounts of FSH and LH in adult sequences. The gonadal hormones are consequently released with resultant manifestations of mature female development. Linear bone growth is enhanced, but the eventual body height is limited by early estrogen-induced epiphyseal closure as in constitutional precocity. The natural history of this type of disorder is dependent on that of the underlying inciting process, and therapy is directed thereto.

Organic female precocious pseudopuberty occurs as a result of increased levels of estrogens from the ovaries, adrenal cortex, and, rarely, from malignant hepatic tumors (Table 20.2), as well as from sources of exogenous estrogens. Occasionally there is an end-organ hyper-responsiveness to normal amounts of estrogen, resulting in occurrence of pseudopubertal changes. In all cases of pseudopuberty, there is no ovulation as the cyclic FSH and LH changes are missing. Ovarian disorders are found in 1–2% of girls with sexual precocity, and there 75% are caused by estrogen-producing tumors or cysts such as granulosa cell tumors, thecal cell tumors, thecomas, luteomas mixed granulosa and thecal tumors, theca lutein cysts, and follicular cysts. Tumors such as teratomas, dysgerminomas, and chorionepitheliomas may be the basis of precocious pseudopuberty by ectopic and noncyclic gonadotropin activation of normal ovarian tissue.

Sexual pseudoprecocity may develop at any time, occasionally as early as the 1st year of life. In most cases, the earliest manifestations are of thelarche, an increase of height and weight, and advanced skeletal maturation. The patients may have a whitish or brownish vaginal discharge and occasionally a frank noncylic vaginal bleeding. Abdominal pain and swelling may be noted, and sexual hair and acne may occur. Rectoabdominal examination (under anesthesia) often discloses the presence of a tumor. In general, thecal tumors are less frequently palpable than granulosa tumors. Most "granulosa cell tumors" are now considered to be mixed granulosa-theca tumors. Only 5% of granulosa cell tumors occur before puberty. The malignancy potential of thecal tumors is about 3%. Ovarian chorionepitheliomas and teratomas may produce gonadotropins, but not cyclically, so that ovulation and menstruation are not induced. The findings of an abdominal mass in a girl with sexual precocity is strong evidence for the presence of an ovarian tumor. The presence of especially large amounts of plasma in urinary estrogens strongly indicates an ovarian tumor. Increased levels of HCG (may be assayed as LH by RIA) suggest a gonadotropin-producing tumor. In the treatment of sexual precocity, all ovarian tumors and cysts should be removed as early as possible. If a teratoma is found, it should be removed along with the uterus and adnexa because of the malignancy potential of this type of lesion.

In the forms of adrenocortical hyperplasia where there are increased gonadal hormones, heterosexual incomplete precocious puberty is seen in females. Purely feminizing adrenocortical tumors are rare and, when found, the direction of clinical manifestations in the female is mainly isosexual. Clinical manifestations include early breast development and early appearance of pubic hair and acne. Vaginal bleeding (noncylic) may occur before age 4 years, and these patients exhibit accelerated skeletal growth. Urinary 17-KS are elevated because of dehydropiandrosterone, which is an intermediate in estrogen and androgen synthesis. Plasma estradiol and estrogen levels are moderately elevated, and urinary pregnanediol may be increased. Treatment of the tumors requires complete removal as early as possible. Management of adrenal hyperplasia associated with biosynthetic defects is considered in Chapter 15.

Exogenous gonadal hormones may induce symptoms and signs of puberty, including statural growth, but without gonadal maturation. Most of the manifestations, except for skeletal changes which depend on the age of the patient and period of exposure, regress on cessation of exposure to the hormones.

LITERATURE CITED

1. Rasmussen, H., and P. Bordier. 1973. The cellular basis of metabolic bone disease. N. Engl. J. Med. 269:25–32.
2. Harris, W. H., and R. P. Heaney. 1969. Skeletal revewal and metabolic bone disease. N. Engl. J. Med. 280:193–202, 253–259, 303–311.
3. Albrink, M. J. 1969. Overnutrition and the fat cell. In P. K. Bondy (ed.), Diseases of Metabolism, pp. 1261–1279. W. B. Saunders Co., Philadelphia.
4. Bray, G. A., M. B. Davidson, and K. W. Walls. 1972. Obesity: A serious symptom. Ann. Intern. Med. 77:773–778.
5. Bacchus, H. 1972. Endocrine profiles in the clinical laboratory. In M. Stefanini (ed.), Progress in Clinical Pathology. Vol. 4, pp. 1–101. Grune & Stratton, Inc., New York.
6. Debons, A. F., J. W. Wallace, and H. Bacchus. 1956. Ketone body metabolism in ascorbic acid deficiency. Am. J. Physiol. 185:31–34.
7. Grumbach, M. M., and J. J. Van Wyk. 1974. Disorders of sex differentiation. In R. H. Williams (ed.), Textbook of Endocrinology, pp. 423–501. W. B. Saunders Co., Philadelphia.
8. Bacchus, H. 1975. Essentials of Gynecologic and Obstetric Endocrinology. University Park Press, Baltimore. 232 p.
9. Federman, D. D. 1967. Abnormal Sexual Development. W. B. Saunders Co., Philadelphia. 206 p.

Subject Index

Acetyl-CoA
  in gluconeogenesis, 8
  oxidative decarboxylation of
    pyruvate to, 2
  transport of, 17
Acid mucopolysaccharides
  biological functions, 220
  clinical disorders, 217–222
  degradation of, 220–222
Acidemia
  isovaleric, 164–165
  methylmalonic, 165
Acidosis
  cerebrospinal fluid, 47
  DPG levels in, 10
  lactic, 47–48
    clinical manifestations, 48
    management, 48
Aciduria, isovaleric, 179
Addison's disease, 95, 373–374
Adenosine monophosphate, cyclic,
  mechanism of action,
  294– 296
Adenylate cyclase
  in glycogen synthesis, 6
  membrane, processes propagated
    by release of, 293–296
Adipose tissue, insulin effects on
  metabolism, 32
Adrenal cortex, 361–394
  biological actions of androgens,
    369
  biological actions of hormones,
    366–369
  biosynthesis of hormones, 363–
    365
  catabolism of aldosterone, 371
  catabolism of biosynthetic inter-
    mediates, 372

catabolism of 17-ketosteroids,
  371–372
catabolism of secretions,
  369–372
clinical disorders of function,
  372–383
clinical syndromes caused by biosynthetic defects in, 383–390
diagnostic procedures, 391–393
diseases of mineralocorticoid excess, 379–383
feminizing tumors, 390
fetal, steroid hormone production
  in, 366
glucocorticoid actions, 366–368
hyperfunction, 377–379
hyperplasia
  caused by desmolase defect,
    389
  caused by hydroxydehy-
    drogenase deficiency,
    385– 389
  caused by hydroxylase defi-
    ciency, 383–385, 389
  laboratory diagnosis, 390–391
  treatment, 389
insufficiency, 372–376
  laboratory diagnosis, 374
  treatment, 375–376
regulation of glucocorticoid secretion, 361–362
regulation of mineralocorticoid
  secretion, 362
renin-angiotensin mechanism,
  362–363
synthesis of androgens by, 366
transport of hormones, 365–366
Adrenal medulla and chromaffin
  system, 395–402
Adrenocorticotropic hormone, assessment of function, 321

Alanine, control of gluconeogenesis
by, 10
Albinism, 174
Albumin, displacement of bilirubin
from, 267
Alcaptonuria, 173, 229–230
Aldose reductase, glucose conversion, 7
Aldosterone, catabolism of, 371
Alkalosis, DPG levels in, 10
Amblyopia, 276
nutritional, 288
Amenorrhea, laboratory diagnosis,
435–437
Amino acid metabolism
acquired disturbances in, 186
aromatic, clinical disorders of,
171–174
branched chain, clinical disorders
of, 179
clinical disorders of, 151–187
defects associated with neurological symptoms, 162–166
Amino acids
classification, 22–23
distribution of, 153–154
essential, 23
metabolism, 22–25
nonessential, 23
sulfur, metabolic disorders of,
180–183
β-Amino acids, clinical disorders of,
184–185
Aminoacidopathies, hereditary, 167
Aminoacidurias
congenital prerenal, 161–186
generalized, in premature and
newborn infants, 186
renal, 168
Anasarca, 276
Androgenic derivatives, actions of,
406–414
Androgens
adrenal, biological actions, 369
role in differentiation of external
genitalia, 482
synthesis by adrenal cortex, 366
Anemia, pernicious, 287–288
Antidiuretic hormone
clinical states associated with increased secretion of, 306–307

syndrome of inappropriate, management, 309–310
Arginase in amino acid metabolism,
25
Argininosuccinase, deficiency, 164
Argininosuccinic acid synthetase
in amino acid metabolism, 25
deficiency, 164
Arthritis
acute gouty, 197–199
mechanism of, 198
prophylactic management,
203–204
treatment of, 203
rheumatoid, 232
Ascorbic acid, 284–286
deficiency, 284–286
Ataxia, 276

Beriberi
childhood, 275
heart disease, 275
Bile acid metabolism, 87–100
Bile acids
altered kinetics in duodenojejunal
diseases, 92
altered kinetics in intestinal
bacterial overgrowth, 92–93
Bile salts
altered kinetics in ileal diseases,
91
disturbances in reabsorption of,
91–92
enterohepatic circulation, 89–90
passive processes in absorption,
90–91
Bilirubin
displacement from albumin, 267
transport in plasma, 257–259
Bilirubin metabolism
clinical disorders of, 255–268
drug effects, 267–268
heme degradation, 255–257
Biotin, 282
deficiency, 282
Bone
actions of vitamin D metabolites
on, 446
metabolic disease, 463–465
PTH action on, 441

Calcitonin, interrelationships
    among metabolic actions of
    PTH, vitamin D, and, 442–446
Calcium, influence of interplay
    among PTH, calcitonin, and
    1,25-DHCC on homeostasis,
    446–447
Cancer of thyroid gland, 359
Carbamylphosphate synthetase
    deficiency, 164
Carbohydrate metabolism
    clinical disorders of, 27–79
    effect of fatty acid oxidation on,
        20–21
    in erythrocytes, 69–74
    hepatic, insulin action, 32
    hormonal control, 33–34
    interrelations with fat and protein
        metabolism, 1–25
    pentose phosphate pathway in,
        3–5
    tests of, 34–37
Carbohydrate starvation, gluconeo-
    genesis in, 10
Carbohydrates, endocrine factors in
    control of homeostasis,
    30–31
Carnitine in acetyl-CoA transport,
    17–18
Carnosinemia, 166, 184
Catecholamines
    activation of adenylate cyclase
        by, 6
    biological effects, 397–398
    biosynthesis of, 395–397
    metabolism of, 397
Central nervous system role in glu-
    cose homeostasis, 30
Cerebrospinal fluid, polyol pathway
    in, 8
Childhood, thyroid function, 353
Cholestasis, 268
Cholesterol
    metabolism, 22
    synthesis, 21
Cholesterol metabolism, 118–120
    altered, diseases associated with,
        119–120
Cholesterologenesis
    endogenous, 119

    regulation in liver and intestinal
        mucosa, 119
Chromaffin system
    and adrenal medulla, 395–402
    clinical disorders, 398–402
Citrate synthetase and citric acid
    cycle, 12
Citric acid cycle
    control mechanisms in, 11–14
    and Embden-Meyerhof pathway,
        2
    functions, 11–14
    in intermediary metabolism, 1
Coenzyme A, presence of panto-
    thenic acid in, 279
Collagen
    biosynthesis, 210–214
    clinical disorders, 207–214
    degradation, 214
    synthesis, 233
Coma
    hyperosmolar, management, 8
    hyperosmolar non-ketotic, 44–47
        complications during manage-
        ment, 46–47
        management, 46
        precipitating causes, 45
        symptomatology, 45
    hypoglycemic, 48–49
Connective tissue complex
    clinical disorders of, 207–234
    effects of drugs and other factors
        on metabolism, 232–233
    inherited disorders of, 227–232
    other disorders of metabolism,
        232–233
Copper
    deficiency, 289–290
    toxicity, 290
    as trace mineral in metabolic
        processes, 289–290
Coproporphyria, hereditary,
    243–244
Coproporphyrinogen oxidation,
    238
Cori cycle, glucose homeostasis, 30
Corticosterone catabolism, 372
Cortisol metabolism in liver,
    370–371
Cortisone, glucose tolerance test,
    36

Cretinism, familial goitrous, 163
Crigler-Najjar syndrome, 264
Cushing's syndrome, 377—379
  caused by adrenocortical neo-
    plasia, 377
  caused by ectopic ACTH produc-
    tion, 377
  caused by excess ACTH, 377
  clinical picture, 377—378
  hirsutism, 434
  laboratory diagnosis, 378—379
  treatment, 379
Cystathionuria, 165—166, 182
Cystinosis, 182
Cystinuria, 185—186
Cytosol, processes propagated by
  participation of, 296—298

Decarboxylation reactions, thiamin,
  275
Deoxycorticosterone catabolism,
  372
11-Deoxycortisol catabolism, 372
21-Deoxycortisol catabolism, 372
Dermopathy, diabetic, 54
Desmolase defect, adrenocortical
  hyperplasia caused by, 389
Diabetes, phosphate, 272
Diabetes insipidus, 305—306
  management, 309—310
  procedures for establishing
    diagnosis, 307—309
Diabetes mellitus, 37—63
  classification, 38
  coma in, 40—49
    hyperosmolar non-ketotic,
      44—47
  dermopathy, 54
  diet therapy, 54—56
  insulin resistance phenomena,
    67—69
    insulin antibodies as cause of,
      68
    treatment of, 68—69
  insulin therapy, 56—57
  ketoacidosis, 40—44
  management, 54—60
    in surgical patients, 60
  natural history and course of,
    38—40
  nephropathy, 49—51
  neuropathy, 54

oral hypoglycemic agents, 57—60
  in pregnancy, 60—63
  diagnosis, 62
  retinopathy, 51—54
Diet, lipids in, 82—87
Diphosphoglycerate, erythrocyte,
  and oxygen delivery to
  tissues, 10—11
Diuresis, osmotic, 41, 44
Dwarfism, pituitary, treatment of,
  326—327
Dysautonomia, familial, 162—163,
  174

Ehlers-Danlos syndrome, 230
Elastin
  clinical disorders, 214—215
  synthesis, 233
Electrolytes, control of, in diabetic
  ketoacidosis, 44
Embden-Meyerhof pathway
  and citric acid cycle, 11
  hemolytic disorders of, 70—71
  in intermediary metabolism, 1—3
Endocrine glands
  changes in parturition, 427
  changes in pregnancy, 426—427
  control of mammary growth and
    lactation, 427
  hypertension, 469—473
Endoplasmic reticulum, cholesterol
  synthesis in, 21
Enzymes, deficiencies of non-
  glycolytic, 74
Epinephrine, stimulation of phosphorylase, 7
Erythrocytes
  carbohydrate metabolism in,
    69—74
  G-6-P dehydrogenase-deficient,
    changes during drug
    administration, 73
  hexose monophosphate shunt,
    71—74
  pyruvate kinase deficiency,
    70—71
Exercise, gluconeogenesis, 10
Eye, treatment of changes in, in
  Graves' disease, 348—350

Fabry's disease, 134—135
Fajans-Conn system, 37

Fat metabolism
  factors controlling, 15—16
  interrelations with carbohydrate
    and protein metabolism, 1—25
Fatty acid metabolism, diseases
    affecting, 122
Fatty acids
  free, synthesis of triglyceride
    from, 15
  mobilization of, 20
  oxidation, 18—19
    effect on carbohydrate metab-
      olism, 20—21
  synthesis, 16—17
    factors controlling, 19—20
  synthesis and degradation,
    121—122
Ferrochelatase, 238
  steroid hormone production in
    adrenals, 366
  steroidogenesis in, 422—426
    control of, 426
Folic acid, 283—284
  deficiency, 283—284
  dietary sources, 283
  in intermediary metabolism of
    nucleoproteins, 283
Fructose diphosphate phosphatase
    in gluconeogenesis, 8

Galactose metabolism, clinical
    disorders of, 76—78
Galactocerebroside metabolism,
    clinical disorders of, 136—138
Ganglioside metabolism, 141—148
  clinical disorders of, 142—148
Gangliosides, biosynthesis and
    degradation of, 142
Gangliosidosis, 144—145
Gastrointestinal tract, abnormalities
    in, 158—159
Gaucher's disease, 132—134
Genitalia, external, role of an-
    drogens in differentiation of,
    482
von Gierke glycogenosis, 6

Glucagon
  and intermediary metabolism, 33
  stimulation of phosphorylase, 7
Glucocorticoid provocative test,
    452

Glucocorticoid secretion regulation
    in adrenal cortex, 361—362
Glucocorticoids in gluconeogenesis,
    10
Gluconeogenesis
  in carbohydrate starvation, 10
  and Embden-Meyerhof pathway,
    2
  increased by fatty acid oxidation,
    21
  irreversible steps in, 8
  pathway of, 8
  process of, 29
Glucose
  conversion of ingested carbohy-
    drate to, 27
  in intermediary metabolism, 1
  role of CNS in homeostasis, 30
  role of kidney in homeostasis, 30
  role of red cell mass in ho-
    meostasis, 30
Glucose-alanine cycle, 10
Glucose -6-phosphatase in carbohy-
    drate metabolism, 4
Glucose 6-phosphate, phosphoryl-
    ation of glucose to, 1
Glucose 6-phosphate dehy-
    drogenase deficiency
  changes during drug administra-
    tion, 73
  clinical considerations, 73—74
Glucose tolerance tests, 34—37
  analysis of, 36—37
  cortisone, 36
  intravenous, 35—36
  oral, 36
Glycerokinase, lack of, 15—16
Glycerol
  in carbohydrate starvation, 10
  released from triglyceride break-
    down, 15
Glycerophosphatide metabolism,
    126—128
Glycine metabolism, clinical dis-
    orders of, 161—168
Glycogen
  biosynthesis, 5—6
    control mechanisms, 6
  breakdown, 6—7
  storage diseases, 74—78

Glyocogen phosphorylase break-
        down of glycogen catalyzed
        by, 6
Glycogen synthetase in glycogen
        synthesis, 5–6
Glycogen synthetase D, 6
Glycogen synthetase I, 6
Glycogenosis I, 6
Glycolysis
    anaerobic, in intermediary metab-
        olism, 1–3
    pathway of, 8
Glycoproteins
    catabolism of, 216–217
    classification of, 217
    clinical disorders, 215–217
    functions of, 216
    synthesis of, 215–216, 233
Glycosphingolipids, neutral, clinical
        disorders, 132–136
Gonadal differentiation, 479–482
Gout, 195–197
    tophaceous, 198–199
Graves' disease, treatment of eye
        changes in, 348–350
Günther's disease, 246–248
Gynecomastia, 413

Hartnup's disease, 163, 175–176
Hemes
    biosynthesis, 236–240
        control of, 238–240
    degradation, 255–257
    structure and function, 236
Hexose, transmucosal transfer, 27
Hexose monophosphate shunt
    in carbohydrate metabolism, 3–5
    in erythrocyte metabolism,
        71–74
    in intermediary metabolism, 1
Hickey-Hare test, 308
Hirsutism
    idiopathic, 390, 434
    laboratory diagnosis, 434–435
    treatment of, 434–435
Histidine metabolism, disorders of,
        170–171
Homocystinuria, 165, 180–182,
        229

Hormones
    adrenocortical
        biological actions, 366–369
        biosynthesis, 363–365
        transport, 365–366
    adrenocorticotropic, 314–315
    control of carbohydrate metabo-
        lism, 33–34
    follicle-stimulating, 313–314
    growth
        assessment of decreased,
            315–321
        assessment of excess, 321
        assessment of functions, 315
    luteinizing, 314
    mechanisms of actions, 293–298
    mineralocorticoid, biological
        actions, 368–369
    neurohypophiseal, chemical and
        physical characteristics,
        300–303
    produced by anterior pituitary,
        312–327
    steroid, production in fetal
        adrenals, 366
    thyroid
        biosynthetic processes in
            production of, 330–334
        formation, 330–332
        metabolic effects, 334–335
        metabolism of, 333
        physiological effects, 335–341
        synthesis of, 330
        transport of, 332–333
    thyroid-stimulating, 314
Hydroxydehydrogenase deficiency,
        adrenocortical hyperplasia
        caused by, 385–389
β-Hydroxyisovaleric aciduria, 166
Hydroxylase deficiency, adreno-
        cortical hyperplasia caused
        by, 383–385, 389
β-Hydroxy-β-methylglutaryl-CoA
        synthesis, 21
17-Hydroxyprogesterone catabo-
        lism, 372
Hyperadrenocorticotropinism,
        pituitary, assessment of,
        321–323
Hyperaldosteronism
    primary, 379–381

secondary, 381–382
treatment, 382–383
Hyperammonia disorders, 164
Hyperbetaalaninemia, 166, 184
Hyperbetalipoproteinemia, serum
    and lipid levels, 107–115
Hyperbilirubinemia
    conjugated, 265–267
    unconjugated, 262–265
Hypercalcemia, differential diag-
    nosis, 453–454
Hyperglycinemia
    clinical disorders with, 168–169
    ketotic, 162
    non-ketotic, 162
Hyperhistidinemia, 163
Hyperlaninemia, 166
Hyperlipoproteinemia, inherited,
    115–118
Hyperlysinemia, 164, 183–184
    persistent, 184
Hyperoxaluria, primary, 169–170
Hyperparathyroidism, 448–458
    clinical manifestations, 448–450
    laboratory diagnosis, 450–454
    medical management, 455–456
    primary, 448
    secondary, 456–458
    treatment of, 455
Hyperprolinemia, 162
Hypertension, endocrine, 469–473
Hyperthyroidism, 341–359
    in infancy, 353
    juvenile, 353–354
    natural course, 345–346
    pediatric aspects, 352–354
    in pregnancy, treatment of,
        351–352
    symptoms, 343–345
    treatment, 347–348
Hypertriodothyroninemia, 342
Hyperuricemia
    hereditary diseases with, 199–200
    secondary, 200–201
    treatment of, 201–203
Hyperuricemic states, 195–197
Hypervalinemia, 165, 179
Hypoglycemia, alimentary, 67
Hypoglycemic syndromes, 63–67
    etiology, 64
    laboratory studies, 64–66

treatment, 66–67
Hypogonadism, male, clinical and
    laboratory features, 407
Hypoparathyroidism, 458–460
    clinical manifestations, 458–460
    laboratory findings, 460
    treatment of, 460
Hypopituitary states, 325
Hypoprothrombinemia, 274
Hypothalamic-hypophysiotropic-
    neurohypophysial system,
    299–310
Hypothalamus and pituitary-thy-
    roid axis, 333–334
Hypothyroidism, 354–359
    clinical signs, 355–356
    differential diagnostic procedures,
        357
    treatment, 355–359

Ileum, altered bile salt kinetics in
    diseases of, 91
Imino acid metabolism, clinical
    disorders of, 183
Infancy
    hyperthyroidism, 353
    thyroid function, 352–353
Infertility, male, 407–414
Insulin
    antibodies as cause of resistance
        phenomena in diabetes, 68
    effect on hepatic carbohydrate
        metabolism, 32
    effects on adipose tissue metabo-
        lism, 32
    effects on muscle metabolism, 32
    and intermediary metabolism,
        31–33
    mechanism of stimulation of
        secretion, 32–33
    release by β islets of pancreas, 27
    resistance phenomena in diabetic
        patients, 67–69
    therapy for diabetes mellitus,
        56–57
    therapy for diabetic ketoacidosis,
        44–45
    for transmembrane transfer of
        carbohydrate, 1

Intestine
  clinical disorders of lipid metabo-
    lism, 93–97
  flora activity, 268
  lipid metabolism, 84–86
  PTH action on mucosal cell, 441
Iodide trapping by thyroid cells,
    330
Iodine
  butanol-extractable, 339
  protein-bound, 338–339
  thyroid, organification of, 331
Iodotyrosines, coupling of, 331
Isoprenoid unit, synthesis, 21

Kayser-Fleischer ring, 290
Keratomalacia, 270
Ketoacidosis, diabetic, 40–44
  complications during manage-
    ment of, 46–47
  management in pregnancy, 63
  polyol pathway in, 8
  precipitating events, 41
  symptoms and signs, 41–42
  treatment, 42–44
Ketogenesis in fat metabolism, 19
Ketolysis in fat metabolism, 19
Ketosis, management, 8
Ketosteroids
  catabolism of, 371–372
  urinary, 390–391
Kidney
  action of vitamin D metabolites
    on, 446
  PTH action on tubule cell, 441
  role in glucose homeostasis, 30
Korsakoff's syndrome, 276
Krabbe's disease, 137–138
Krebs citric acid cycle: see Citric
    acid cycle
Krebs-Henseleit cycle and urea
    synthesis, 24
Kussmaul respirations in diabetic
    ketoacidosis, 42
Kwashiorkor, 186

Lactate
  conversion of pyruvate to, 2
  oxidation of, 2
Lactation, endocrine control of,
    427

Lactic dehydrogenase, conversion
  of pyruvate to lactate
  catalyzed by, 2
Lactoflavin, 278–279
Lanosterol, conversion of squalene
  to, 21
Lesch-Nyhan syndrome, 200
Lipase, hormone-sensitive, 16
Lipid metabolism, 81–150
  intestinal, 84–86
    clinical disorders, 93–97
Lipid storage disorders, 148–149
Lipidosis sphingomyelin, patho-
    physiology, 132–138
Lipids
  dietary, 82–87
  malabsorption, diagnosis of,
    97–100
  transport in serum, 100–118
    clinical disorders of, 106–107
Lipogenesis and gluconeogenesis, 8
Lipoic dehydrogenase in mitochon-
    dria, 2
Lipoic transacetylase in mitochon-
    dria, 2
Liver
  cortisol metabolism in, 370–371
  fatty infiltration of, 123–124
  insulin action on carbohydrate
    metabolism, 32
  lipid transport to, 86–87
  metabolic aciduria with disease
    of, 186
  phosphorylase, 7
  porphyria, 240–246
Lysine intolerance, 164

Malic enzyme, carboxylation of
  pyruvate by, 2
Malonyl-CoA system in fatty acid
  synthesis, 18
Manganese
  deficiency, 292
  functions, 291
  toxicity, 292
  as trace mineral in metabolic
    processes, 291–292
Maple syrup urine disease, 179
Marfan syndrome, 227–229
Menstrual cycle, 418–419
Metabolism

adipose tissue, insulin actions, 32
intermediary
  and glucagon, 33
  and insulin, 31–33
  interrelations among carbohy-
    drate, fat, and protein metab-
    olism, 1–25
  muscle, insulin actions, 32
β-Methylcrotonylglycinuria, 166
Mevalonic acid synthesis, 21
Mineralocorticoid excess, diseases
  of, 379–383
Mineralocorticoid secretion, regulation in adrenal cortex, 362
Minerals, trace, 289–292
Mucopolysaccharidoses
  genetic, 223–227
    nature of metabolic defect,
      223–226
    methods of laboratory diagnosis,
      226–227
Muscle phosphorylase, 7
Mutase system deficiency, 179

Nephropathy, diabetic, 49–51
Neurological symptoms, defects in
  amino acid metabolism
  associated with, 162–166
Neuropathy, diabetic, 54
Niacin, 276–278
  biological functions, 276
  deficiency, 277–278
  dietary sources, 276
Nicotinamide adenine dinucleotide,
  reduced, reoxidation of, 2
Niemann-Pick disease, pathophysiology, 132–138
Nitrogen fixation, process of, 24
Nuclear receptors, processes
  propagated by participation
  of, 296–298

Obesity, 466–469
  drug therapy, 469
  methods of control, 467–468
Ornithine transcarbamylase
  deficiency, 164
  in urea cycle, 25
Osteogenesis imperfecta, 230–231
Osteoporosis, postmenopausal, 465
Ovaries, 417–437

clinical investigation of disorders,
  428
differentiation of, and oogenesis,
  480–481
disorders caused by defects in
  gonadotropin secretion, 431
endocrine disorders, 429–437
functions, 417
intrinsic disorders causing hypofunction, 430
menstrual cycle, 418–419
polycystic diseases, 429–434
steroid synthesis in, 419–421
syndromes of hyperfunction,
  432–433
Oxalacetate formation in citric acid
  cycle, 2
Oxalosis, 169–170
Oxygen delivery to tissues and
  2,3-DPG, 10–11
Oxyhemoglobin dissociation curve,
  10
Oxytocin, characteristics, 301

Pancreas, insulin release, 27
Pantothenic acid, 279–280
  chemical structure, 279
Parathyroid glands, 439–461
  clinical disorders, 447
Parathyroid hormone
  biological actions, 440–442
    on bone, 441
    on gastrointestinal mucosal cell,
      441
    on renal tubule cell, 441
  interrelationships among meta-
    bolic actions of calcitonin,
    vitamin D, and, 442–446
Parturition, endocrine changes in,
  427
Pellagra, hereditary, 163, 175–176
Pentose phosphate pathway
  in carbohydrate metabolism, 3–5
  in intermediary metabolism, 1
Pertechnate ion, thyroid uptake,
  338
Phenformin, therapy with, 47–48
Phenylketonuria, 162, 173
Pheochromocytoma
  clinical features, 398–399
  clinical investigation, 399–400

Pheochromocytoma (*cont.*)
treatment of, 400–402
variants, 400
Phosphate, tubular reabsorption,
451-452
Phosphoenolpyruvate carboxykinase in gluconeogenesis, 8,
10
Phosphofructokinase in glycolysis,
8
Phospholipid metabolism, 124–138
Phosphorylase
liver, 7
muscle, 7
Phosphorylase kinase in glycogen
breakdown, 7
Pituitary gland
anterior, 311–327
control of, 311–312
hormones produced by, 312–
327
hypothalamic neurohormones
regulating, 301–302
laboratory diagnosis of disorders of, 315-325
assessment of gonadotropic
functions, 323
assessment of thyrotropic function, 324
treatment of diseases of, 325–327
Pituitary-thyroid axis and hypothalamus, 333–334
Plasma, bilirubin transport in,
257–259
Polyol pathway, 7–8
in cerebrospinal fluid, 8
in diabetic ketoacidosis, 8
Porphobilinogen deaminase, 238
Porphyria
acute intermittent, 240–242
erythropoietic, 246–250
congenital, 246–248
hepatic, 240–246
Porphyria cutanea tarda, 244–246
Porphyria variegata, 242–243
Porphyrin metabolism
clinical disorders of, 235–253
descriptions of, 240–253
Porphyrins
biosynthesis, 236–238

physical and chemical properties,
235–236
synthesis, drugs affecting,
250–253
Pregnancy
diabetic mellitus in, 60–63
diabetogenic factors, 61–62
endocrine changes, 426–427
in maternal system, 426–427
steroidogenesis during, 421–426
thyrotoxicosis, 350–351
treatment of hyperthyroidism in,
351–352
Progesterone, catabolism, 372
Prolactin, 313
assessment of pituitary release of,
324
Propionyl-CoA carboxylase deficiency, 179
Protein
definitions in nutrition of,
154–155
hepatic acceptor, competition
for, 267
pathological changes in nutrition
of, 156–161
synthesis, 156–161
conditions affecting mechanism
of, 159–160
Protein metabolism
changes associated with disease
and various physiological
states, 159
changes in individual organs and
tissues, 160–161
clinical disorders of, 151–187
interrelations with fat and protein
metabolism, 1–25
Protein-polysaccharides, synthesis,
233
Prothrombin formation in liver,
274
Protoporphyria, erythropoietic,
248–250
Pseudoxanthoma elasticum,
231–232
Purine biosynthetic, reutilization,
and feedback pathways,
191–193
drug effects, 195

Purine metabolism, 189–193
  clinical disorders of, 189–206
Pyridoxin, 280–282
  deficiency, 281–282
  functions, 281
Pyrimidine metabolism, clinical
    disorders of, 189–206
Pyruvate
  anaplerotic reactions involving, 2
  in Embden-Meyerhof pathway, 2
Pyruvate carboxylase in gluconeo-
    genesis, 8, 10
Pyruvate decarboxylase in mito-
    chondria, 2
Pyruvate dehydrogenase complex in
    mitochondria, 2
Pyruvate kinase
  deficiency in erythrocytes, 70–71
  in glycolysis, 8

Radioiodide, triiodothyronine
    suppression of increased
    thyroid uptake of, 337
Radioiodine, thyroid uptake,
    336–337
Red cell mass, role in glucose
    homeostasis, 30
Refsum's disease, 148
Renin-angiotensin mechanism in
    adrenal cortex, 362–363
Respiratory chain and citric acid
    cycle, 12
Retinopathy, diabetic, 51–54
Riboflavin, 278–279
  biological functions, 278–279
  chemical structure, 278
  deficiency, 279
Rickets, 272
Riley-Day syndrome, 162–163, 174

Sarcosinemia, 162
Schilling test, 288
Scurvy
  adult, 286
  infantile, 285
Serum
  lipid transport, 100–118
  lipoprotein fractions, 101–106
Sex chromosomes, 476–479

Sexual differentiation
  anomalous, 488
  in female, 490–493
  disorders of, 469, 474–475
  hormonal, 482
Sexual precocity
  in females, 494–497
  in males, 488–489, 494
Sodium tolbutamide response test,
    36
Sorbitol, polyol pathway, 7
Spermatogenesis, testicular differ-
    entiation, 479–480
Sphingolipid metabolism, 129–138
Sphingolipodystrophies, summary
    of, 147
Sphingomyelin
  biosynthesis and degradation, 131
  pathophysiology of lipidosis,
    132–138
Sphingomyelin metabolism, clinical
    disorders, 131
Squalene, conversion to lanosterol,
    21
Stein-Leventhal syndrome,
    429– 434
  hirsutism, 435
Steroidogenesis
  control of in fetal life, 426
  in fetoplacental unit, 422–426
  during pregnancy, 421–426
  protein synthesis in control of,
    296
Steroids, synthesis in ovaries,
    419–421
Sulfatide metabolism, 138–141
  clinical disorders of, 139–141
Sulfite oxidase deficiency, 166
Sweaty feet syndrome, 164–165

Tay-Sachs disease, 145
Testes, 403–415
  differentiation of, and spermato-
    genesis, 479–480
  endocrine activity, 404–406
  function, 403
  tumors, 413–414
Testosterone, actions of, 406–414
Thiamin, 274–276
  decarboxylation reactions, 275

Thiamin, (*cont.*)
  deficiency, 275-276
  dietary sources, 274–275
Thyroid gland, 329–359
  assessment of function, 336–341
  autoregulation, 334
  cancer, 359
  function at birth and infancy,
    352–353
  function in childhood, 353
  hormone binding by serum
    proteins, 339–340
  intrauterine function, 352
  long-acting stimulator, 341
  regulation of activity of, 333–334
  uptake of pertechnate ion, 338
Thyrotoxicosis in pregnancy,
  350–351
Thyroxine, serum, 339
Transsulfuration pathway, 180
Tricarboxylic acid cycle
  anabolic functions, 14
  catabolic functions, 13
Triglyceride metabolism, 122–124
  disorders of, 123–124
Triglyceride synthesis, 16
Tryptophan metabolism, clinical
    disorders of, 174–175
Tryptophanuria, congenital, 163
Tumors
  feminizing adrenocortical, 390
  of testes, 413–414
Tyrosinemia, 173
Tyrosinosis, 173

Urea cycle
  metabolic disorders involving,
    176–178
  and ornithine transcarbamylase,
    25
Urea synthesis, Krebs-Henseleit
    cycle, 24
Uric acid
  metabolic and clinical aspects,
    193–195
  renal clearance, 194–195
Uridine diphosphoglucose in
    glycogen synthesis, 5
Uroporphyrinogen III cosynthase,
    238

Uroporphyrinogen decarboxylase,
  238

Vasopressin
  characteristics, 300–301
  clinical disorders associated with
    changes of secretion of,
    305–307
  deficiency, 305–306
    causes, 305–306
    differential diagnosis, 306
  exogenous, responsiveness to,
    308–309
  physiological considerations,
    303–309
Virilization, laboratory diagnosis,
  434–435
Vitamin A, 269–271
  chemical structure, 269
  deficiency, 269
  excess, 270–271
Vitamin B$_1$, 274–276
Vitamin B$_2$, 278–279
Vitamin B$_6$, 280–282
Vitamin B$_{12}$, 286–288
  deficiency, 287
Vitamin C, 284–286
Vitamin D, 271–272
  action of metabolites on bone,
    446
  actions of metabolites on kid-
    neys, 446
  biological actions of active
    metabolites on gastrointesti-
    nal tract, 445–446
  biosynthesis, 271
  deficiency, 271–272
  fat-soluble, structure, 271
  interrelationships among meta-
    bolic actions of PTH, calci-
    tonin, and, 442–446
Vitamin E, 272–273
  dietary requirement, 273
Vitamin K, 273–274
  daily requirement, 273
  deficiency, 274
Vitamins, 269–288

Wernicke's encephalopathy, 276
Whipple's disease, 96

Wilkerson system, 37
Wilson's disease, 290, 291
Wolman's disease, 148

Xanthinuria, hereditary, 204

Zinc
    dietary sources, 290
    toxicity, 291
    as trace mineral in metabolic
        processes, 290–291
Zincuria, 291